CONCEPTS IN

MEDICAL

RADIOGRAPHIC

IMAGING

Circuitry, Exposure & Quality Control

CONCEPTS IN

MEDICAL

RADIOGRAPHIC

IMAGING

Circuitry, Exposure & Quality Control

Marianne Tortorici, Ed.D., RT(R)
Professor
University of Nevada, Las Vegas

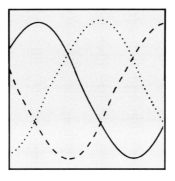

Line Drawings by Joseph A. Tortorici

Photographs by Marianne Tortorici

W.B. SAUNDERS COMPANY
Harcourt Brace Jovanovich, Inc.
Philadelphia   London   Toronto   Montreal   Sydney   Tokyo

W. B. SAUNDERS COMPANY
Harcourt Brace Jovanovich, Inc.

The Curtis Center
Independence Square West
Philadelphia, Pennsylvania 19106

Library of Congress Cataloging-in-Publication Data

Tortorici, Marianne R.

Concepts in medical radiographic imaging: circuitry, exposure and quality control / by Marianne Tortorici; line drawings by Joseph A. Tortorici; photographs by Marianne Tortorici.

p.   cm.

ISBN 0–7216–3117–7

1. Radiography, Medical—Methodology.   2. Diagnostic imaging—Methodology.   I. Title.

[DNLM: 1. Biomedical Engineering.   2. Quality Control.
3. Radiography—instrumentation.   4. Radiography—standards.   5. X-Ray Film—standards. WN 150 T699c]

RC78.T685 1992

616.07'54—dc20

DNLM/DLC   91-21828

Editor: Lisa A. Biello
Designer: Paul Fry
Production Manager: Linda R. Garber
Manuscript Editors: Terry Russell and Amy Norwitz
Illustration Coordinator: Peg Shaw
Indexer: David Prout

Concepts in Medical Radiographic Imaging:
Circuitry, Exposure & Quality Control   ISBN 0–7216–3117–7

Printed in the United States of America.

Last digit is the print number: 9   8   7   6   5   4   3   2   1

DEDICATION

I would like to dedicate this text to the imaging faculties and support staffs at the University of Nevada, Las Vegas (UNLV) and Morehead State University (MSU), who provided me the means to write this text by covering my classes and giving me release time and "mechanical" support during my faculty exchange at MSU and my sabbatical leave from UNLV.

CONTRIBUTORS

Barbara L. Barker, M.S.
Assistant Professor of Radiologic Technology
Morehead State University
Morehead, Kentucky
SILVER RECOVERY

William J. Dallas, Ph.D.
Professor of Radiology
Professor of Optical Sciences
Department of Radiology
College of Medicine, University of Arizona
Health Sciences Center
Tucson, Arizona
DIGITAL IMAGING OVERVIEW

Jacklynn Scott Darling, M.S.
Assistant Professor of Radiologic Technology
Morehead State University
Morehead, Kentucky
SILVER RECOVERY

Joan K. MacDonald, M.S., ARRT(N)
Assistant Professor/Nuclear Medicine Program Director
University of Nevada, Las Vegas
Las Vegas, Nevada
ATOMIC STRUCTURE OF MATTER
FILM, FILM PROCESSING AND PHOTOGRAPHIC TECHNIQUES
SENSITOMETRY AND PROCESSOR QUALITY CONTROL

Kevin M. McNeill, M.S.
Research Specialist
Radiology Research Laboratory
Department of Radiology
College of Medicine, University of Arizona
Health Sciences Center
Tucson, Arizona
FUNDAMENTALS OF COMPUTER TECHNOLOGY

Michael Mixdorf, M.Ed., RT(R)
Assistant Professor
Department of Radiological Sciences
University of Nevada, Las Vegas
Las Vegas, Nevada
GEOMETRIC IMAGE QUALITY
PHOTOGRAPHIC IMAGE QUALITY
REJECT FILM ANALYSIS

Alan L. Ryan, B.S.
Western Division Sales Manager
National Medical Computer Services
San Diego, California
COMPUTERIZING ADMINISTRATIVE TASKS

PREFACE

This text is an outgrowth of many years of teaching experience. It presents a discussion of radiographic techniques, circuitry and quality control in a logical order. Although there are many excellent texts covering these subjects, no one text contains a consolidated discussion of these areas. The material in this text is inclusive without being too brief or overly informative on any one subject.

The results of a research study performed by me and a clinical psychologist found that technologists learn best by practical experience. In support of that finding, this textbook is written in conjunction with *Concepts in Medical Radiographic Imaging: Laboratory Manual*. The textbook provides information regarding the concepts of medical radiographic imaging, and the laboratory manual provides practical experience in understanding the various ideas presented in the text. All experiments in the laboratory manual have been performed and tested by students at the University of Nevada, Las Vegas for several years.

Because this text is designed for student radiographers studying radiographic techniques, circuitry or quality control, likely it will be used for more than one class or academic semester. I believe this will help decrease student expenses while maintaining quality education.

MARIANNE TORTORICI
Las Vegas, Nevada

ACKNOWLEDGMENTS

This text was completed through the efforts of many people, most of whose names do not appear in the text because they are the hundreds of students I encountered over the years. All asked pointed questions, provided constructive criticism and tested the numerous theories and laboratory procedures. I thank all of them for contributing to my knowledge and growth as well as for providing a foundation for students currently training to become radiographers.

I would like to express my gratitude to Natalie Anderson, the editor responsible for my signing a contract to write this text. Natalie served as one of the greatest advocates of this project. It was her words of wisdom and her belief in me and the project that encouraged me to continue working during those times of frustration and doubt.

My appreciation is extended to Lisa Biello, editor-in-chief of Health-Related Professions at W.B. Saunders Company, and to Joanna Sadowska, formerly of W.B. Saunders Company. Both people were extremely helpful in answering my numerous questions and providing guidance and assistance during the development of this text.

I am especially thankful to my brother, Joseph Tortorici, who did all the illustrations in the text. He dedicated hundreds of hours to developing them on computer and ensuring their accuracy. This was a large task considering he lives on the eastern U.S. coast and I lived in the West. I deeply appreciate his visits to Nevada, computer and all in tow, to work with me on the illustrations.

Many of the photographs and some of the illustrations are courtesy of commercial companies. I would like to thank American Medical Sales, Beckman Industrial Corporation, Eastman Kodak Company, E.I. DuPont de Nemours & Company, Fisher Scientific, Fuji Photo Company, General Electric Medical Services, IMG Photo Products, Liebel-Flarsheim, National Medical Computer Services, Radiation Measurements Inc., Phillips Medical Systems, and the United States Bureau of Reclamation for providing me with the necessary photographs, illustrations or information.

A special thanks goes to Mary Klein, Vicki Gooss and Kay Kisner from Humana Hospital Sunrise, Las Vegas, Nevada, and Roger Olson from Mountain Diagnostics, Las Vegas, Nevada who assisted me in taking radiographs and photographs used throughout the text. I would like to thank them for their patience and time dedicated to ensuring that my needs were met.

CONTENTS

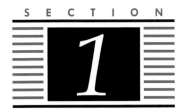

SECTION 1

CIRCUITRY AND
EQUIPMENT

Prior to practicing radiography in a clinical environment, students should have a working knowledge of how radiation is produced and the basic use of conventional radiographic equipment. The chapters in this section discuss the basic concept of electricity. After the reader has learned about electrical units, their function, and how electricity is produced, specific aspects of electrical components related to the production of radiation, e.g., transformers, are discussed. Also included in this section are chapters on specialized conventional imaging equipment of tomography and image intensification. Unlike other texts this includes information on quality control (QC), and specific chapters that discuss QC or chapters in which learning is reinforced by practical laboratory experience contain cross references to laboratory experiments in the laboratory manual, *Concepts in Medical Radiographic Imaging*.

Because imaging departments have become so computerized, highlights of this section include discussions about the fundamentals of computer technology, digital imaging, and computerizing administrative tasks. These introductory chapters provide students a basis from which to pursue their study.

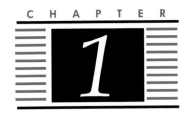

C H A P T E R

1

ATOMIC STRUCTURE
OF MATTER

MARIANNE TORTORICI and **JOAN K. MACDONALD**

INTRODUCTION

Matter is anything that occupies space and has inertia. Consequently, by definition, all things on earth are made of matter. Matter may be found in the form of an element or a compound. An element is composed of atoms with identical numbers of protons in the nucleus and is unable to be divided by normal means. A compound is composed of two or more elements. The smallest unit in which a compound maintains its physical and chemical properties is the molecule. The smallest unit in which an element maintains its physical and chemical properties is the atom.

This chapter discusses the basic structure of the atom. Knowing the basic structure of the atom is useful in understanding other concepts of radiology. Of particular interest in this text are the concepts of electrodynamics, the production of electricity, rectification, film processing, the production of x-rays and radiation interaction with matter.

THE ATOM

Niels Bohr, a Danish scientist, described the atom as a miniature solar system. This theory, although quite an oversimplification, is still used today for basic understanding of atomic structure. At the center of the atomic "solar system" is the nucleus, and the "planets" that orbit the nucleus are electrons (Figure 1–1).

NUCLEUS

The nucleus of the atom houses almost the entire mass of the atom. It contains the nucleons: protons and neutrons. The proton is positively charged, whereas the neutron has no charge. The law of electrical charges states that like charges repel. Thus, it seems logical to assume that the protons would repel each other. However, the protons and neutrons are held together in the nucleus by a nuclear force. This force is extremely strong and overcomes the electrical force of repulsion of the protons. Another feature of nuclear force is that it occurs at short distances, no greater than 10^{-15} m. Consequently, the nucleus of an atom is extremely small.

PROTON

As stated previously, the proton is positively charged and is located in the nucleus of an atom. The proton has a mass of 1.67×10^{-24} g. Because the mass of an atom is so small, it is common to

3

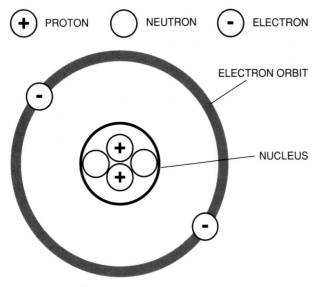

Figure 1-1. Diagram of a helium atom.

describe mass in atomic mass units (amu). Carbon-12 is used as the standard for the amu; 1 amu is equivalent to 1/12 the weight of carbon-12. The atomic mass unit is an average of the element's various masses; therefore, the atomic mass unit is rarely a whole number. A proton has a mass of 1.00728 amu.

A common abbreviation used for the proton is p. In diagrams of an atom, the proton is often symbolized as a circle with a + in the center. The counterpart (oppositely charged particle) of the proton is the electron. The proton is about 1836 times larger than an electron.

NEUTRON

Like the proton, the neutron is located in the nucleus of an atom. It has no charge. The mass of a neutron is about the same as that of a proton: 1.67×10^{-24} g, or 1.00867 amu. A common abbreviation for the neutron is n. In diagrams of an atom, the neutron is often symbolized as a blank or hollow circle.

ELECTRON

Electrons carry a negative charge and orbit the nucleus. The electron is abbreviated as e⁻. In dia-

grams, the electron is identified as a circle with a − in the center. Electrons are much smaller than nucleons and have a mass of 9.11×10^{-28} g, or 0.00549 amu. Electrons revolve around the nucleus at a specific distance and energy level called a shell. An atom may have as many as seven shells. The shells are identified by letters. The first shell is called the K shell. The remaining shells are L, M, N, O, P and Q. The maximum number of electrons in a shell is 2 times the square of the shell location from the nucleus, or $2n^2$. For example, the L shell is the second (2) shell from the nucleus; thus, the maximum number of electrons in the L shell is 8, or $2(2)^2 = 2(4) = 8$.

The electron is attached to the nucleus as a result of electron binding energy. Electron binding energy decreases as the distance from the nucleus increases. For example, the electron binding energy of the K shell is greater than that of the L shell, as more energy is required to remove the inner shell electrons. Generally, the more electrons in the atom (the sum of electrons in all shells), the greater the overall electron binding energy. For example, the electron energy in the K shell of an atom having 2 shells (K and L) and 10 electrons is usually less than the electron energy in the K shell of an atom with 4 shells (K, L, M and N) and 38 electrons.

SCIENTIFIC ELEMENT NOTATION

There are 106 known elements. These elements are expressed using symbols. For example, Ba represents barium, Fe refers to iron and W is tungsten. To list all the element symbols here is impractical. Some periodic tables list the name of the element under the symbol. The best method of determining what symbol represents which element is memorization.

In addition to an element's symbol, three other items are used to describe an element. They are atomic number, mass number and valence. The atomic number (Z) is the number of protons in the nucleus. It is important because it identifies the chemical behavior of the element. The atomic number is written as a subscript to the left of the element symbol. The atomic mass number, or relative atomic weight (A), represents the mass of the atom. It is obtained from the number of nucleons (by adding the number of protons and neutrons). The mass number is written as a superscript to the left of the element symbol. Valence represents the number of electrons in the outermost shell needed for the atom to become stable (to obtain 8 electrons in the outer shell). The valence represents the atom's ability to combine with other atoms. Atoms that easily donate electrons have a positive valence number corresponding to the number of electrons donated. For example, an atom with 1 electron has a valence of +1. Conversely, an atom that accepts electrons has a negative valence relative to the number of electrons it accepts to stabilize. Thus, an atom with 7 electrons in the outer shell has a valence of −1. The valence is written as a superscript to the right of the element symbol. The following is the scientific identification of helium:

$$^4_2He^{+2}$$

PERIODIC TABLE

The elements may be listed in a chart according to their atomic number. Dmitri Mendeleev, a Russian chemist, is credited with developing the system of organizing the elements. His system is referred to as the periodic table (Figure 1–2). In this table, elements are arranged from that with the lowest atomic number to that with the highest. The first 92 elements in the chart occur naturally. The remaining elements are artificial (synthetic).

The chart is divided into horizontal rows and vertical columns. The horizontal rows are called periods and include elements with the same number of electron shells. The vertical columns are referred to as groups. The elements within each group have the same number of electrons (and chemical reactions) in their outermost shell.

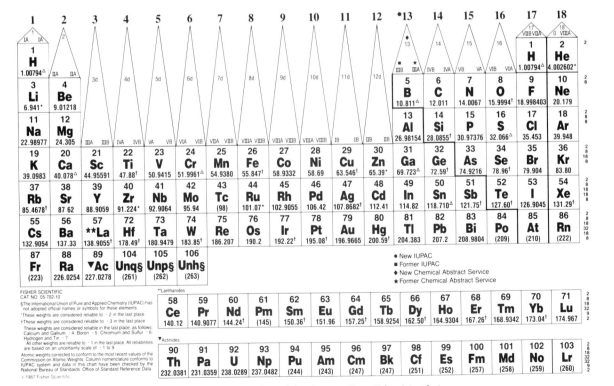

Figure 1–2. Periodic chart of the elements. (From Fisher Scientific.)

There are two relatively important numbers within each element box. The whole number is the atomic number. The mixed number represents the atomic mass unit. The location of these numbers may vary depending on the chart.

TYPES OF ATOMIC ARRANGEMENTS

The neutral atom has no charge. Thus, the number of protons and electrons is equal. Neutrons carry no charge, so they are not considered when determining the charge of the atom. It is possible for atoms of the same element to differ in the number of protons, neutrons or mass number. However, if the ratio of neutrons to protons becomes too unbalanced, the nucleus attempts to achieve a more balanced state (to stabilize) by releasing various types of radiation; such an atom is referred to as radioactive.

Atoms of the same element with a different mass number (A) and the same atomic number (Z) are called isotopes. Recall that the mass number represents the sum of the number of protons and neutrons and that the atomic number is the number of protons. Thus, an isotope has the same number of protons but a different number of neutrons ($A - Z$ = neutrons). The following are examples of hydrogen isotopes:

$$_1^1H \quad _1^2H \quad _1^3H$$

The first isotope is hydrogen (1 proton), the second isotope is deuterium (1 proton and 1 neutron) and the last isotope is radioactive tritium (1 proton and 2 neutrons).

Another type of atomic arrangement is the isobar. Isobars have the same mass numbers but different atomic numbers. Consequently, the number of neutrons also differs. The following are three isobars:

$$_5^{12}B \quad _6^{12}C \quad _7^{12}N$$

The first element is boron, the second element is carbon and the third element is nitrogen.

Isotones are a third type of atomic arrangement. Isotones have the same number of neutrons but different atomic number and mass number. Three isotones are as follows:

$$_5^{11}B \quad _6^{12}C \quad _7^{13}N$$

Table 1–1. SUMMARY OF ATOMIC ARRANGEMENTS

Arrangement	Z (Protons)	Neutrons (A − Z)	A (n + p)
Isotope	Same	Different	Different
Isobar	Different	Different	Same
Isotone	Different	Same	Different
Isomer	Same	Same	Same

Z = atomic number; A = mass number; n = neutrons; p = protons.

The first element is boron, the second is carbon-12 and the third is nitrogen-13.

Isomers have the same atomic number and mass number. The difference rests with the energy state of the nucleus. It is sometimes difficult to understand the differences among the various atomic arrangements. Table 1–1 is a summary of the atomic arrangements.

CHART OF THE NUCLIDES

Recall that the periodic table presents general information on all 106 known elements. It does not, however, yield information on the more than 2500 nuclides known at the date of this publication. A chart of the nuclides lists all nuclides according to their symbols and atomic, neutron and mass numbers. A multitude of information can be found on these charts, such as nuclear stability, radioactive origin (synthetic or artificial), modes and energies of radioactive decay and physical half-lives of radioactive nuclides. The following is a brief discussion of the chart of the nuclides. The examples are extremely condensed. To explain the voluminous amount of information demonstrated on the chart is beyond the scope of this text.

Figure 1–3 shows the general, gridlike structural arrangement of the chart. The atomic numbers (Z) are represented on the vertical axis, the number of neutrons (N) on the horizontal axis and the nuclide's symbol and mass number within each box of the grid. Stable nuclides are usually represented by the color gray, whereas radioactive ones are either white or a combination of white and black, green, yellow, orange or blue. The color choice for the radionuclides denotes naturally occurring or artificially produced radionuclides and the radio-

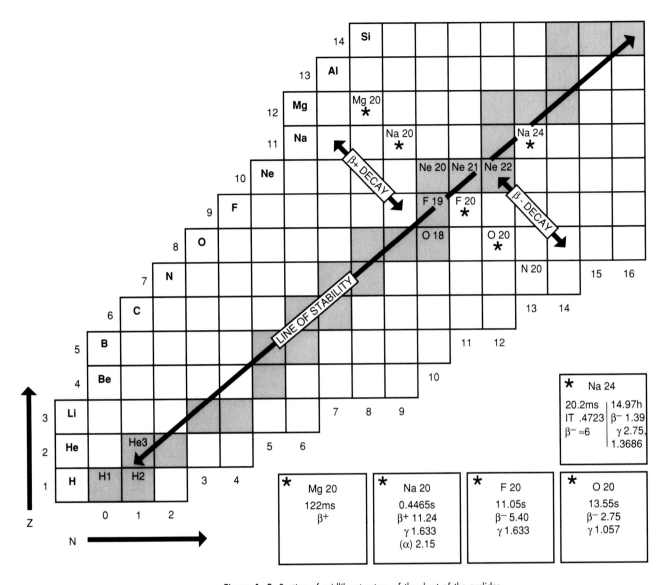

Figure 1–3. Section of gridlike structure of the chart of the nuclides.

nuclide's half-life (the time it takes for one-half of the original atoms to emit various forms of energy or decay).

Note that the stable nuclides create a diagonal line across the chart. This is referred to as the line of stability. Those nuclides residing outside this border are radioactive. Nuclides with a relative imbalance of protons and neutrons attempt to achieve stability by either losing or gaining nucleons, thus getting closer to the line of stability. This line actually ends at bismuth-83 (^{83}Bi), as all nuclides with a higher atomic number are radioactive. (^{83}Bi is not identified in Fig. 1–3.)

The radionuclides lying above the line of stability are inclined to have more protons than neutrons. To achieve stability, they essentially lose the extra protons in the form of positive beta particles (β+, or positrons). Stated another way, they undergo positive beta decay. For example, ^{20}Mg (magnesium) emits a beta particle and becomes ^{20}Na (sodium), which in turn also emits a positron to become stable ^{20}Ne (neon). These nuclides all have the same mass number but a different atomic number and are therefore isobars.

Nuclides lying below the line of stability are too rich in neutrons. They try to achieve balance by emitting neutrons in the form of negative beta particles (β−, or negatrons). This is called negative beta decay. For example, ^{20}O (oxygen) emits a negative beta particle and becomes ^{20}F (fluorine), which in turn emits a negatron to become stable ^{20}Ne. These nuclides are also isobars, as they have the same mass number but a different atomic number.

Because both types of beta emission (positive and negative) produce isobars, beta decay is often referred to as an isobaric transition. Note that isobars occur in a particular structural arrangement within the chart, as they lie along a diagonal line running from the upper left corner to the lower right corner.

Another important method of reaching stability is through alpha decay. Alpha particles (α) are essentially the nucleus of a helium atom, which consists of 2 neutrons and 2 protons. This type of decay primarily occurs in radionuclides of high atomic numbers, as they have a relatively large imbalance of neutrons to protons. Although not identified in Figure 1–3 the decay product of an alpha emitter can be located on the chart by counting down 2 boxes and then moving 2 boxes to the left from the original nuclide.

Isomers differ primarily in their energy states, implying that one state is usually higher in energy than another. The extra energy in this case is often released in the form of a gamma (γ) ray (similar to x-rays). Because both nuclides have the same atomic and mass numbers, they are identified on the chart by dividing the box into sections. The higher state, often referred to as the metastable state, is found in the left side of the box and is generally represented by writing a lower case m (metastable) after the mass number. For example, the box for ^{24}Na is divided into two sections. The metastable state, on the left, is usually identified by the initials IT (isomeric transition). It is written as ^{24m}Na. That state with the lower energy is called the ground state and it is noted on the right side of the box. It is referred to simply by the element symbol and the mass number, e.g., ^{24}Na. Figure 1–4 shows an enlargement of the box for ^{135}Ba (barium). Note that it has two isomeric states, one radioactive (^{135m}Ba) and one stable (^{135}Ba). Although a discussion of all the information contained within this box is beyond the scope of this text, it is shown to demonstrate the chart's complexity.

Recall that isotones have the same number of neutrons but different atomic and mass numbers. Similar to the case with isobars, isotones also form a particular structural arrangement within the chart of the nuclides. Nuclides within each column are

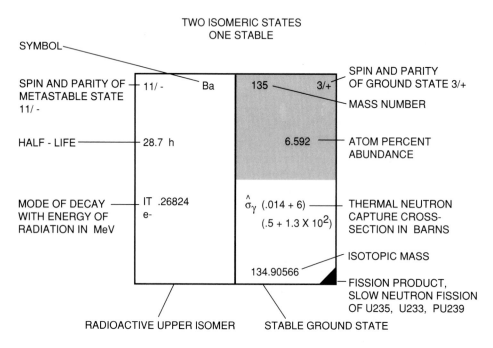

Figure 1—4. Enlargement of ^{135}Ba from chart of the nuclides.

isotones. ^{20}Ne, ^{19}F and ^{18}O are examples of isotones, as they all lie in the column indicating that they have 10 neutrons.

BONDING

Bonding occurs when two or more elements attach themselves to one another. Two common forms of bonding are ionic and covalent. In ionic bonding, one element gives up an electron to another element. The result is often that both elements have an imbalance in the number of protons and electrons. When the numbers of protons and electrons are not the same, the element displays a charge relative to the charge of the subatomic part with the highest frequency (proton or electron). For example, if there are more protons $(+)$ than electrons $(-)$, then the element has a positive charge. Charged atoms are called ions.

The second type of bonding is covalent. In this type of bonding, the outer shell electrons share electrons. Thus, electrons in the outer shell orbit both elements.

Bibliography

Ball, JL and Moore, AD. Essential physics for radiographers (2nd edition). Boston: Blackwell Scientific Publications, 1986.

Bushong, SC. Radiologic science for technologists (4th edition). St. Louis: Mosby, 1988.

Graham, BJ and Thomas, WN. An introduction to physics for radiologic technologists. Philadelphia: Saunders, 1975.

Kelsey, CA. Essentials of radiology physics. St. Louis: Warren H. Green, 1985.

Oman, RM. An introduction to radiologic science. New York: McGraw-Hill, 1975.

Selman, J. The fundamentals of x-ray and radium physics (7th edition). Springfield, IL: Thomas, 1985.

Sprawls, P. The physics and instrumentation of nuclear medicine. Baltimore: University Park Press, 1981.

Walker, F, Miller, D and Feiner, F. Chart of the nuclides. San Jose: General Electric, 1984.

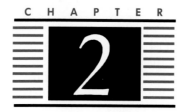

MAGNETISM

INTRODUCTION

Magnetism is the ability of a material to attract iron. The phenomenon of magnetism has been known for thousands of years. However, it was not until the 1800s that the characteristics of magnetism were employed to human advantage. Today, magnetism is used in many areas of everyday life, including the production of electricity, the use of compasses and the separation of materials (by electromagnet). The most recent medical use of magnetism is in magnetic resonance imaging (MRI).

As with so many physical concepts, it is possible to write a book on magnetism and its uses. This text limits discussion of magnetism to the laws and characteristics that relate to electricity. Further discussion of the relationship of electricity and magnetism is located in Chapter 3, Electromagnetism. Information regarding the relationship of magnetism and MRI is beyond the scope of this text.

THEORY OF MAGNETISM

It is theorized that the atoms or molecules of a magnetic material contain a north and a south pole (dipole). Because they are dipolar, each atom or molecule contains all the properties of a magnet. Thus, when a magnetized material is broken, each piece contains a north and a south pole, becoming a magnet (Figure 2–1). The atoms or molecules tend to cluster in a group. The groups form a domain.

Each electron within a domain spins on its axis and orbits the atom's respective nucleus. When atoms are in an unmagnetized state, the direction of electron movement is disoriented (random). Conversely, when atoms are in the magnetized state,

the electrons become organized and follow a specific orientation (Figure 2–2). The number of organized domains is increased as the strength of the magnet increases. When all the domains are aligned, the material is said to be saturated.

MAGNETIC FIELD

There is an invisible force surrounding a magnet. This force is called a magnetic field. The magnetic field consists of flux lines (Figure 2–3). Because the lines cannot be seen, they are demonstrated by inference. This is achieved by using a compass or iron filings. The presence of a magnetic field deflects the needle of a compass. The advantage of using a compass to detect a magnetic field is that the compass can identify direction (Figure 2–4). Flux lines can be demonstrated with iron filings on a piece of paper. The paper is placed over the magnet. A thin layer of iron filings is sprinkled on the paper and the paper is tapped gently with a pencil. The filings are attracted to the flux lines, outlining the position of the lines.

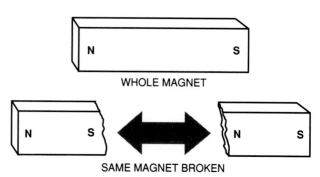

Figure 2–1. Breaking a magnet results in two individual magnets.

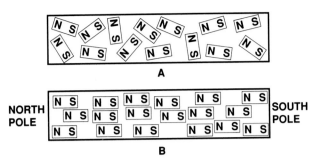

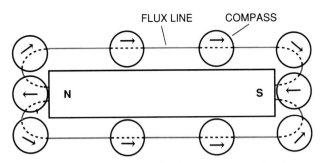

Figure 2–2. Domain orientation. *A*, Unmagnetized state; *B*, magnetized state.

Figure 2–4. Compass showing flux line (magnetic field) direction.

One characteristic of flux lines is the manner in which they travel. Flux lines travel parallel to each other. On the exterior aspect of the magnet, the flux lines travel from the north pole of the magnet to the south pole. Within the magnet, flux line flow is from the south pole to the north pole.

The strength of the magnetic field depends on the number and concentration of flux lines. The number of flux lines may be measured using the centimeter-gram-second (cgs) scale or the International System of units (SI) scale. The cgs unit used to measure magnetic strength is the maxwell (Mx). One maxwell is equivalent to 1 flux line. The magnetic strength SI unit is the weber (Wb). One weber is equal to 10^8 Mx. The concentration of the flux lines is often referred to as flux density. The cgs unit for flux density is the gauss (G), and the SI unit is the tesla (T). One tesla is equal to 10^4 G. Concentration of the flux is a ratio of the number of flux lines (measured in maxwells or webers) for a specific area (Figure 2–5). For example, 1 G = 1 Mx/cm^2 or 1 T = 1 Wb/m^2. The greatest magnetic strength is located at the poles of the magnet.

A second characteristic of magnetic flux is that flux lines flowing in the same direction repel,

whereas those moving in the opposite direction attract (Figure 2–6).

Another characteristic of flux lines is that flux lines are distorted when a magnetic material is placed in the field and are unaffected when a nonmagnetic material is positioned in the flux path (Figure 2–7).

LAWS OF MAGNETISM

There are three laws of magnetism. One law states that all magnets have two poles: north and south. Another law, related to polarity, states that like poles attract and unlike poles repel. Thus, if two magnets are placed near each other with either the north or the south poles of the magnets facing each other, the magnets will repel. Conversely, if the two magnets are positioned so the north pole of one magnet faces the south pole of the other magnet, the magnets will attract. The third law of magnetism refers to the force of attraction or repulsion. This law states that the strength of the force

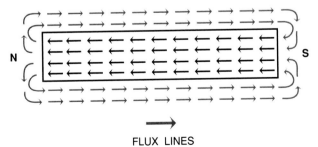

FLUX LINES

Figure 2–3. Magnetic field surrounding a magnet.

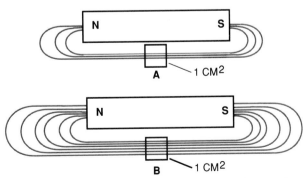

Figure 2–5. Strength of magnetic field for 1 cm^2 area; there are fewer flux lines in *A* than in *B*, resulting in a stronger magnetic field in *B*.

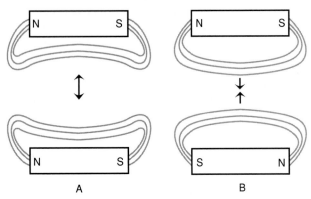

Figure 2—6. A, Flux lines traveling in same direction repel. B, Flux lines flowing in opposite directions attract.

varies directly with the product of the pole strength and is inversely proportional to the distance between the poles. Thus, increasing polarity increases the force. For example, if the pole of one magnet is 15 G and a second magnet has 5 G strength, the force is 75 G (15 × 5 = 75). Doubling the strength of the second magnet to 10 G doubles the force to 150 G, or 15 × 10 = 150. An example of the effect of distance on strength is that two magnets with a force of 1.8 T and separated by 1 cm demonstrate a force of 0.3 T when the distance between them is increased to 3 cm, or $(1/3)^2 × 1.8 = 1/9 × 1.8 = 0.3$.

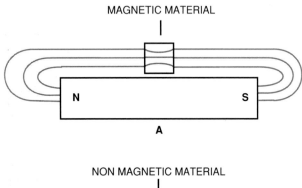

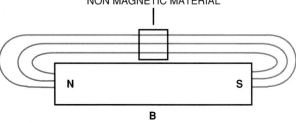

Figure 2—7. Flux lines are distorted by magnetic material (A) and unaffected by nonmagnetic material (B).

CLASSIFICATION OF MATTER RELATIVE TO MAGNETISM

Matter may be classified relative to magnetic traits. The traits used are permeability and reluctance. Permeability refers to the ease with which a material is magnetized (ability to create magnetic flux). Reluctance is the degree of opposition (resistance) a material exhibits to being magnetized.

The standard used for permeability is air. This is often referred to as relative permeability and is expressed as 1. The higher the permeability number is, the easier the matter is to magnetize.

Reluctance is the opposite of permeability. The higher the reluctance the material displays, the more resistance it exhibits to being magnetized. When a material with a high reluctance is placed in a magnetic field, the flux lines flow in the air around the material (Figure 2–8). This occurs because air has a low reluctance relative to the high reluctance material. Thus, flux lines follow the route of least resistance.

On the basis of a matter's permeability or reluctance, the material is classified as being nonmagnetic or magnetic. Nonmagnetic material is unaffected by a magnetic field. Examples of nonmagnetic matter are wood, glass and plastic. Magnetic materials are further categorized (see below).

CATEGORIZATION OF MAGNETIC MATERIAL

Magnetic material is divided into three categories: paramagnetic, diamagnetic and ferromagnetic. Paramagnetic material has the ability to become slightly magnetic in the presence of a strong magnetic field. The paramagnetic material takes on the opposite polarity of the magnetic pole magnetizing it, e.g., a north magnetizing pole produces a south pole in the paramagnetic material. These materials have a permeability that is relative (1) or slightly

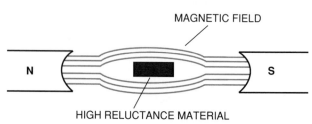

Figure 2—8. Flux lines follow the route of least resistance.

Table 2–1. CHARACTERISTICS OF MAGNETIC MATERIAL

Material	Permeability	Reluctance	Retentivity
Diamagnetic	<1	Very high	None
Paramagnetic	1	High	None
Ferromagnetic	>1	Low	High or low

higher than relative. Examples of paramagnetic material are chromium, platinum and tungsten. Diamagnetic materials also become slightly magnetized in the presence of a strong magnetic field. However, unlike paramagnetic material, diamagnetic material takes on the same polarity as that of the magnetic field (the pole of magnetic field repels the pole of diamagnetic material). The permeability of these materials is less than 1 (negative). Copper, bismuth, silver and gold are examples of diamagnetic material. Ferromagnetic material is easily magnetized. The material takes on the opposite polarity of the magnetic pole magnetizing it. Ferromagnetic materials have a permeability of greater than 1. These materials make the strongest magnets. Examples of ferromagnetic material are iron, nickel and cobalt.

The ability of a ferromagnetic material to retain its magnetism (residual magnetism) after being removed from a magnetic field is called retentivity. Materials with a low retentivity (temporary magnet), e.g., soft iron, lose their magnetic field rapidly. Materials that retain their magnetism for a long time (high retentivity), e.g., compass needle, are called permanent magnets. Paramagnetic and diamagnetic materials have no retentivity (no residual magnetism). Table 2–1 lists the characteristics of magnetic materials.

METHODS OF MAGNETIZING A MATERIAL

One technique used to magnetize a material is to place the material in a magnetic field. Three common magnetic field sources are the earth, electricity and a permanent magnet. The earth has a magnetic field of about 0.5 G. Thus, it is considered a magnet. Some elements found in the earth e.g., lodestone, have become magnetized because they have rested within the earth's magnetic field for thousands of years. These materials are called natural magnets. A more recent method used to make magnets is by

electricity. An electrical current has a magnetic field surrounding it. Thus, if a ferromagnetic material is placed in a magnetic field, it becomes magnetized. This method is important relative to x-ray circuitry and is discussed in Chapters 3, Electromagnetism, and 7, Transformers. Permanent magnets have a magnetic field surrounding them. Placing a ferromagnetic material in a magnetic field magnetizes the ferromagnetic material.

In addition to placement in a magnetic field, mechanical means may be used to magnetize a material. A common mechanical method is heating or hammering a piece of steel while it lies near a magnet. This causes the steel to become a magnet.

LABORATORY EXPERIENCE

In *Concepts in Medical Radiographic Imaging: Laboratory Manual*, Laboratory 1, Magnetism, is dedicated to demonstrating basic magnetic principles and phenomena. This laboratory contains three experiments. The first experiment employs a compass to demonstrate the existence of a magnetic field and iron filings to illustrate characteristics of magnetic flux and polarity. The experimenter maps the lines of force surrounding a magnet. The second experiment demonstrates the law of magnetism that states that like poles attract and unlike poles repel. In the third experiment, the experimenter is provided with several unknown materials and is requested to use a magnet to identify which materials are magnetic and which are nonmagnetic.

Bibliography

Ball, JL and Moore, AD. Essential physics for radiographers (2nd edition). Boston: Blackwell Scientific Publications, 1986.

Bushong, SC. Magnetic resonance imaging physical and biological principles. St. Louis: Mosby, 1988.

Bushong, SC. Radiologic science for technologists (4th edition). St. Louis: Mosby, 1988.

Curry, TS, Dowdey, JE and Murry, RC. Christensen's Introduction to the physics of diagnostic radiology (3rd edition). Philadelphia: Lea & Febiger, 1984.

Graham, BJ and Thomas, WN. An introduction to physics for radiologic technologists. Philadelphia: Saunders, 1975.

Hazen, ME. Experiencing electricity and electronics, electron flow version. Philadelphia: Saunders, 1989.

Kelsey, CA. Essentials of radiology physics. St. Louis: Warren H. Green, 1985.

Oman, RM. An introduction to radiologic science. New York: McGraw-Hill, 1975.

Multi-media. Radiation physic series, lesson 2, section D. Slide/Audio tape. Denver: Multi-media, 1983.

Selman, J. The fundamentals of x-ray and radium physics (7th edition). Springfield, IL: Thomas, 1985.

Wilson, JD. Physics: A practical and conceptual approach. Philadelphia: Saunders, 1989.

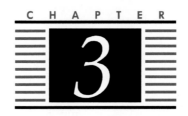

ELECTROMAGNETISM

INTRODUCTION

For hundreds of years, magnetism and electricity were studied as unrelated entities. As stated in Chapter 2, Magnetism, people have been aware of magnetic phenomena for thousands of years. For example, compasses were used to navigate ships as early as the 14th century. During this time, the study of electricity also occurred. Experimentation was limited to static electricity. It was not until the early 1800s that it was discovered that electricity and magnetism were related. The study of the relationship of electricity and magnetism is appropriately called electromagnetism.

This chapter describes the basic phenomena of electromagnetism. The various uses of electromagnetism, e.g., in transformers, are discussed in the respective chapters of this text.

OERSTED'S DISCOVERY

A Danish experimenter, Hans Christian Oersted, is credited with discovering that a magnetic field surrounds a moving electrical current. Oersted demonstrated this phenomenon in 1820 by placing a compass near a straight wire conductor. After positioning the compass near a conductor with no current flow, Oersted noted that the compass pointed to the earth's magnetic north pole. However, when he passed an electrical current through the conductor, the compass pointed toward the conductor, proving that a magnetic field existed around a moving current.

The direction of the magnetic flow may be determined by using a compass (Figure 3–1). If a compass is unavailable, magnetic field direction can be dem-

onstrated by applying the left hand thumb rule. This rule states that if a conductor is grasped by the left hand so that the thumb is pointing in the direction of electron flow (toward the positive charge), the fingers point in the direction of the magnetic field flow (Figure 3–2). It should be noted that there is also a right hand thumb rule. The difference between the right and left thumb rules is in the direction the thumb points. As stated previously, the thumb points in the direction of electron flow (toward the positive charge) in the left hand thumb rule. For the right hand thumb rule, the thumb points toward the current flow (toward the negative charge). Thus, regardless of

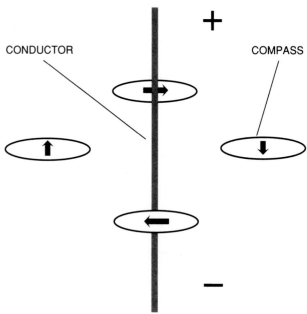

Figure 3–1. Compass demonstrating the direction of a magnetic field surrounding a moving current.

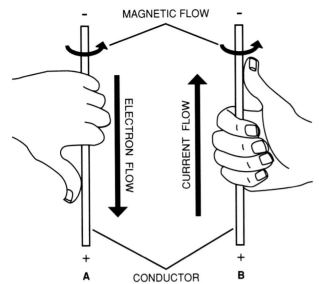

Figure 3-2. Direction of magnetic field as demonstrated by the left hand thumb rule (A) and the right hand thumb rule (B).

the hand used, as long as the rule is applied correctly, the direction of the magnetic field flow is demonstrated (Figure 3-2).

Electricity is able to flow through a straight or a coiled wire conductor. The magnetic field in a coiled conductor follows the left hand thumb rule. A conductor containing multiple coils is called a solenoid. The magnetic fields of the coils overlap inside the loop and flow together. This allows the solenoid to simulate a bar magnet with north and south poles (Figure 3-3). Placing a soft iron core in a solenoid concentrates the magnetic flux lines and increases the magnetic field. A solenoid with a soft iron core inside is called an electromagnet. Two advantages of an electromagnet are the ability to turn the current on and off and the ability to regulate the intensity of the current by adjusting the position of the core in the solenoid.

PRODUCING A CURRENT

Several years after Oersted discovered that a magnetic field surrounded an electrical current, Michael Faraday demonstrated that magnetism could be used to induce an electrical current. Faraday, a British scientist, discovered that the relationship of a conductor and a magnetic field is such that a current may be induced in a conductor by

varying the strength of the magnetic field. There are three primary methods of changing the magnetic field to induce a current:
1. Have a magnetic field move over a stationary conductor
2. Move a conductor over a stationary magnetic field
3. Have both the magnet and the conductor stationary and vary the strength of the magnetic field, e.g., with alternating current.

The magnitude of the current is directly proportional to the number of magnetic flux lines cut by the conductor per second. Four factors influence the number of magnetic flux lines cut:
1. The strength of the magnetic field. The stronger the field is, the more flux lines are able to be cut per second, increasing the current.
2. The speed of the conductor. The faster the conductor moves across the magnetic field, the more lines are cut per second, increasing the current.
3. The angle of the plane of the conductor. A maximum amount of flux lines are cut when the plane of the conductor is perpendicular to the magnetic field. Thus, the closer the plane of the conductor is to 90 degrees, the greater is the current produced.
4. The number of turns of the conductor. The more turns the conductor has, the greater the current.

LENZ'S LAW

Heinrich Lenz, a German physicist, discovered that an induced current flows in a direction such that it opposes the action that induces it. For example, if the north pole of a magnet is inserted into a coiled wire conductor, the magnetic field increases in the wire, producing a current. Recall that a solenoid acts like a magnet having a north and south pole. Lenz's law states that the current is in the opposite direction of (opposes) the magnetic field (magnet) inducing it. Consequently, to oppose the north pole of the magnet, the coiled wire as-

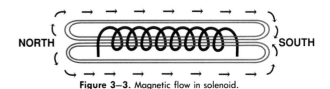

Figure 3-3. Magnetic flow in solenoid.

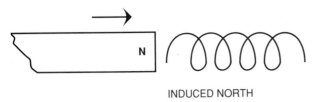

INDUCED NORTH

Figure 3—4. Lenz's law.

sumes the same polarity as the end of the magnet entering the coil. Figure 3–4 illustrates this effect. There are two types of induction: self and mutual.

As the name implies, in self-induction, the magnetic field induces an opposing action in its own coil. This produces a current that opposes the current produced by the magnet. Mutual induction requires two coiled conductors. One conductor (source or primary coil) has an alternating current passing through it. The primary coil current creates a changing magnetic field. Placing a second coiled conductor (secondary coil) near the primary coil induces a current in the secondary coil. Self-induction and mutual induction are useful in transformers.

LABORATORY EXPERIENCE

In *Concepts in Medical Radiographic Imaging: Laboratory Manual*, Laboratories 3, Electromagnetism, and 6, Production of Electricity, are relevant to this chapter. There are two experiments in the Electro-magnetism laboratory. The first experiment duplicates Oersted's demonstration that a magnetic field surrounds a straight wire conductor. The second experiment employs a compass to identify the magnetic north and south ends of a solenoid.

The Production of Electricity laboratory duplicates Faraday's experiment to demonstrate the method of inducing a current in a conductor. This laboratory contains two experiments to demonstrate the induction of an electrical current in a conductor by the cutting of magnetic lines of force. Two methods (experiments) are used to produce electricity. One experiment produces electricity by moving a magnet through a stationary coiled wire. The second experiment induces a current by moving the coiled wire over a stationary magnet. A third experiment demonstrates two factors, the number of turns of the conductor and the speed of the conductor, that affect the strength of the current.

Bibliography

Ball, JL and Moore, AD. Essential physics for radiographers (2nd edition). Boston: Blackwell Scientific Publications, 1986.

Bushong, SC. Radiologic science for technologists (4th edition). St. Louis: Mosby, 1988.

Graham, BJ and Thomas, WN. An introduction to physics for radiologic technologists. Philadelphia: Saunders, 1975.

Oman, RM. An introduction to radiologic science. New York: McGraw-Hill, 1975.

Multi-media. Radiation physic series, lesson 3, section C. Slide/Audio tape. Denver: Multi-media, 1983.

Selman, J. The fundamentals of x-ray and radium physics (7th edition). Springfield, IL: Thomas, 1985.

Wilson, JD. Physics: A practical and conceptual approach. Philadelphia: Saunders, 1989.

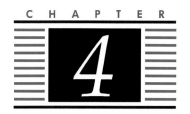

ELECTRICAL SYMBOLS

AND DIAGRAMS

INTRODUCTION

An electrical circuit often contains several electronic parts. The number of components increases with the complexity of the circuit. The construction and design of circuits are described by drawing an illustration of the circuit. The circuit diagrams use symbols to represent the various electrical components. Originally, the symbols were drawn to represent the appearance of the object. As the science of electronics grew, it became impractical to draw a pictorial representation of the numerous electrical components. Today, there are thousands of electrical symbols, many of which have little resemblance to the true shape of the part. To avoid misinterpretation of the object a symbol represents, efforts have been made to standardize symbols and diagrams.

Standardization of symbols is important to maintain a universal understanding of the meaning of color codes, printed circuits, enclosure requirements, etc. In the United States, the two most common resources for defining standard symbols are the American Standards Association and the United States government.

This chapter presents the electrical symbols used throughout this text and in the laboratory manual. The symbols are used to represent electrical components, except when the construction of the part needs emphasis. In these instances, the standard symbol is replaced by a pictorial example of the part being described. The logic symbols used for computers are found in Chapter 15, Fundamentals of Computer Technology. The logic symbol is often located next to the corresponding logic circuit diagram.

ELECTRICAL SYMBOLS

BATTERY

The battery symbol is often employed in the laboratory manual associated with this text. The symbol is composed of two vertical lines, each having a perpendicular horizontal line exiting at the center (Figure 4–1). The longer vertical line represents the positive side of the battery. The shorter vertical line refers to the negative battery terminal. The horizontal line is the path the current travels. The battery symbol is used to refer to a single battery cell. Multiple symbols are used to identify two or more batteries. Generally, a maximum of four symbols are used to represent multiple batteries regardless of the number of batteries employed in the circuit.

CAPACITOR

A capacitor stores electricity. Numerous symbols are used to represent the capacitor (Figure 4–2). The capacitor is often represented by two parallel lines.

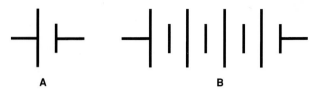

Figure 4–1. *A*, Single cell battery symbol. *B*, Multiple batteries.

RESISTOR

A resistor symbol is a zigzag line (Figure 4–3A). The most common number of peaks to the zigzag is three. The resistance of a resistor is measured in ohms. The amount of ohms of the resistor may be identified by having a number and ohm symbol (the Greek letter omega, Ω) next to the resistor symbol.

Another type of resistor symbol is a long cylinder with rings around the left side and lines exiting each end of the cylinder (Figure 4–3A). The rings are labeled by color, e.g., red and brown. The color represents the ohms of the resistor. Discussion of how to calculate ohms by color code is located in Appendix A.

Resistors may have a fixed ohm value or may vary in ohms. A resistor that can change the ohm value is called a variable resistor. Figure 4–3B is an example of a variable resistor symbol.

SWITCHES

A switch is used to open or close a circuit. There are several type of switches, including mechanical, rotary, fixed, moving and sliding. Figure 4–4 presents examples of switches.

RECTIFIER

There are two types of rectifiers: the diode tube and the solid state. The diode tube has a cathode,

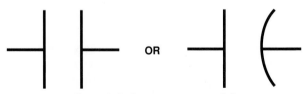

Figure 4–2. Common capacitor symbols.

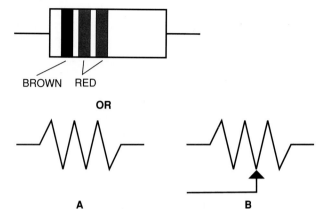

Figure 4–3. *A*, Resistor symbols. *B*, Variable resistor.

which emits an electron cloud, and an anode (Figure 4–5A); these are encased in a glass envelope. The symbol for a cathode looks like the end of a pencil; the anode is represented by a line at a 45 degree angle to the cathode. The anode and cathode are drawn within a circle. The circle represents the glass envelope.

The x-ray tube is a type of diode tube and is represented by the diode symbol. This text diverges from the typical diode symbol and illustrates the filament of the cathode of the x-ray tube as a coiled wire and demonstrates the anode as a picture. This version is drawn for emphasis (Figure 4–5B).

A solid state rectifier has a solid arrow representing the cathode and a perpendicular line for the anode (Figure 4–6). Electron flow is in the direction opposite that of the arrow. The arrow points in the direction of current flow.

TRANSFORMER

Transformers are used to increase or decrease voltage. They use two coiled wires to perform this function (refer to Chapter 7, Transformers, for more specific information on their function). The wires are often wrapped around a core. Transformers may have no core (air instead of core material) or may have some form of magnetic core (Figure 4–7).

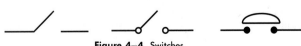

Figure 4–4. Switches.

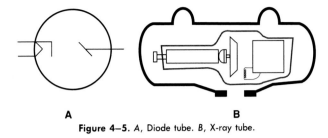

Figure 4–5. A, Diode tube. B, X-ray tube.

The coiled wires of a transformer may be parallel to one another, triangular (called delta) or Y shaped (referred to as wye or star). Figure 4–8 shows the symbols used to represent each coiled configuration.

METERS

It is possible to measure volts (potential difference), amperes (current) or ohms (resistance) in a circuit. This is achieved by using specialized instruments designed to measure the respective unit (refer to Chapter 6, Measuring Volts, Ohms and Amperes for more information on the use of meters). A meter is represented by a circle. A designation is placed in the circle to identify the meter type (Figure 4–9).

ELECTRICAL DIAGRAMS

Previous discussion related to symbols used for different components of an electrical circuit. An electrical circuit may consist of one or more of these components (or other items not mentioned here). An electrical diagram is an illustration representing the manner in which various components are connected. Components are most often placed in parallel or in series within the circuit. In a series circuit, the items are connected one after the other (in a continuous line). Items in a parallel circuit are arranged so that the current is divided among the

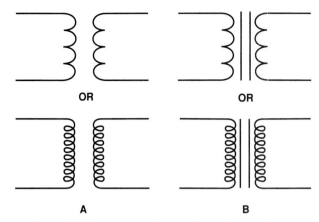

Figure 4–7. Transformer symbols. A, Air core; B, magnetic core.

various items. Figure 4–10 presents examples of simple parallel and series circuits. Refer to Chapter 5, Electrodynamics, for an in-depth discussion of parallel and series circuits and their relationship to potential difference (volts), current (amperes) and resistance (ohms).

LABORATORY EXPERIENCE

In *Concepts in Medical Radiographic Imaging: Laboratory Manual,* Laboratories 2, Electrical Symbols and Diagrams, and 4, Resistors, are relevant to this chapter.

There are three procedures in the Electrical Symbols and Diagrams laboratory. The first procedure is used to provide a means for the researcher to memorize various electrical symbols using flash cards that have a symbol on the front and the name of the symbol on the back. The experimenter memorizes the symbol on each card. The front of the cards are shown to the learner one at a time. The

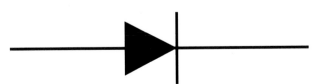

Figure 4–6. Solid state rectifier.

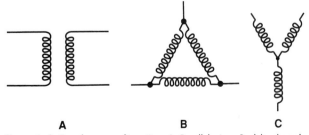

Figure 4–8. Transformer configuration. A, Parallel wires; B, delta shaped; C, star (wye) formation.

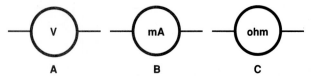

Figure 4–9. *A, Voltmeter. B, Milliammeter. C, Ohmmeter.*

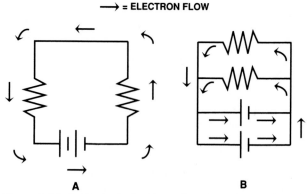

Figure 4–10. *A, Simple circuit with two batteries and two resistors in series. B, Simple circuit with two batteries and two resistors in parallel.*

learner continues to see the cards until he/she is able to identify all the symbols correctly. The second procedure requires the learner to construct a circuit from a circuit diagram. In the last procedure, the experimenter views a constructed circuit and must draw a diagram to represent the circuit.

In the Resistors laboratory, the researcher uses the color code located on a resistor to determine the ohm range of the resistor. After mathematically calculating the ohms, the researcher uses an ohmmeter to measure the exact amount of resistance of the resistor. Because this experiment requires use of a meter, the instructor may wish the student to perform Laboratory 5, Multitesters, before the Resistors laboratory.

Bibliography

Baer, CJ. Electrical and electronic drawing (2nd edition). New York: McGraw-Hill, 1966.

Bushong, SC. Radiologic science for technologists (4th edition). St. Louis: Mosby, 1988.

Snow, CW. Electrical drafting and design. Englewood Cliffs, NJ: Prentice Hall, 1976.

ELECTRODYNAMICS

INTRODUCTION

From the beginning of time, electricity coexisted with humankind. At that time, the most common form of electricity was lightning. The electricity produced by lightning is created by nature. Thousands of years passed before society learned to produce its own electricity. Today, there are thousands of conveniences provided by electricity, e.g., the production of light and the use of stoves and refrigerators. Often, individuals take electricity for granted. It is not until one experiences a loss of electricity, e.g., loss of power due to an electrical storm, that one's dependence on it is fully appreciated.

There are two common forms of electricity—the fixed electrical charge and electricity in motion. The former is termed static electricity. The latter is often referred to as electrical current. The study of electricity in motion is electrodynamics.

This chapter concentrates primarily on electricity in motion. It contains information about basic laws and theories of electricity. Discussion includes basic components of electricity, methods of producing electricity, Ohm's law, parallel circuits and series circuits. The concepts presented here serve as a foundation for the chapters that consider applications of these theories, e.g., kilovoltage and quality control. For a discussion on the methods used to produce electricity, refer to Electromagnetism, Chapter 3.

FUNDAMENTALS OF ELECTRICITY

Current is the flow of electricity created by electrical charges and a force. Electrical charges are either negative or positive. The positive electrical charge is the proton, whereas the negative charge is the electron. A positive to negative flow of current is called conventional current. Electron current is characterized by a negative to positive current flow. In this text, any mention of current refers to electron current unless otherwise stated.

A minimum of two conditions must exist for current to flow. They are a force to move the current and a medium in which the current can flow. The force is referred to as electromotive force (EMF) or potential difference and is measured in volts (V). The medium may be almost anything. Common mediums are vacuum, air and solids. The medium for current flow contains its own atoms (with the exception of a vacuum), which tend to hinder current flow. This hindrance to current flow is called resistance and is measured in ohms. The higher the resistance, the less the current flow.

One factor affecting the amount of resistance is the type of material used to conduct the current. The resistance for a particular medium is a constant and is referred to as the medium's resistivity. Mediums with no resistivity, e.g., titanium and niobium, are called superconductors. These substances allow a free flow of current. Materials with a low resistivity, e.g., copper and silver, are referred to as conductors. These materials serve as an excellent vehicle for current flow. High resistivity materials are called insulators. A good insulator prevents the flow of current. Some materials have both low and high resistivity. In these materials, the type of resistivity depends on the conditions applied to the medium. These mediums, e.g., silicon and germanium, are called semiconductors. Semiconductors are useful in regulating the direction of current flow (see Chapter 8, Rectification, for more information on semiconductors).

Recall that electrical charges are required for a current flow. All atoms contain electrical charges. If the atom contains an equal amount of negative and positive charges, it is neutral. Neutral atoms have no current flow. Any imbalance in charges, e.g., more positive charges than negative, provides favorable conditions for current flow. Charges are similar to magnetism. As is the case in magnetism (in which unlike poles attract), in electricity, unlike charges attract each other. Conversely, like charges repel each other.

Current flow is from an area of electron excess (more negatively charged) to an area of electron deficiency (less negatively charged). The flow in solids is concentrated on the outer surface of the medium. In solids having a bend or curve, e.g., copper wire connected to various electrical components, the greatest magnitude of the charge is at the curved surface or point of the medium.

As mentioned earlier, a force is needed to move the current. Positively charged particles have a force that is directed outward from the proton. The electron has an inward force. The closer the negative and positive charges are, the greater the force is. Force (F) is inversely proportional to the square of the distance (d) of the charges, or $F = 1/d^2$. Force is also related to charge. Its relationship is directly proportional to the product of the charges (q), or $F = q_1q_2$. Recall that the type of medium (k) influences the flow of current. Thus, in addition to distance and charge, medium is a factor on force.

Combining the concepts of distance, charge and medium results in Coulomb's law. This law is represented mathematically as

$$F = k\,\frac{q_1q_2}{d^2}$$

DIRECTION OF CURRENT FLOW

Current flow may be in one direction or it may periodically reverse directions. Current that flows in one direction is called direct current. The term alternating current is used to describe current that changes directions. The direction of current represents its waveform. It is possible to graph the waveform.

When plotting the waveform, the horizontal line of the graph (*x* axis) represents time, usually in fractions of a second. The vertical line of the graph (*y* axis) is the amplitude, which is often measured in potential difference (volts). The location of the graph relative to the horizontal line indicates the direction of the current. A graph above the horizontal line represents positive current direction. Conversely, a graph below the horizontal line refers to a negative flow of current. Points on the horizontal line indicate that there is no flow of current.

Figure 5–1A is a graph of direct current. Notice that the graph is parallel to the horizontal line. The height of the line is the maximum potential differ-

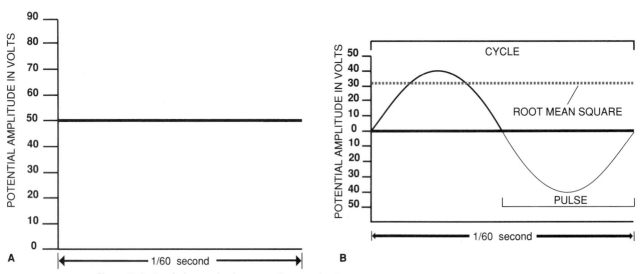

Figure 5–1. Graph showing the direction and magnitude of current. A, Direct current; B, alternating current.

ence. The location relative to the horizontal line indicates the current's direction.

Alternating current is represented graphically in Figure 5–1B. This type of graph is called a sine wave. Each curve that begins at zero (on the horizontal line) and ends at zero is a pulse. Two consecutive pulses equal one complete cycle. Because the amplitude of the current varies, the effective potential difference is not the peak of the pulse but an average of the amplitude changes. The effective potential difference is the root-mean-square.

The rate at which electricity is generated (better known as frequency) is expressed in a unit called hertz (Hz). This unit is the number of cycles per second (cps). The term frequency is interchangeable with cycles per second. In the United States, electricity operates at a frequency of 60 Hz, or 60 cps. Many other counties generate electricity at 50 cps.

COMPONENTS OF ELECTRICITY

Electricity consists of a flow of current. Most electrical circuits contain a potential difference and resistance. The potential difference pushes the current through the conductor. The resistance hinders the flow of electricity. Resistance exists primarily in solid materials. There is no resistance in superconductive materials. The following discussion expands on the concepts of current, potential and resistance.

POTENTIAL

Electrical potential is the means used to move electrons. An electrical circuit contains one point that has a high negative charge and a second point with a less negative charge. Recall that current flows when the electrons move from the point of excessive (high negative) charge to the point of deficient (less negative) charge. The difference between these charges is called potential difference and represents the amount of potential needed to move the charge (electrons) from one point to another.

Potential difference is sometimes referred to as EMF. The name electromotive force is misleading, as it implies it represents a force. EMF refers to a type of energy that is changed from its original form to electricity. The type of EMF referred to in this text is measured in volts. The symbol used to represent potential difference (EMF) is E; the symbol used to represent the unit volt is V.

CURRENT

As mentioned previously, current is a flow of charges. Current is defined as 1 coulomb (C) per second (1 C = 6.25×10^{18} electrons). The rate of flow (number of coulombs per second) determines the size of the current. Current needs a potential difference to move the charges and a medium in which to travel. The relationship of current to potential difference is discussed below under Ohm's Law.

The unit used to measure current is the ampere. The symbol used to represent ampere is A, whereas the symbol for current is I.

RESISTANCE

Any hindrance to the flow of current is called resistance. Resistance is measured in ohms. The Greek letter omega (Ω) is used to represent ohms, and the symbol R refers to resistance. In addition to the type of medium used as a conductor, three other factors affecting the amount of resistance are length, temperature and cross-section. Resistance is directly proportional to the length of the conductor and temperature. This means the longer the conductor or the higher the temperature, the greater the resistance. The converse is also true. Recall that the flow of electrons is on the outer surface of a conductor. The larger the cross-section of the conductor is, the more area there is for the current to flow. Thus, resistance is inversely proportional to the cross-section, or the larger the cross-section, the less the resistance. The following is a mathematical representation of the relationship of resistance factors:

$$R = \rho \, \frac{L(T)}{A}$$

where ρ is the medium, L is length, T represents temperature and A is cross-section.

OHM'S LAW

Georg Simon Ohm, a German physicist, established a mathematical relationship of current to potential and resistance. This relationship is referred to as Ohm's law. Because superconductors have no resistance, Ohm's law does not apply to these circuits. Ohm's law states that current is directly related to potential and inversely related to resistance. The mathematical formula is

$$I = E/R$$

By using algebraic rules, it is possible to determine the relationship of potential to resistance and current. The result is

$$I = E/R$$
$$IR = E$$

Algebraic rules also apply to determine the relationship of resistance to potential and current. The result is

$$I = E/R$$
$$IR = E$$
$$R = E/I$$

Ohm's law is useful in calculating the current, potential or resistance of the entire electrical circuit or a portion of the circuit. Capital letters are used when Ohm's law is used for the entire circuit (as in the preceding Ohm's law formula). Lower case letters are used with a subscript to represent a portion of the circuit. For example, to calculate the amount of ohms over the first resistor in a circuit with three resistors,

$$r_1 = e_1/i_1$$

POWER

Electrical power is measured in watts (W). Watts are the product of voltage and resistance, or $W = EI$. Recall that voltage is the product of current and resistance, $E = IR$. Because $IR = E$, it is possible to substitute IR for E in the watts formula. This results in the following:

$$W = (IR)I$$
$$W = I^2R$$

SIMPLE ELECTRICAL CIRCUITS

There are two basic types of electrical circuits: series and parallel. A series circuit is constructed so that all the components are in the same path or attached in a series (Figure 5–2A). Parallel circuits have components that are bridged across a common connection to the potential source (Figure 5–2B).

SERIES CIRCUIT

In a series circuit, the current has only one path. Consequently, the current is a constant for a given circuit. When one component in a series circuit, e.g., light bulb, burns out the circuit is opened and the remaining components do not function. Thus, it is advantageous to place a circuit breaker or fuse in series.

In a series circuit, resistance and voltage can be calculated by using Ohm's law. The total resistance (R_T) is the sum of the individual resistances. This is represented mathematically as

$$R_T = r_1 + r_2 + \ldots r_n$$

In Figure 5–2A, the current is 4 A. Individual resistances in Figure 5–2A are 2 Ω, 4 Ω and 5 Ω for an R_T of 11 Ω, or $2 + 4 + 5 = 11$.

The total voltage (E_T) is the sum of the individual voltages, or

$$E_T = e_1 + e_2 + \ldots e_n$$

It is possible to calculate the individual voltages in Figure 5–2A by using the known resistance and current values. The following are the individual voltage calculations for Figure 5–2A:

$$e_1 = i_1r_1$$
$$e_1 = (4)2 = 8$$

$$e_2 = i_2r_2$$
$$e_2 = (4)4 = 16$$

$$e_3 = i_3r_3$$
$$e_3 = (4)5 = 20$$

On the basis of the preceding calculations, the total voltage is 44 V, or $8 + 16 + 20 = 44$. When the

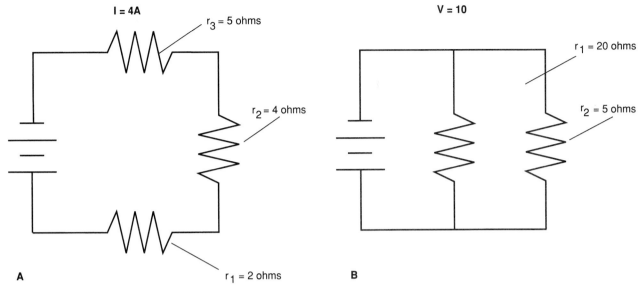

Figure 5–2. A, Series circuit; B, parallel circuit.

total resistance and current are known in a series circuit, rather than calculating the individual voltages and summing them, one can calculate total voltage by multiplying I_T by R_T. In Figure 5–2A, this is $E_T = 4(11) = 44$ V.

PARALLEL CIRCUIT

In a parallel circuit, the voltage is divided equally among the branches and is constant for a given circuit. When one component in a parallel circuit, e.g., light bulb, burns out the circuit remains closed and the remaining components continue to function. A common use of parallel circuits is in strings of lights.

In a parallel circuit, resistance and current can be calculated by using Ohm's law. The total resistance (R_T) is inversely proportional to the sum of the reciprocal of the individual resistances. This is represented mathematically as

$$1/R_T = 1/r_1 + 1/r_2 + \ldots 1/r_n$$

In Figure 5–2B, the voltage is 10. Individual resistances in Figure 5–2B are 20 Ω and 5 Ω for a R_T of 4 Ω, or

$$1/R_T = 1/20 + 1/5$$
$$1/R_T = 1/20 + 4/20$$

$$1/R_T = 5/20$$
$$5R_T = 20$$
$$R_T = 20/5$$
$$R_T = 4$$

The total resistance in a parallel circuit cannot be greater than the smallest resistance value.

The total current (I_T) is the sum of the individual currents, or

$$I_T = i_1 + i_2 + \ldots i_n$$

It is possible to calculate the individual currents in Figure 5–2B by using the known resistance and voltage values. The following are the individual current calculations for Figure 5–2B:

$$i_1 = e_1/r_1$$
$$i_1 = 10/20 = 0.5$$

$$i_2 = e_2/r_2$$
$$i_2 = 10/5 = 2$$

On the basis of the preceding calculations, the total current is 2.5 A, or 0.5 + 2.0 = 2.5. When the total resistance and voltage are known in a parallel circuit, rather than calculating the individual currents and summing them, one can calculate total current by dividing E_T by R_T. In Figure 5–2A, this is $I_T = 10/4 = 2.5$ A.

In *Concepts in Medical Radiographic Imaging: Laboratory Manual*, Laboratories 7, Ohm's Law; 8, Series Circuits; and 9, Parallel Circuits are relevant to this chapter.

The Ohm's law laboratory is designed to demonstrate the basic law relating to electrical potential, current and resistance. There are two experiments. In the first procedure, the experimenter measures the current and resistance and calculates the voltage of a series circuit. The second procedure requires the investigator to measure the voltage and resistance and calculate the current.

The Series Circuits laboratory also has two experiments. In the first procedure, the experimenter constructs a series circuit consisting of two resistors. The current, resistance and voltage are measured. Ohm's law is used to determine if the measured values coincide with the formula. The second experiment requires the investigator to connect two light bulbs in series. Each bulb is unscrewed one at a time and the effect on the other bulb is observed.

The Parallel Circuits laboratory is similar to the Series Circuits laboratory, the difference being in the construction of the circuit. The experimenter constructs a parallel circuit with three resistors.

There are two experiments in the laboratory. In the first procedure, the current, resistance and voltage are measured. The experimenter determines if the measured values coincide with the Ohm's law formula. The second experiment requires the investigator to connect two light bulbs in parallel. Each bulb is unscrewed one at a time and the effect on the other bulb is observed.

Bibliography

Ball, JL and Moore, AD. Essential physics for radiographers (2nd edition). Boston: Blackwell Scientific Publications, 1986.

Bushong, SC. Radiologic science for technologists (4th edition). St. Louis: Mosby, 1988.

Graham, BJ and Thomas, WN. An introduction to physics for radiologic technologists. Philadelphia: Saunders, 1975.

Hazen, ME. Experiencing electricity and electronics, electron flow version. Philadelphia: Saunders, 1989.

Hendee, WR, Chaney, EL and Rossi, RP. Radiologic physics, equipment and quality control. Chicago: Year Book Medical, 1976.

Kelsey, CA. Essentials of radiology physics. St. Louis: Warren H. Green, 1985.

Oman, RM. An introduction to radiologic science. New York: McGraw-Hill, 1975.

Multi-media. Radiation physics series, lesson 3, section A. Slide/tape (audio). Denver: Multi-media, 1983.

Selman, J. The fundamentals of x-ray and radium physics (7th edition). Springfield, IL: Thomas, 1985.

Wilson, JD. Physics: A practical and conceptual approach. Philadelphia: Saunders, 1989.

C H A P T E R

6

MEASURING VOLTS, AMPERES AND OHMS

INTRODUCTION

Electricity consists of current, potential difference and resistance. Current (I) is a flow of electrical charges. It is measured in a unit called an ampere (A). An ampere is equal to 1 coulomb (6.24 × 10¹⁸ electrons) per second. The amount of work required to move one unit of current from one point in a circuit to another is potential difference, or electromotive force (EMF), E. The unit for potential difference is the volt (V). One volt is the potential that is required to cause 1 A of electric current to flow through 1 ohm (Ω) of resistance. Resistance (R) is the hindrance to the flow of current. The ohm is the unit for resistance. One ohm is the resistance that permits the flow of 1 A of current when the applied potential is 1 V.

The preceding electrical units may be in fractional or multiple form. The prefix attached to the electrical unit determines its value. An example of a fractional prefix is milli- which has a value of $\frac{1}{1000}$, or 10^{-3} of the unit. Thus, 1 mA is equal to $\frac{1}{1000}$, or 10^{-3}A; 1 mV is equivalent to $\frac{1}{1000}$, or 10^{-3}V; and 1 mΩ has a value of $\frac{1}{1000}$, or $10^{-3}\Omega$. An example of a multiple unit value is kilo- which has a value of 1000 times, or 10^3 of the unit. One kiloampere represents 1000, or 10^3A; 1 kV equals 1000, or 10^3V and 1 kΩ has a value of 1000, or $10^3\Omega$.

Instruments are able to measure these electrical units. Measuring units is useful in diagnosing problems, testing an electrical device or proving electri-

cal theories. This chapter is designed to provide information on common types and uses of electrical measuring instruments. In practice, the technologist is not required to measure volts, amperes or ohms. However, the accompanying laboratory manual contains approximately 10 laboratory procedures in which instrumentation is employed to substantiate the electrical theories presented in this text. Consequently, individuals performing the laboratories should read this chapter before attempting to complete the laboratories.

BASIC METER COMPONENTS

The first electrical meter (galvanometer) was developed in 1881 by Jacques d'Arsonal, a French scientist. It was large and cumbersome. In 1882, Edward Weston, an English inventor, improved on the d'Arsonal galvanometer. Today, there are many different types of meters, which are easily used and transported.

Meters may be designed to measure a specific electrical unit, e.g., volt, or may be capable of measuring several electrical units (Figure 6–1). Meters with the capability of measuring several electrical units are referred to as multimeters or multitesters.

The multimeter has a dial or switch to select the unit to be measured. Also, multimeters employing an analog scale (see below for explanation of analog

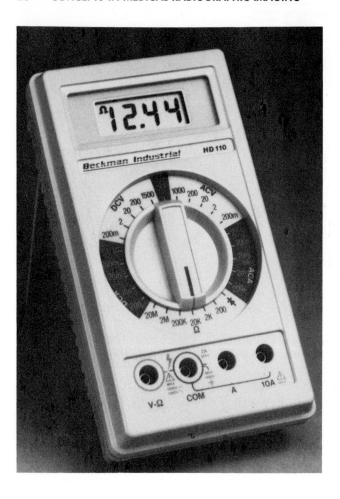

Figure 6–1. Multimeter for measuring voltage (ACV/DCV), amperage (ACA/DCA) and ohms. (From Beckman Industrial.)

scale) have several scales for readout. The scales are labeled relative to what they measure, e.g., alternating current voltage (ACV). The user must match the correct scale to the unit being measured.

The readout for meters may be analog (scale) or digital (Figure 6–2). Analog meters use a scale with a mirror. The mirror is used to superimpose the actual scale pointer (needle) on its reflection. This eliminates the parallax effect. The parallax effect occurs when the angle of the user and the scale pointer is less than 90 degrees. When the user reads the scale at an angle of less than 90 degrees, the location of the pointer appears in an area other than the true reading (the reading will be higher or lower than the actual value).

The advantages of an analog meter are that it is less expensive than the digital meter, capable of reading slow voltage changes and less susceptible to errors caused by electromagnetic fields. The dig-

ital meter is more accurate than the analog meter and the readout is easy to understand (no parallax effect). Table 6–1 compares analog and digital meters.

Meters use leads for measuring an electrical unit. One end of the lead is inserted in the meter and the other end is positioned in the electrical circuit (the lead to the circuit connector). The lead's meter end is usually much shorter than the lead to the circuit connector end. The lead's meter end may be a banana plug or a fork lug (Figure 6–3). The banana plug is cylindrical and is inserted in a hole in the meter called a jack. The fork lug is U shaped and is attached to the pressure terminal (screw with a nut) of the meter. The lead to the circuit connector may be movable or fixed (Figure 6–4). Movable connectors are called probes and are pointed on the end. Fixed connectors usually have an alligator clip tip.

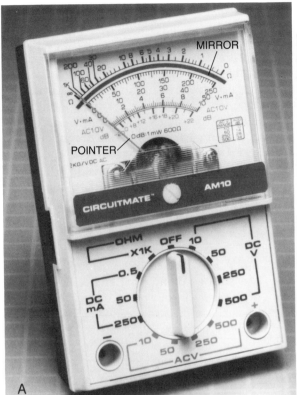
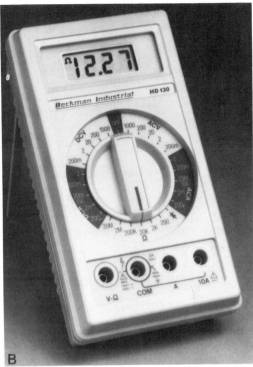

Figure 6–2. Multitester readouts. A, Analog scale; B, digital. (From Beckman Industrial.)

PRECAUTIONS BEFORE USING A METER

Before a meter is used, several items should be checked or tasks need to be performed. Many meters look similar but function differently. Too often individuals tend to bypass the instruction manual and learn things by trial and error. In the case of meters, misuse of the instrument may cause serious damage to the instrument or injury to the user. Consequently, before using a meter for the first time, the operator should read the instruction manual. Also, anytime the user is uncertain about the operation of the meter, he/she should refer to the instruction manual for clarification.

If the meter measures ohms, it contains a battery. Meters with several ohm ranges may have more than one battery. The user should check the batteries' power level. Battery type and location are identified in the instruction manual. If the meter is stored for a long period of time, the batteries should be removed to avoid potential meter damage caused by battery leakage.

The lead ends are usually insulated with a hard or soft plastic shield. The insulation protects the user against electrical shock. The insulation should be checked for fraying or kinks. Also, probes sometimes have plastic insulations that screw onto the

Table 6–1. ANALOG AND DIGITAL METER COMPARISON		
Item	**Analog**	**Digital**
Accuracy	±1–3% of actual value	±1% of actual value and 1 or more counts of last digit (significant number)
Readout error	Parallax effect	None
Ohm's zeroing	Yes	No
Voltage reading	Good for slowly changing voltage	Best for steady voltage
Electromagnetic field effect	Little	May be significant

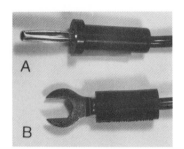

Figure 6–3. Meter leads. *A,* Banana end; *B,* fork lug.

metallic point. These should be checked to ensure they are screwed on tight.

Some meter readouts are best used in the horizonal position, whereas others are used in the vertical position. The user should place the meter in the proper readout position. The instruction manual identifies the best readout position.

GUIDELINES FOR METER USE

Several guidelines or rules should be adhered to when using a meter. After following the proper precautions before meter use, one can turn the meter on. The pointer or digital readout should be on zero. If it is not, the user must zero the meter. The procedure for zeroing the meter is located in the instruction manual.

Meters have a minimum to maximum range in which they can be employed. The operator should never use a meter to measure units exceeding the maximum limits of the instrument. This may cause damage to the meter or harm to the user. Also, the user should check to ensure that the meter is set on the correct unit, e.g., ohms. In the case of multiple ranges of a unit, e.g., R × 1, R × 10, R

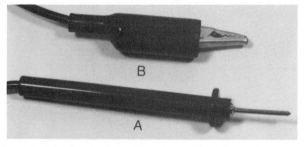

Figure 6–4. Lead to circuit connectors. *A,* movable (probe); *B,* fixed (clip).

× 100, R × 1000 ranges for ohms, set the instrument on the highest range. If the instrument is set on a range lower than the circuit output, the meter needle moves off scale. This may damage the meter. If the electrical output is less than the set range, the needle may not move or moves slightly. In this case, to obtain a reading, change the setting to the next lower range. For example, if no reading is obtained on the R × 1000 Ω range, reset the range to R × 100. On analog meters, continue resetting the range until the pointer is deflected at least one-third of the scale. For digital meters, continue re-setting the range until a readout is obtained. Never change from one range to another while the meter is connected to the circuit.

To obtain a readout, the lead to circuit connectors must be in the correct position in the circuit (see Measuring Potential Difference, Measuring Current and Measuring Resistance sections for information on lead connector positions). Because the human body has resistance, it can act as an electrical conductor. Consequently, it is important that the user hold the insulation portion of the leads when obtaining a readout. Also, it is important that polarity be observed during direct current measurements. This means that the negative side of the meter must be connected to the negative side of the circuit. The leads are color coded to help identify polarity. Usually, a red color signifies the positive lead and a black color identifies the negative lead.

MEASURING POTENTIAL DIFFERENCE

A voltmeter is used to measure potential difference (volts). Two kinds of voltages may be measured: the direct current voltage (DCV) and the alternating current voltage (ACV). The respective voltmeter must be selected to measure alternating or direct current voltage. For measurements in a direct current circuit, polarity must be observed. Polarity is not a factor when measuring voltage in an alternating current circuit. For measurements using a multimeter, the correct knob settings must be selected. Regardless of the type of meter employed for measurement, the lead connectors are positioned in the same manner.

Voltage is measured in a closed circuit (a circuit with a current flow). The voltmeter is connected in

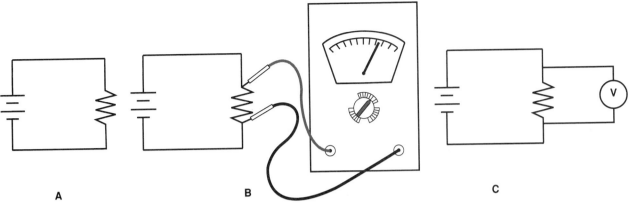

Figure 6–5. A, Circuit prior to connecting a voltmeter to measure the voltage over the resistor. B, Voltmeter connected to the circuit to record the resistor voltage. C, Circuit diagram to read voltage over the resistor.

parallel over the area being measured. Figure 6–5A is a diagram of a circuit before connecting a voltmeter to measure the potential difference over the resistor. Voltage is measured by placing the leads of the meter in parallel to the part being measured (Chapter 5, Electrodynamics, describes parallel circuits in more detail). Figure 6–5B represents the voltmeter position for measuring the potential difference over the resistor. Figure 6–5C is the electrical circuit diagram used to demonstrate measuring voltage over a resistor.

The circuit represented in Figure 6–5 uses direct current. Figure 6–6 shows the knob setting for Figure 6–5. The potential difference in Figure 6–6 is 5 V. This is obtained by locating the correct readout scale on the meter. The correct scale is determined by looking at the voltage knob range selection and choosing the appropriate readout scale. In this example, there are four DCV readout scales:

0–10
0–50
0–125
0–250

To determine the most appropriate scale, the readout scale is matched to the voltage range selected or to any multiple or fraction of the voltage range. In this example, there is a match scale, the 0–10. Notice that any scale can be used to obtain the true voltage.

For example, the 0–50 scale represents a multiple of five times the set voltage range of 0–10. In Figure 6–6, the pointer reads 25 V if the multiple 0–50

scale is used as the readout. Because the 0–50 scale is a multiple of the set voltage range (0–10), the readout of 25 must be divided by the multiple factor 5. Dividing 25 by 5 results in a voltage reading of 5, the same as that obtained using the 0–10 scale.

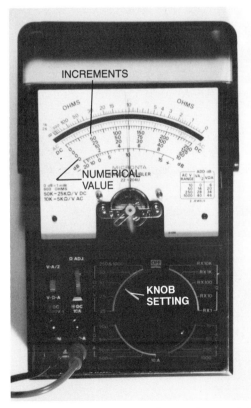

Figure 6–6. Meter setting for Figure 6–5 demonstrating a readout of 5 V.

It becomes obvious that the second example readout (0–50) results in the same answer but is more time consuming and more complicated. Consequently, it is wise to obtain a readout by matching the readout scale exactly with the voltage range selected. The 0–50 readout scale example is used here because it is common that an exact match readout scale does not exist on the meter. This leaves the user no option but to use a multiple or fractional readout scale. The easiest multiple scale to use is one in which the multiple factor is 10, 100, 1000, etc. In these type of multiples, the true readout is obtained by moving a decimal point to the left relative to the multiple. In a multiple of 10, record the multiple readout value and move the decimal one position to the left. For example, if the multiple readout is 250 with a multiple factor of 10, the true readout is 25. If fractional scales are used, e.g., $\frac{1}{10}$ and $\frac{1}{100}$, then the fractional readout is divided by the fraction (remember that to divide fractions, invert them and multiply). For example, if the readout is 25 on a fraction scale of $\frac{1}{10}$, then the true readout is 250 (25 divided by $\frac{1}{10}$ = 25 × 10/1 = 250).

MEASURING CURRENT

Current is measured by an ammeter. Two kinds of amperage may be measured: the direct current amperage (DCA) and the alternating current amperage (ACA). The respective ammeter must be selected to measure alternating or direct current. For measurements in a direct current circuit, polarity must be observed. Polarity is not a factor when measuring current in an alternating current circuit. For measurements using a multimeter, the correct knob settings must be selected. Regardless of the type of meter employed for measurement, the lead connectors are positioned in the same manner.

Current is measured in an open circuit (a circuit with *no* current flow). Connecting the ammeter in series over the area being measured completes the circuit. Figure 6–7A is a diagram of the circuit before connecting the ammeter to measure the current over the resistor. Current is measured by placing the leads of the meter in series to the part being measured (Chapter 5, Electrodynamics, describes series circuits in more detail). Figure 6–7B represents the ammeter position for measuring the current over the resistor. Figure 6–7C is the electrical circuit diagram used to demonstrate the measurement of current flow of the resistor.

The circuit represented in Figure 6–7 uses direct current. Figure 6–8 shows the knob setting for Figure 6–7. The current in Figure 6–8 is 200 mA. The reading was obtained by matching the current range selection of 500 mA with the direct current readout scale of 0–50. Because the 0–50 scale is $\frac{1}{10}$ the set current range, the fractional readout of 20 was multiplied by 10 for a true readout of 200 mA.

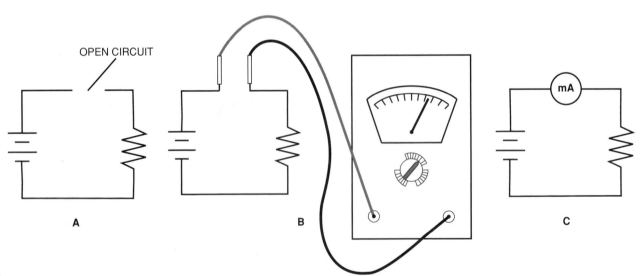

Figure 6–7. A, Circuit prior to connecting an ammeter to measure the current over the resistor. B, Ammeter connected to the circuit to record the resistor current. C, Circuit diagram to read current over the resistor.

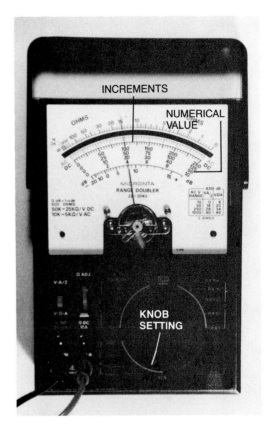

Figure 6–8. Meter setting for Figure 6–7 demonstrating a readout of 200 mA.

MEASURING RESISTANCE

Resistance is measured with an ohmmeter. For measurements using a multimeter, the correct knob settings must be selected. Before the ohms measurement, the meter may need to be zeroed by touching the leads together and adjusting the pointer, if necessary. Regardless of the type of meter employed for measurement, the lead connectors are positioned in the same manner.

Resistance is measured in an open circuit (a circuit with *no* current flow). Because the ohmmeter con-

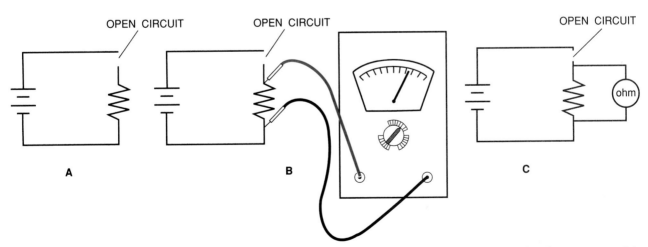

Figure 6–9. *A,* Circuit prior to connecting an ohmmeter to measure the resistance over the resistor. *B,* Ohmmeter connected to the circuit to record the resistor resistance. *C,* Circuit diagram to read resistance over the resistor.

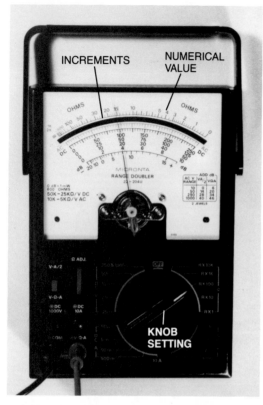

Figure 6–10. Meter setting for Figure 6–9 demonstrating a readout of 1500 Ω.

ter position for measuring the resistance over the resistor. Figure 6–9C is the electrical circuit diagram used to demonstrate the measurement of the ohms of a resistor.

Figure 6–10 shows the knob setting for Figure 6–9. The resistance in Figure 6–10 is 1500 Ω. This was obtained by multiplying the factor identified on the ohm range (R × 100) by the readout number on the ohm scale. In this example, the readout number was 15 and the multiple factor was 100 for a readout of 1500 Ω, or 15 × 100 = 1500.

LABORATORY EXPERIENCE

Several laboratories in *Concepts in Medical Radiographic Imaging: Laboratory Manual* entail the use of meters. Before performing these laboratories, the researcher must be competent in the use of meters. Laboratory 5, Multitesters, provides the learner the practical experience of recording volts, milliamperes and ohms. The laboratory is designed to use a multimeter, but individual meters to measure volts, amperes and ohms, respectively, may be employed. The Multitesters laboratory requires the experimenter to construct elementary parallel and series circuits. Some instruction or guidance may be needed for individuals inexperienced in the construction of parallel and series circuits.

Bibliography

Hazen, ME. Experiencing electricity and electronics, electron flow version. Philadelphia: Saunders, 1989.
Shelton, JK. Diagnostic testing of static electrical equipment. New York: Wiley, 1983.

tains its own battery source, connecting the meter in parallel over the area being measured completes a circuit. Figure 6–9A is a diagram of the circuit before connecting the ohmmeter to measure the resistance over the resistor. Resistance is measured by placing the leads of the meter parallel to the part being measured. Figure 6–9B presents the ohmme-

7

TRANSFORMERS

INTRODUCTION

Electricity enters a building from a power plant at either 120 or 220 V. X-ray machines and many other types of electrical equipment operate in part or wholly at potentials (voltages) above or below those provided by the power supply. The usual voltage range of conventional (nonmammography) radiography is 40,000–120,000 V. It becomes readily apparent that the incoming voltage must be increased substantially to produce x-rays.

The two most common means for lowering the potential of alternating current are the use of resistors and transformers. A resistor lowers the potential of an electrical current by wasting enough energy that the remaining energy is at a lower voltage. The wasted energy is dissipated as heat. A large amount of heat emanating from a resistor may be difficult or impossible to disperse without damage to equipment or danger to the equipment operator. Transformers, on the other hand, may be designed to either increase or decrease potential of an alternating current without a major loss of energy.

This chapter is dedicated to transformers. Information is provided on transformer construction, laws, losses and use within the x-ray machine.

TRANSFORMER CONSTRUCTION

A transformer is a device used to increase or decrease voltage. It consists of an input side (primary coil), output side (secondary coil) and core (Figure 7–1). A high voltage transformer is immersed in oil, which serves as an insulator and helps cool the transformer.

The electrical current that is supplied to a trans-

former (input side) is known as the primary current and the coil that receives the primary current is known as the primary coil. The current that leaves the transformer (output side) is known as the secondary current and the coil from which the secondary current travels is known as the secondary coil.

The coils are wound around the core and are insulated. The primary coil contains the incoming voltage. The current from the primary coil is induced in the secondary coil (see Mutual Induction and Self-induction below). Recall that a coiled wire placed around an iron core increases the strength of the magnetic flux. The manner in which the coils are wound around the core and the configuration of the core is discussed further below.

TYPES OF TRANSFORMER CORES

Transformer cores are used to increase the magnetic flux. They are made of a material with high permeability (magnetizes easily) and low retentivity (demagnetizes rapidly). This material is usually some form of iron. There are three common types of transformer core configurations. From least efficient to most efficient, they are open, closed and shell (Figure 7–2).

The open core is the simplest configuration. In this design, each of the coils (primary and secondary) has a core of its own. This design is inefficient because it has a large amount of leakage flux.

One configuration that reduces leakage flux is the closed core. In this design, the core is square or donut shaped. The primary coil is usually wound around one side of the core. Located opposite the primary coil winding is the secondary winding.

The most efficient core configuration is the shell.

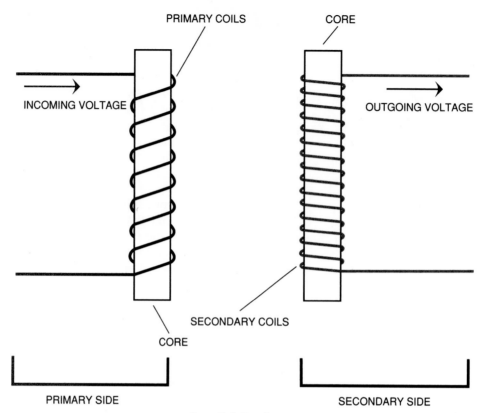

Figure 7–1. Transformer.

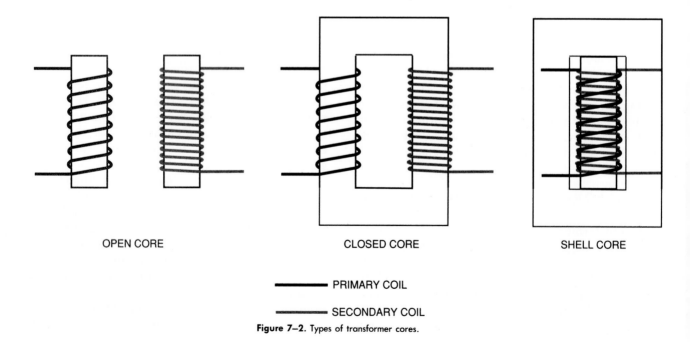

Figure 7–2. Types of transformer cores.

In this design, the primary and secondary windings are wrapped around the center of the shell.

MUTUAL INDUCTION AND SELF-INDUCTION

Recall that Oersted proved that a magnetic field surrounded an electrical current. Also, Faraday demonstrated that an electrical current can be induced in a conductor by placing the conductor in a fluctuating magnetic field. When an alternating current is applied to the primary side of a transformer, the current intensity changes, creating a variability in the magnetic field. Placing the secondary coil near a primary coil with an alternating current flow causes the magnetic field of the primary coil to induce a current in the secondary coil. This process is called mutual induction.

Another method of inducing a current is self-induction. Self-induction utilizes one coil, which acts as both a primary and a secondary coil (see Autotransformers section). Current flow is a function of the manner in which the conducting wires are connected. In self-induction, the magnetic field cuts the coil, producing a current. The primary difference between mutual induction and self-induction is in the number of coils.

STEP-UP AND STEP-DOWN TRANSFORMERS

As mentioned previously, transformers may increase or decrease voltage. Transformers that increase voltage are called step-up transformers and those decreasing voltage are referred to as step-down transformers. The voltage induced in the secondary coil is directly proportional to the number of turns in the coil. The ratio of the number of turns (turns ratio) in the primary and secondary sides of the transformer determine if it is a step-up or step-down type. The turns ratio is expressed mathematically as N_s/N_p, where N_s is the number of turns on the secondary side and N_p is the number of turns on the primary side. An answer greater than unity (1) reflects a step-up transformer. Answers less than unity represent step-down transformers. For example, a transformer with 10 turns in the primary side and 100 turns on the secondary side is a step-up transformer, or $N_s/N_p = 100/10 = 10$.

WINDINGS

In a step-up transformer, the voltage on the primary side is less than that on the secondary side. However, the current on the primary side is greater than the current on the secondary side. If the diameters of the windings are the same for the primary and the secondary side, the larger current on the primary side produces more heat (increasing resistance). Recall that the larger the cross-section of a conductor, the lower the resistance. Thus, to reduce the resistance of the primary coil, its cross-section must be greater than that of the secondary coil. The converse is true for step-down transformers.

TRANSFORMER LAWS

There are two transformer laws. One relates to the relationship of voltage and the number of turns in the transformer. This is referred to as the transformation ratio. The other refers to power.

TRANSFORMATION RATIO

The voltage output is proportional to the turns ratio. The voltage in the secondary side times the number of turns in the primary side is the same as the voltage of the primary side multiplied by the number of turns in the secondary side. This is expressed mathematically as

$$E_s/E_p = N_s/N_p$$

where E_s is the voltage in the secondary side and E_p represents primary side voltage. By using algebraic laws, the previous formula may be rearranged to determine the value of E_s. The resulting formula is

$$E_s = E_p (N_s/N_p)$$

TRANSFORMER POWER

Power in a transformer abides by the law of conservation of energy. That is, power cannot be created or destroyed (however, it is possible to change the form of energy). The input power of a transformer is equal to the output power. Transformer power is measured in watts. This is expressed as IE or I^2R (because $E = IR$, then $IE = I(IR) = I^2R$). The ideal transformer is 100% efficient. Unfortunately, there is a conversion of output energy, usually in the form of heat. This energy conversion reduces the actual amount of output voltage (see Transformer Efficiency below).

TRANSFORMER EFFICIENCY

Several factors result in a loss of power (see discussion of these losses under Transformer Losses).

As mentioned previously, the power input must equal the power output. This is expressed mathematically as

$$E_pI_p = E_sI_s$$

where I_p is the current on the primary side and I_s refers to the current on the secondary side.

The percentage of transformer efficiency is determined by dividing the output power by the input power. This is represented mathematically as

$$\text{Efficiency} = E_sI_s / E_pI_p \ (100)$$

For example, a transformer having an output of 90 W and an input of 100 W is 90% efficient, or 90/100 (100) = 90%. The efficiency can never exceed 100%.

TRANSFORMER LOSSES

There are two areas of the transformer in which losses occur: the windings and the core. Losses in the windings are termed copper losses. There are two types of core losses. They are eddy currents and hysteresis losses.

COPPER LOSSES

Windings are made of a material that contains some resistance to electricity. This resistance increases as the intensity of the current (amperes) increases. The resistance is manifest in the form of heat. The heat results in power loss of the transformer called copper losses. It is possible to reduce copper losses by using a large diameter wire for windings carrying large currents.

EDDY CURRENTS

As the windings carry the alternating current, there is an associated alternating magnetic flux. The changing magnetic flux created by the alternating current induces currents in the core. These currents are called eddy currents. Eddy currents produce heat, decreasing the efficiency of the transformer. It is possible to reduce eddy currents by laminating the core.

A laminated core is constructed of individual layers or plates of iron. The layers are insulated. The insulation prevents eddy current flow between the layers. It is important that the layers be firmly attached to one another. Failure to attach the layers firmly may result in humming of the transformer. The humming occurs because the magnetic fields in the layers repel each other. This causes the layers to separate slightly. When the current reaches zero, there is no magnetic field and the layers return to their original shape. The constant movement of the layers results in the humming sound.

HYSTERESIS LOSSES

Alternating current moves in one direction and then the opposite direction. This constant movement induces magnetic domains in the core, which correspond to the direction of the current. Consequently, the magnetic domains are rearranging themselves first in one direction and then in another direction. This movement creates a transformer loss in the form of heat. This type of transformer loss is called hysteresis. It is possible to reduce hysteresis by using a core with low retentivity.

AUTOTRANSFORMERS

Transformers constructed with individual primary and secondary coils have a fixed rate for changing the output voltage. That is, the turns ratio cannot be changed unless the construction of the transformer is altered. In conventional radiography, there is a need to vary the amount of kilovoltage relative to the part undergoing radiographic examination. Consequently, a need exists to provide a means of regulating the voltage. This is accomplished by using an autotransformer.

An autotransformer allows the user to vary the output voltage. Autotransformers are used for low voltage changes and should not be used for high voltage. This is achieved by having one winding act as both the primary and the secondary coil (Figure 7–3). The number of turns on the secondary coil is determined by the location of the movable contact. Recall that the number of turns (turns ratio) is proportional to the voltage output. The mathematical representation of the transformation ratio for an autotransformer is

$$E_s / E_p = N_t / N_p$$

where N_t represents the number of turns tapped on the secondary side of the transformer. By using algebraic laws, the previous formula may be rearranged to determine the value of E_s. The resulting formula is

$$E_s = E_p (N_t / N_p)$$

For example, if the number of turns tapped on an autotransformer is 12, the incoming voltage is 110 and the number of primary turns is 9, then E_s is approximately 146, or $E_s = E_p (N_t / N_p) = 110 (12/9) = 146$.

A special type of autotransformer is the Variac (General Radio Corporation). The Variac is cylin-

drical and has a contact arm that slides over the windings (Figure 7–4).

TRANSFORMER USE IN THE X-RAY CIRCUIT

There are many transformers in an x-ray circuit. Three types are significant enough to mention here. One is the autotransformer, another is the high tension transformer and the last is the filament transformer.

The autotransformer is used to select the kilovoltage. It is located between the power supply and the high tension transformer. The high tension transformer receives its input voltage from the autotransformer. The high tension transformer increases the voltage received from the autotransformer, usually by a factor of 1000. For example, if the operator selects 75 kV, the contact on the autotransformer moves to a point to step down the incoming voltage to 75 V. The current (now 75 V) travels to the high tension transformer, where it is increased to 75,000 V.

The filament transformer is a step-down transformer. It is used to provide a small amount of voltage to the cathode of the x-ray tube for thermonic emission (see Chapter 10, Production of X-rays).

LABORATORY EXPERIENCE

Two laboratories are associated with this chapter. Laboratory 10 is Step-up and Step-down Transformers; Laboratory 11 is Transformer Power and Efficiency.

Laboratory 10 is used to demonstrate the effective transformer ratio of a step-up and step-down transformer. This is achieved by using the transformation ratio. The experimenter measures the output voltage, records the input voltage and uses the information provided with the transformer to determine the turns ratio. This information is used to determine the effective transformer ratio for step-up and step-down transformers.

In the Transformer Power and Efficiency laboratory, as the name implies, the researcher determines the power and efficiency of a transformer. This is

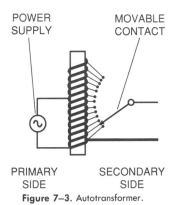

Figure 7–3. Autotransformer.

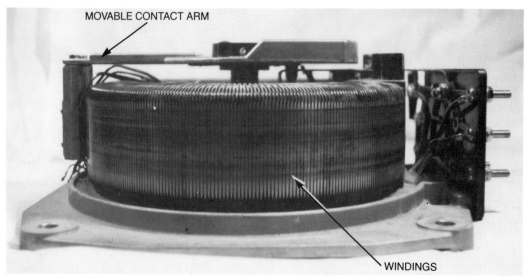

Figure 7–4. Cylindrical autotransformer.

achieved by measuring the current and voltage on the primary and secondary sides of the transformer. The experimenter compares the results with those from the watts formula (see Chapter 5, Electrodynamics) and the transformer efficiency formula.

Bibliography

Ball, JL and Moore, AD. Essential physics for radiographers (2nd edition). Boston: Blackwell Scientific Publications, 1986.

Bushong, SC. Radiologic science for technologists (4th edition). St. Louis: Mosby, 1988.

Chesney, DN and Chesney, MO. X-ray equipment for student radiographers (3rd edition). Boston: Blackwell Scientific Publications, 1984.

Curry, TS, Dowdey, JE and Murry, RC. Christensen's Introduction to the physics of diagnostic radiology (3rd edition). Philadelphia: Lea & Febiger, 1984.

Curry, TS, Dowdey, JE and Murry, RC. Christensen's Physics of diagnostic radiology (4rd edition). Philadelphia: Lea & Febiger, 1990.

Graham, BJ and Thomas, WN. An introduction to physics for radiologic technologists. Philadelphia: Saunders, 1975.

Hazen, ME. Experiencing electricity and electronics, electron flow version. Philadelphia: Saunders, 1989.

Oman, RM. An introduction to radiologic science. New York: McGraw-Hill, 1975.

Selman, J. The fundamentals of x-ray and radium physics (7th edition). Springfield, IL: Thomas, 1985.

Sprawls, P. Principles of radiography for technologists. Rockville, MD: Aspen, 1990.

RECTIFICATION

CURRENT FLOW

The electricity used in homes and businesses originates in a power plant. Large generators are employed for the production of this electricity (Figure 8–1). After it is generated, the electricity is transported from the power plant to homes and businesses through a series of power lines and transformers. The type of current generated and delivered to homes and businesses is alternating current (AC).

AC occurs when the flow of electrons changes direction (moves back and forth). In the United States, current changes direction 60 times per sec-

ond (refer to Chapter 5, Electrodynamics, for a more involved discussion of AC). Not all electrical flow alternates. Another type of current flow is direct current (DC). In direct current, electrons flow in one direction only. A battery is a typical example of a DC source.

During x-ray production, the x-ray tube operates most efficiently on DC. Because the incoming current from the power plant to the x-ray machine is AC, there is a need to change AC to DC. The method used to change AC to DC is called rectification.

There are two methods to rectify an AC. One method is to suppress the negative impulse of the sine wave; the other is to change the negative impulse to positive. Suppressing the negative impulse is achieved by self-wave or half wave rectification of single phase x-ray machines. Changing the negative impulse to positive is accomplished by full wave rectification by either a single or a three phase x-ray machine.

METHODS OF RECTIFICATION

SUPPRESSING THE NEGATIVE IMPULSE

Self-Wave Rectification

The simplest method of suppressing the negative impulse is to allow the x-ray tube to rectify the current. Because the x-ray tube itself does the rectifying, this type of rectification is appropriately called self-wave rectification. An x-ray tube is a type of diode vacuum tube. To understand how self-wave rectification is achieved, a brief explanation

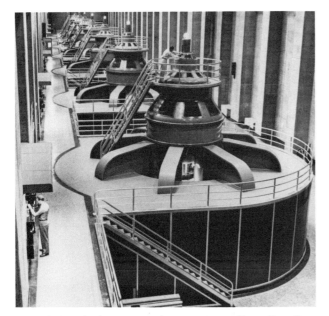

Figure 8–1. Hydroelectric power plant generators at Hoover Dam. (From U.S. Bureau of Reclamation.)

of a diode vacuum tube follows (a more in-depth explanation of the x-ray tube is located in Chapter 10, Production of X-rays).

A diode tube contains two electrodes. One electrode consists of a coiled wire (filament) and focusing cup. This coiled wire and focusing cup are called the cathode. The other electrode is a metallic plate located opposite the cathode and is termed the anode. The cathode and anode are sealed in a vacuum glass. In addition to variations in the physical appearance of the cathode and the anode, the primary difference between the two is that the cathode has a small electrical current passing through it. This current heats the filament, causing an emission of electrons, or electron cloud, near the cathode (Figure 8–2). Emission of electrons by heat is called thermonic emission.

Rectification occurs when high voltage is applied to the cathode and the anode. High voltage traveling during the positive portion of the sine wave produces a large negative charge on the cathode and a large positive charge on the anode. This large potential difference between the cathode and the anode causes the electrons from the electron cloud to be attracted to the anode at a high speed (Figure 8–3A). When a high voltage traveling during the negative part of the sine wave is applied to the cathode and the anode, the polarity of the electrodes reverses. That is, the cathode assumes a positive charge and the anode assumes a negative charge. Because there is no electron cloud at the anode, there is no flow of electrons (Figure 8–3B). The resulting sine wave output graph is a series of positive impulses (representing electron flow) separated by spaces (straight line plot) representing no current flow (Figure 8–3C).

Self-wave rectification is advantageous because the equipment needed to rectify the current is inexpensive, simple, relatively small and easily maneuvered. In the early years of radiology, self-wave rectification was especially popular because it could be used for mobile and dental (low power) radiography. The primary disadvantage of self-wave rectification is that care needs to be taken never to heat the anode to the point of electron emission. If the anode emits electrons, there may be a flow of current from the anode to the cathode during the negative part of the sine wave. This current would cause overheating and melt the cathode, destroying the x-ray tube. Thus, the continual changing of polarity (charges) of the cathode and the anode in the x-ray tube decreases the efficiency and life span of the tube.

Half Wave Rectification

As time progressed, it was discovered that the negative part of the sine wave could also be suppressed by placing diode tubes (valve tubes) between the high tension transformer and the x-ray tube of the x-ray circuit. The advantage of using valve tubes instead of the x-ray tube to rectify the current is that the valve tubes increase the life span of the x-ray tube. Rectification using valve tubes is called half wave rectification and can be accomplished with one or two valve tubes. Figure 8–4 is a simplified diagram of the x-ray tube with two valve tubes. During the positive portion of the sine wave, electrons flow through one valve tube to the x-ray tube and return through another valve tube (Figure 8–4A). Electrons do not flow during the negative impulse (Figure 8–4B) because there is no electron cloud at the anode of the valve tube.

The sine wave diagram for half wave rectification appears the same as that for self-wave rectification; i.e., a series of positive impulses separated by gaps (Figure 8–4C).

CHANGING THE NEGATIVE IMPULSE TO POSITIVE

Full Wave Rectification

The second method used to change AC to DC is by making the negative impulse positive. This is

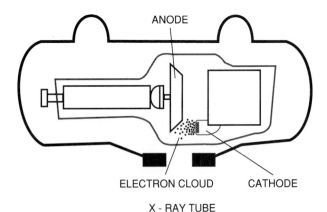

X - RAY TUBE

Figure 8–2. Electron cloud, or thermonic emission.

ABORATORY EXPERIENCE

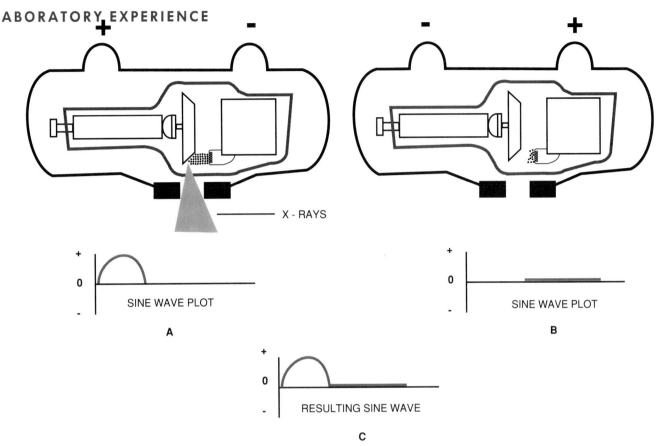

Figure 8–3. Self-rectification. A, Positive impulse resulting in x-ray production. B, Negative impulse, no x-ray production. C, Resulting sine wave output.

achieved by using four valve tubes or several modules of solid state rectifiers. The primary difference between electron travel in a valve tube and that in a solid state rectifier is that electron travel in valve tubes is through a vacuum tube, whereas electron flow using solid state rectifiers is through solid materials. As a result, solid state rectifiers have the following advantages over valve tubes:

1. Solid state rectifiers are smaller and hence require less space.
2. Solid state rectifiers have no filaments; thus, there is no need for transformers to heat the filament. This results in smaller generators, which can be used to produce full wave rectification in mobile units.
3. There are no filaments to burn out in solid state rectification, increasing the life span of the rectifiers.
4. There is a lower forward voltage drop and less

reverse current with solid state, which creates more economical use of power.

Because most modern x-ray machines use solid state rectifiers, this discussion concentrates on solid state rectification. Before the use of solid state rectifiers in the x-ray circuit is explained, a brief discussion of the physics principles behind solid state rectification is in order.

The fundamental physics concept that applies to solid state rectification is the principle of conductivity. A material falls into one of three conductive categories: (1) conductors, (2) nonconductors (insulators) and (3) semiconductors. Recall that current is the flow of electrons. Materials classified as conductors, e.g., copper, readily allow the flow of electrons. The atoms of these materials have loosely bound electrons in their outer shell. Application of a small amount of energy (volts) allows easy movement of these electrons within the material, result-

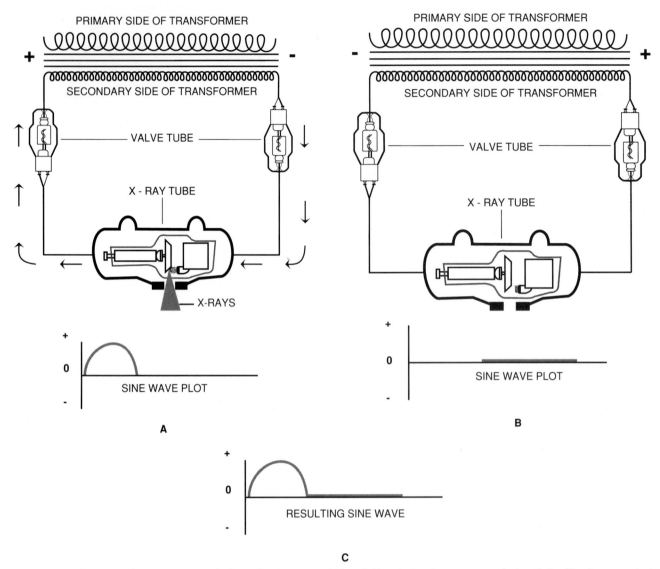

Figure 8–4. Half wave rectification. *A*, Positive impulse resulting in x-ray production. *B*, Negative impulse, no x-ray production. *C*, Resulting sine wave output.

ing in an electrical current. Nonconductors, e.g., wood, hinder the flow of electrons. These insulators have atoms with tightly bound electrons in their outer shell. Application of energy in insulators has no effect on creating an electron flow. The tight binding of electrons in the material inherently resists or hinders electron movement from one atom to another atom. Semiconductors contain conductive and resistive materials. The type of material used in making a semiconductor determines if it conducts or resists the flow of electrons. The material common to both the conductive and the resis-

tive material in solid state rectifiers is silicon. Impurities added to silicon determine if the material conducts or resists the flow of electrons. The concept of having a conductive and a resistive material is to simulate the cathode and the anode of a vacuum tube.

Simulation of the cathode is accomplished by mixing a small amount of arsenic with silicon. This mixture creates an excess of loosely bound electrons, giving the atom the ability to give up or donate electrons to another atom. Arsenic and silicon combination is referred to as an N-type (think of the N as atoms with negative charges or electrons) semiconductor. Because N-type semiconductors donate electrons, they are also referred to as donor material or a donor atom.

Anode simulation is achieved by combining a small amount of gallium with silicon. This mixture creates a deficiency of tightly bound electrons in the atom, giving the atom the capability of receiving electrons from another atom. The gallium and silicon mixture is called a P-type (think of the P as atoms with a positive charge) semiconductor. Because P-type semiconductors receive electrons, they may also be referred to as acceptor material or an acceptor atom. These materials are said to have holes that can migrate in a material and be filled by migrating electrons from other atoms.

Recall that in a diode vacuum tube, the electron flow is from cathode to anode. In a solid state rectifier, electron flow is from N-type material to P-type material. Placing an N-type material with a P-type material in a specific order makes it possible to direct the flow of electrons. The path in which one would like to direct electron flow determines the position of the rectifiers within the circuit. Figure 8–5 shows solid state electron flow.

Figure 8–5 is a diagram of a solid state diode. The diode contains N-type and P-type material. The area where the N-type and P-type material meet is called the N-P junction. The diode is connected to a voltage source. When the negative terminal of the voltage source is connected to the N-type material and the positive terminal of the voltage source is connected to the P-type material (Figure 8–5*A*), there is a flow of electrons. This occurs because the N-type material donates its electrons to the P-type material. Thus, electrons flow through the N-P junction. Conversely, in Figure 8–5*B*, connecting the positive terminal of the voltage source to the N-type material and the negative terminal of the voltage source to the P-type material results in no electron flow. This occurs because the N-type electrons are attracted to the positive terminal and the P-type material's holes migrate to the negative terminal. In this case, the N-P junction acts as a barrier prohibiting the flow of electrons.

The symbol used to represent a solid state diode is a solid arrow resting against a perpendicular line (Figure 8–6). As can be seen from Figure 8–6, the arrow represents the anode and the perpendicular line is symbolic of the cathode. Electron flow is

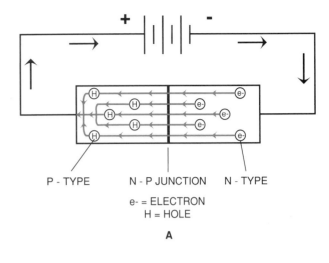

P - TYPE   N - P JUNCTION   N - TYPE

e- = ELECTRON
H = HOLE

A

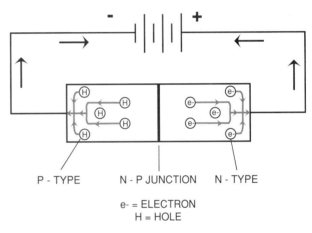

P - TYPE   N - P JUNCTION   N - TYPE

e- = ELECTRON
H = HOLE

B

Figure 8–5. Conductivity of solid state. A, Electron flow; B, no electron flow.

toward the anode. This symbol is used to demonstrate the electron flow in the x-ray circuit.

It should be noted that x-ray circuits require the application of thousands of volts. No individual solid state diode can withstand these high voltages. However, by placing a stack of solid state diodes together in series (Figure 8–7) and enclosing them in an insulated case, it is possible to design a system that can withstand thousands of volts.

A stack of diodes is called a rectifier module (Figure 8–8). These modules come in different sizes. The number of modules needed in an x-ray circuit depends on the number of volts each module can withstand and the amount of voltage of the x-ray generator. In the following discussion regarding

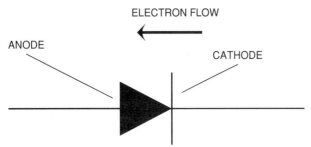

Figure 8–6. Solid state rectifier symbol.

full wave rectification of single and three phase equipment, one solid state diode symbol is used to represent a bank of modules.

Single phase, full wave rectification alters the x-ray circuit by changing the negative portion of the sine wave to positive. This is achieved by placing several solid state rectifier modules between the high tension transformer and the x-ray tube. Figure 8–9 is a diagram of the positions of the rectifiers relative to the x-ray tube and the high tension transformer.

Recall that electron flow is in the direction of the anode (opposite direction to that of the arrow part of the diode symbol). When the incoming voltage occurs during the positive portion of the sine wave, the electron flow is through diode 1 (D1) to the x-

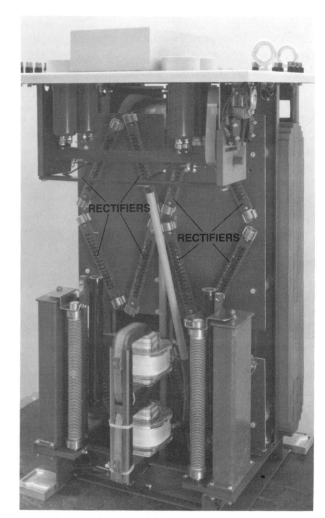

Figure 8–8. Rectifier modules. (From GE Medical Systems.)

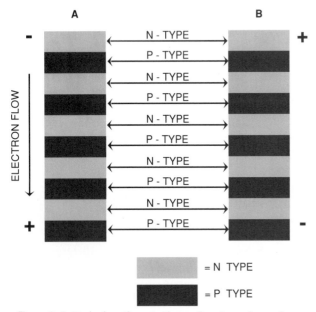

Figure 8–7. Stack of rectifiers. *A,* Electron flow; *B,* no electron flow.

ray tube and exits through D3 (Figure 8–9*A*). No electrons flow through D4 because the N-P junction acts as a barrier to the electron flow. The resulting output sine wave is a positive impulse. During the negative portion of the incoming sine wave, electron flow is from D2 to the x-ray tube and returns through D4. In this instance, the N-P junction of D3 acts as a barrier, preventing any flow of electrons. The output sine wave is a positive impulse. Notice that the incoming voltage changes direction (polarity of the high tension transformer), whereas the direction and polarity of the x-ray tube are constant. In the x-ray tube, the cathode is always negative and the anode is always positive. Thus, during both portions of the sine wave, the x-ray

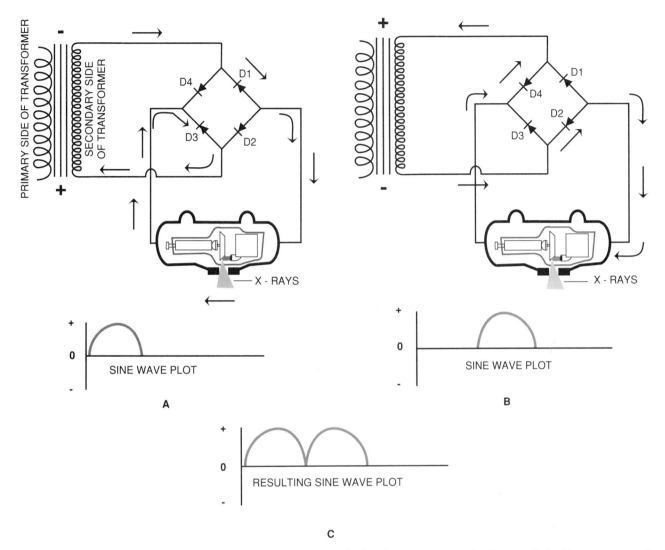

Figure 8–9. Full wave rectification. A, Flow of current during positive sine wave. B, Flow of current during negative sine wave. C, Resulting sine wave output.

tube is energized by a pulsating DC and is constantly producing x-rays.

Full wave rectification is more advantageous than half wave or self-wave rectification. The principal advantage of full wave rectification is that it permits greater heat load capacity of the x-ray tube. The increased x-ray tube capacity enables the user to employ larger milliamperage and kilovoltage settings. Because of the need for additional circuitry not used in self-wave or half wave rectification, full wave rectification has the disadvantages of being more expensive, heavier, larger and more complex.

Three Phase Rectification

Although single phase, full wave rectification is a great improvement over half wave or self-wave rectification, the voltage does reach zero. X-rays produced near zero are of low intensity and have no diagnostic value. When the sine wave is traced, the voltage starts at zero, rises to a maximum and drops back to zero. This variation in voltage is called a ripple. Thus, it can be said that single phase, full wave rectification has a 100% ripple (from zero to zero). The actual amount of energy produced is an average or mean of the sine wave

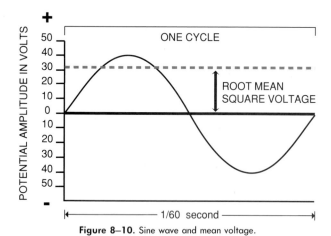

Figure 8–10. Sine wave and mean voltage.

(Figure 8–10). X-ray energy changes in intensity relative to the sine wave. It is estimated that the peak kilovoltage obtained on a single phase, full wave rectified unit occurs 75% of the time. In an effort to decrease the amount of energy lost using single phase units, scientists sought a way to build a more efficient x-ray machine. The result was a three phase unit. Before discussion of the types of rectification in three phase units, a review of how they operate is appropriate.

Three phase equipment represents an incoming current of three single phase sine waves. Each sine wave is out of phase by one-third cycle, or 120 degrees (Figure 8–11). Thus, phase 2 begins 120 degrees after phase 1 and phase 3 starts 120 degrees after phase 2 (and 240 degrees from phase 1).

This out-of-phase sequence occurs in such a way that one phase is at zero, while another phase is approaching the negative maximum and the last phase is just past the positive portion of the sine wave. The location of a specific phase relative to the sine wave changes with the passage of time. The phase at zero is inactive (has no electron flow), while the other two are providing current to the circuit. This concept is used later to demonstrate three phase rectification.

Because three phase circuits represent three single phases, there is a need to provide components, such as exposure switches and kilovoltage controls, for each phase. The transformers contain three windings, one for each phase. These windings may be in the shape of a star (also called a wye, or Y) or delta (Greek letter Δ) (Figure 8–12).

Modern three phase x-ray machines may rectify current by using 6 or 12 banks of rectifiers. The main difference between the 6 and 12 bank rectifiers is in the number of sets of windings on the secondary side of the transformer. The 6 bank has one set of secondary windings, whereas the 12 bank has two sets of secondary windings (each set contains 6 banks of rectifiers).

Units with 6 banks commonly employ a delta winding in the primary side and a star secondary winding (Figure 8–13).

Twelve bank x-ray machines have a primary delta winding and two star secondary windings or one star and one delta secondary winding (Figure 8–14).

As previously stated, in a three phase unit, one of the three phases is at zero and is inactive, while the other two are conducting current.

The voltages in the three windings change in accordance with the sine wave. Thus, the specific pair of windings supplying current to the rectifier banks varies. Only two banks of rectifiers have an electron flow at any one time. The specific pair of rectifiers permitting electron flow is directly related to which pair of windings is energized. The following discussion of rectification refers to Figure 8–15

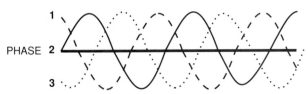

Figure 8–11. Three phase sine wave.

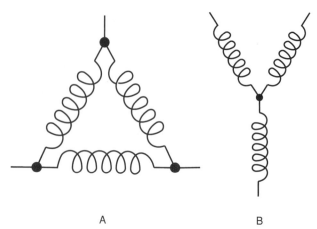

Figure 8–12. Transformer winding design. A, Delta; B, star, or wye.

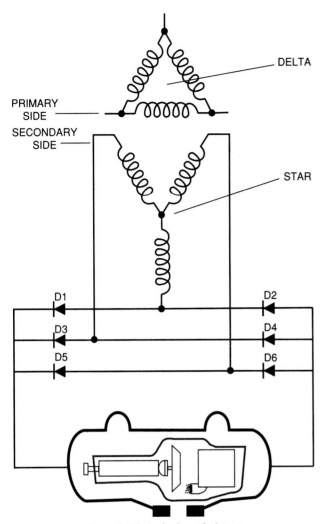

Figure 8–13. Six bank rectified circuit.

this happens, A becomes inactive, leaving B and C to conduct.

The flow of electrons when B and C are active depends on which winding is positive and which is negative. In the case in which B is negative and C is positive, the sequence of flow is from B to D2 to the x-ray tube and returning to C through D5 (Figure 8–15C). As the polarity changes (C becomes negative and B is positive), electron flow changes

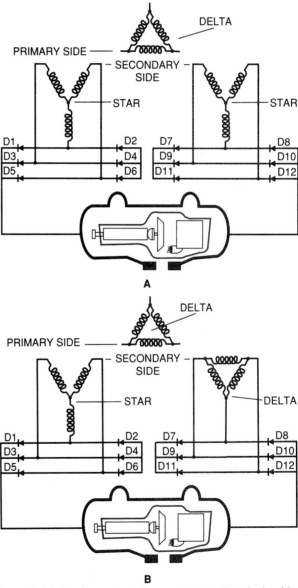

Figure 8–14. Transformer circuit diagram. *A,* Unit with 12 banks, delta primary winding, and two star secondary windings. *B,* Unit with 12 banks, delta primary winding, and one star and one delta secondary winding.

(it is recommended that the reader correlate Figure 8–15 with the following text describing electron flow).

When winding A is negative, B is positive and C is inactive, the electron flow starts at A, passes through D4, travels to the x-ray tube and returns to B via D1 (Figure 8–15A). The N-P junction acts as a barrier for all other rectifiers. During the second half of the sine wave, the polarity changes. Winding A assumes a positive charge and B is negative. The current flow begins at B, passes through D2 to the x-ray tube and returns to A using D3 (Figure 8–15B). Eventually with time, the voltage in winding A reaches zero, while the voltage in C increases to a point at which it is greater than that in A. When

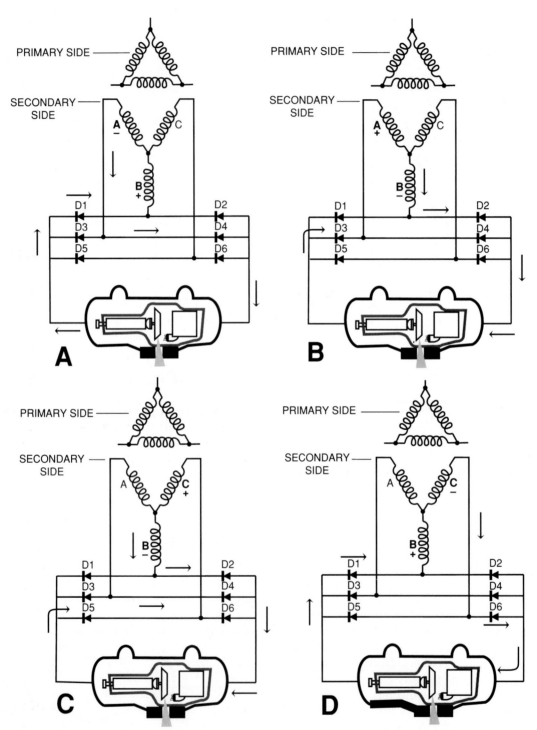

Figure 8–15. Current flow in six bank rectifier. *A*, A is negative and B is positive. *B*, B is negative and A is positive. *C*, B is negative and C is positive. *D*, C is negative and B is positive.

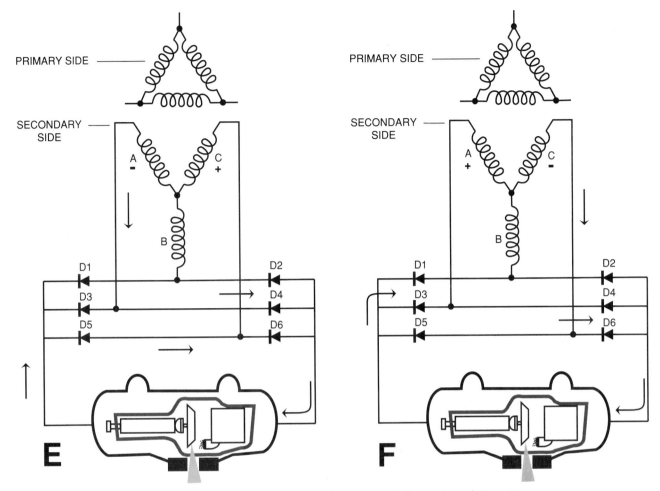

Figure 8–15 *Continued. E,* A is negative and C is positive. *F,* C is negative and A is positive.

so that it starts at C, travels through D6, continues to the x-ray tube and returns through D1 to B (Figure 8–15*D*). As the sine wave continues to travel, eventually B becomes inactive, leaving A and C to conduct.

The flow of electrons when A is negative and C is positive is from A to D4 to the x-ray tube through D5 and returning to C (Figure 8–15*E*). As the polarity of A and C changes, electron flow originates at C, travels through D6 to the x-ray tube and returns to A through D3 (Figure 8–15*F*). A summary of electron flow relative to which windings are active can be found in Table 8–1.

The corresponding sine wave for a three phase, six bank rectified unit changes the three formerly negative impulses to positive (Figure 8–16), resulting in six useful impulses per cycle (1/60 second).

The use of a six bank rectified, three phase unit can reduce the 100% ripple found in single phase units to about 13.5% (Figure 8–17). This means the x-ray voltage never reaches zero. As a result, the

Table 8–1. FLOW OF CURRENT IN THREE PHASE, SIX RECTIFIER UNIT

Negative	Positive	Current Flow
A	B	A → D4 → x-ray tube → D1 → B
B	A	B → D2 → x-ray tube → D3 → A
B	C	B → D2 → x-ray tube → D5 → C
C	B	C → D6 → x-ray tube → D1 → B
A	C	A → D4 → x-ray tube → D5 → C
C	A	C → D6 → x-ray tube → D3 → A

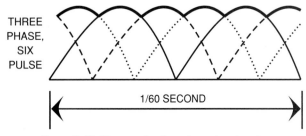

Figure 8–16. Sine wave for three phase, six pulse unit.

effective kilovoltage with a six bank rectified unit occurs about 87% of the time.

The 12 bank rectifier, three phase x-ray machine may result in either 6 or 12 useful impulses. The type of secondary windings determines whether a 12 bank unit has 6 or 12 useful impulses. In general, the two star secondary windings are used in six impulse rectification. The one star and one delta secondary windings are used in 12 pulse rectification. An in-depth discussion of the differences when a 12 bank unit produces 6 or 12 pulses is beyond the scope of this text. The importance of mentioning the 12 bank unit rests with the effect on ripple. A 12 bank, 12 pulse unit has a 3.5% ripple effect (Figure 8–18). This means that the x-ray machine operates at approximately 97% effective kilovoltage.

For simplicity, the terminology used to identify the type of generator and rectifying combination is referred to as 1 pulse, 2 pulse, 6 pulse or 12 pulse. These terms relate to self-wave (or half wave) rectification; single phase, full wave rectification; three phase, 6 bank or 12 bank units producing 6 useful impulses; and a 12 bank unit producing 12 useful impulses, respectively.

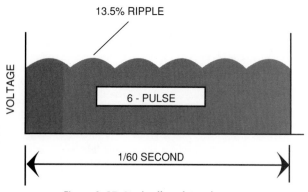

Figure 8–17. Ripple effect of six pulse unit.

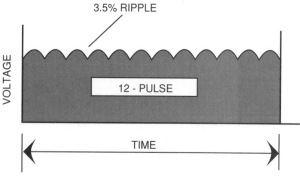

Figure 8–18. Ripple effect of 12 pulse unit.

Three phase equipment has several advantages over full wave, single phase machines. These advantages include (1) ability to use a higher milliamperage, (2) a substantial decrease in exposure time, (3) a high quality x-ray and (4) greater x-ray quantity. The ability to use a higher milliamperage and lower time is useful in gastrointestinal radiography and angiographic procedures. The high quality and high quantity x-ray beam seems to have generated disagreements among scientists regarding radiation absorption by the patient. Some scientists appear to contend that a higher beam quality has fewer low energy x-rays, resulting in less radiation absorption by the patient. Other investigators seem to believe that, after adjusting the radiographic technique to obtain comparable radiographic contrast and densities between single and three phase units, the radiation absorption by the patient is the same.

TEST FOR RECTIFIER FAILURE

Should the radiographer suspect a rectifier failure on a single phase x-ray unit, it is possible to determine rectifier function by performing a simple test. The test is called a spinning top test. Tests for rectifier failure on three phase machines require much more sophisticated testing equipment (usually an oscilloscope). These tests should be performed by qualified service personnel. The following discussion concentrates on the spinning top test.

A spinning top consists of a metallic disk that is mounted on a base (see Figure 9–10). The disc is radiopaque, except for a small hole near its periphery. The hole permits passage of the x-ray beam. When the disc is placed on the base, it can be freely rotated. To use a spinning top, the mounted disc is placed on a corner of a cassette and rotated (spun). An exposure is made while the top is spinning. This procedure is repeated until the cassette is completely exposed (usually a total of four exposures). The radiograph displays a series of dots (see Figure 9–11).

Each dot represents a single pulse of x-ray photons (or a single pulse of electron flow). The number of dots is determined by multiplying the exposure time by the useful impulses per second. The exposure time is set by the operator. The number of useful impulses per second is a function of the current frequency and type of rectification. For example, a 60 cycle per second (cps) current frequency that is half wave rectified has one useful impulse per cycle. Thus, for 1 second there are 60 useful impulses (60 cps × 1 useful impulse/cycle = 60 useful impulses/second). Because full wave rectification has 2 useful impulses/cycle, there are 120 useful impulses in 1 second (60 cps × 2 useful impulses/cycle = 120 useful impulses/second). The following is an example of how to calculate the number of dots expected on a radiograph.

Given,

Exposure time of 1/20 second

Full wave rectified unit

60 cps

Then,

1. Useful impulses = 60 cps × 2 useful impulses/cycle = 120 useful impulses
2. number of dots on radiograph = 1/20 second × 120 useful impulses = 6 dots

Assessment of the dots determines the functional accuracy of the rectifiers. Before evaluating the dots as a unit, it is important to understand the meaning of one dot.

A dot represents a variation of radiographic densities. The darkest part of the dot is the middle. The densities decrease in intensity toward its periphery. Figure 9–12 shows the relationship of the radiographic dot to the sine wave.

It can be seen that, as the sine wave increases, the density of the radiograph increases (gets darker). A normal spinning top test should demonstrate the correct number of dots and have the appropriate distribution of density within the dot. Therefore, on a properly functioning full wave rectified unit using an exposure time of 1/20 second, six dots of uniform density should be demonstrated. If one or more of the rectifiers is not functioning, there is a decrease in the amount of current within the x-ray circuit. During the decreased phase of the sine wave, the radiographic dot density is also decreased. As a result, on a spinning top test, malfunctioning rectifiers tend to appear with the correct number of dots, but every other dot is decreased in density.

LABORATORY EXPERIENCE

Readers may expand their knowledge of rectification by performing Laboratory 12, Rectification, and the spinning top test experiment of Laboratory 13, Timer Tests, in *Concepts in Medical Radiographic Imaging: Laboratory Manual*.

In the Rectification laboratory, the experimenter constructs and determines the amount of voltage of nonrectified, half wave and full wave rectified circuits. The purpose is to provide the experimenter with practical experience in determining the effect of diodes on AC voltage.

The spinning top experiment is designed to provide the experimenter with practical experience in achieving quality control and assessing the accuracy of the rectifiers. This laboratory is also used to test time accuracy, which may be performed after studying Chapter 9, X-ray Timers and Quality Control.

Bibliography

Bushong, SC. Radiologic science for technologists (4th edition). St. Louis: Mosby, 1988.

Chesney, DN and Chesney, MO. X-ray equipment for student radiographers (3rd edition). Boston: Blackwell Scientific Publications, 1984.

Curry, TS, Dowdey, JE and Murry, RC. Christensen's Introduction to the physics of diagnostic radiology (3rd edition). Philadelphia: Lea & Febiger, 1984.

Curry, TS, Dowdey, JE and Murry, RC. Christensen's Physics of diagnostic radiology (4th edition). Philadelphia: Lea & Febiger, 1990.

Graham, BJ and Thomas, WN. An introduction to physics for radiologic technologists. Philadelphia: Saunders, 1975.

Oman, RM. An introduction to radiologic science. New York: McGraw-Hill, 1975.

Selman, J. The fundamentals of x-ray and radium physics (7th edition). Springfield, IL: Thomas, 1985.

X-RAY TIMERS AND QUALITY CONTROL

INTRODUCTION

The length of time (exposure time) it takes to produce x-rays in radiographic procedures is usually a fraction of a second. This exposure process involves the starting of the exposure, a method to time its duration and a means of stopping the exposure. The starting and stopping of the exposure is performed by a switching mechanism that directs the flow of current. The duration of the exposure is a function of a timing device. Because exposures are often fractions of a second, the length of time that switches or timers take to perform their function should be minimal. Also, the time that switches or timers take to reset between exposures (repeat or recycle time) should be minimal. This is especially critical in rapid filming, e.g., angiography.

This chapter discusses the various types of switches and timers used in the x-ray circuit. The latter part of the chapter includes information on timer quality control tests.

SWITCHES

The starting and stopping of an exposure is the function of a switch. The switch begins and ends the exposure by controlling the flow of current in the circuit. Closing the circuit allows current to flow and starts the exposure. Opening the circuit stops the flow of current and subsequent exposure.

The current flow is regulated on either the primary or the secondary side of the high tension transformer. Switches placed on the primary side of the high tension transformer experience low voltage and high amperage. Conversely, switches on the secondary side of the high tension transformer are exposed to high kilovoltage and low amperage. The construction of a switch determines its position in the x-ray circuit. The most common types of switches are mechanical contact and electronic.

Regardless of the type of switch employed, certain features are common to all switches. One feature is response time. That is, a certain amount of time is needed for the switch to perform its function (open or close the circuit). Some switches have a significant length of response time, whereas the response time of others is so short that it is considered negligible. Another characteristic of switches is the length of time needed to reset itself (recycle or repeat) between exposures. As with response time, some switches have a long recycle time, whereas others have a recycle time so short that it is almost instantaneous. Lastly, the combination of response time, recycle time and construction determine the switch's minimum accurate exposure time. Table 9–1 is a summary of the features of common types of exposure switches.

MECHANICAL CONTACT SWITCH

The mechanical contact is the simplest type of switch. It is spring loaded and operates on the

Table 9–1. EXPOSURE SWITCH FEATURES

Type	Minimum Exposure Time	Response Time	Recycle Time	Location Relative to Transformer	Comments
Mechanical contact	0.008 (1/120) S	Lag	Slow	Primary side	Tends to arc Contains movable parts Electromagnetic Spring loaded Stop/start at 0 in sine wave
Electronic (thyratron)	0.001 (1/1000) S	Instantaneous	Excellent	Secondary side	Triode tube Need another switch Stop/start any place on sine wave Need heat at cathode
Electronic (silicon controlled rectifier or thyristor)	0.001 S	Instantaneous	Excellent	Primary side	Solid state No heat at cathode Small in size

principle of electromagnetism. The mechanical contact switch is always located on the primary side of the high tension transformer. The following is a description of how the mechanical switch operates.

When the x-ray exposure button is depressed, current flows, creating a magnetic field around the wire. The magnetic field attracts the copper contact pieces, closing the circuit (Figure 9–1A). Release of the exposure button stops the current flow and subsequent magnetism. When this occurs, a spring pulls the contacts apart, opening the circuit (Figure 9–1B).

The spring of the mechanical contact switch must be strong enough to stop the exposure (pull the contacts apart) without delay. Also, to ensure accurate repetitive exposure times, the spring must be consistent in its function from one exposure to the next. Consequently, the spring must retain its shape and strength with increased use (exposures).

Because the mechanical contact switch has movable parts, it requires some time to respond, which creates a delay between exposures (recycle time). Thus, the mechanical contact switch is not conducive to serial filming, e.g., angiography. Also, sometimes an electrical arc (spark) occurs with higher voltages. This may damage the switch, decreasing its life span and adversely affecting the switch's accuracy. Care must be taken to avoid sudden surges of high voltage. Thus, it is recommended that the mechanical switch be synchronized with the sine wave (start and stop at zero).

ELECTRONIC SWITCHES

There are two types of electronic switches. One type, the thyratron, is a gas filled triode tube. The other, thyristor or silicon controlled rectifier, is made of solid state material. The triode tube is placed on the secondary side of the high tension transformer. Solid state electronic switches are located on the primary side of the high tension transformer. Both switches are advantageous because they can open and close the circuit at any point in the sine wave. This is extremely useful in serial filming. Also, the response time of electronic switches is so short, at 0.001 (1/1000) second (1 ms), it is considered instantaneous.

As stated previously, the thyratron is a gas filled triode tube. It contains three electrodes (thus the name triode): the cathode, the anode and the grid (Figure 9–2). The anode has a positive charge, whereas the cathode is negatively charged. The grid carries a charge (negative) whose strength can be varied. The grid is located close to the cathode and regulates current flow. A normal current flow is for

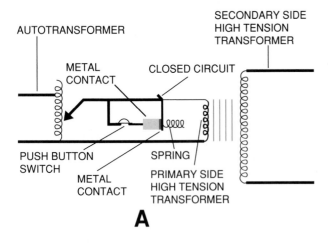

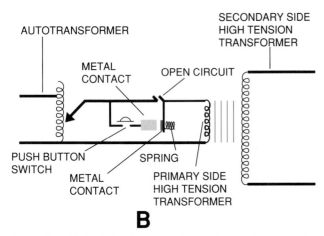

Figure 9–1. Mechanical contact switch. A, Closed circuit; B, open circuit.

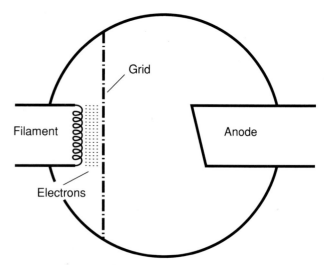

Figure 9–2. Triode tube.

electrons to travel from the cathode to the anode. However, the negative charge on the grid repels the electrons (negative charge) of the cathode, preventing the flow of current (it acts as a switch in the off position). Current is made to flow by decreasing the charge of the grid (the charge becomes less negative). This enables the electrons from the cathode to escape the weaker negative field of the grid and travel to the anode (the switch is in the on position). A triode tube is often used in conjunction with another thyratron or electromagnetic switch.

MANUAL TIMING DEVICES

Recall that switches are used in conjunction with timers. A discussion of the various types of timers

and their function follows. Most timing devices are rather simple in operation. However, the automatic timer is more complex and is discussed below under Automatic Timing Devices. Table 9–2 lists some features of common types of timers.

MECHANICAL TIMER

The simplest form of timer is the mechanical timer. This device operates like a spring wind clock.

Table 9–2. TIMER FEATURES

Type	Accuracy	Comment
Mechanical	0.05 (1/20) S	Use with low energy x-ray units
		Not recommended for short exposure
		Spring loaded
		Technologist regulates exposure length
Synchronous	0.017 (1/60) S	Not good for serial filming
		Open and close at 0 in sine wave
		Technologist regulates exposure length
Electronic	0.001 (1/1000) S	Good for serial filming
		Technologist regulates exposure length
Automatic	0.001 S	Provides uniform density
		Equipment regulates exposure length

The mechanical timer employs a spring to regulate the length of exposure. To set the timer, the operator turns a dial to the desired length of exposure. This winds a spring. When the exposure is made, current flows to the x-ray tube and the spring begins to unwind. The exposure is terminated when the spring is completely unwound. The tighter the spring is wound, the longer the duration of the exposure.

The mechanical timer is used for low power x-ray units, e.g., units for dental radiography. This type of timer is most reliable with long exposure times. It is accurate to 0.05 (1/20) second. The usual time range is 0.05 to 20 seconds.

SYNCHRONOUS TIMER

Synchronous timers are more accurate than mechanical timers. The synchronous timer uses a motor that rotates at the same frequency as that of the electrical current used to operate it. In the United States, that is 60 cycles per second (cps). These types of timers open and close the circuit at zero in the sine wave. Thus, in the United States, the minimum exposure time of a synchronous timer is 0.017 (1/60) second.

An advantage of the synchronous timer is that it provides a much shorter exposure time than the mechanical timer. However, the synchronous timer has a long recycle time, making it inappropriate for rapid serial filming.

ELECTRONIC TIMER

The most sophisticated manually set timer is the electronic timer. This timer uses a capacitor, a thyratron and a variable resistor. Capacitors may be charging or discharging.

The charging capacitor builds up a charge to a specified level. When the capacitor is fully charged, it becomes conductive and discharges. A discharging capacitor begins with a full charge. As current is applied to the capacitor, it discharges. The capacitor continues to discharge until it reaches a preselected level. It then becomes conductive and is recharged to its full capacity.

The amount of current entering the capacitor determines how long it takes for the capacitor to charge or discharge. The more current entering the capacitor, the shorter the time to charge or discharge the capacitor. Thus, by regulating the current, the charging or discharging time can be controlled. In an x-ray unit, the current is regulated by increasing or decreasing the resistance (variable resistor) of the circuit. The higher the resistance, the less the current flow and the longer the time for the capacitor to charge or discharge.

Figure 9–3 diagrams the components of a simple electronic timer. To energize this timer, the operator depresses the exposure button on the x-ray unit. When the exposure button is depressed, two events occur simultaneously. One event is that current flows to a switch, which closes the circuit, resulting in the x-ray tube's being energized. This begins the

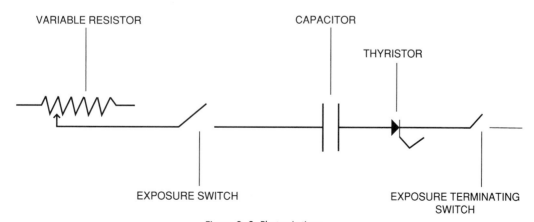

Figure 9–3. Electronic timer.

production of x-rays. The other event is that the capacitor begins to charge or discharge (depending on the type of capacitor). When the capacitor reaches its preset level, it conducts current to the thyratron, which sends a signal to a switch to terminate the exposure. The duration of the exposure is determined when the operator sets the time station on the x-ray machine. This adjusts the variable resistor (alters the resistance) to control the length of time it takes for the capacitor to reach its preset level.

Electronic timers are advantageous because they are accurate up to 1 ms. Also, they have short recycle times, making it possible to perform rapid serial filming.

AUTOMATIC TIMING DEVICES

With manual timing devices, the technologist determines the time of the x-ray exposure. The time is usually selected from a technique chart. The technologist measures the patient and reads a chart to identify the desired settings. Many variables are involved in this process, e.g., the exact location of the area to measure, making this system unreliable. For automatic timing devices, the technologist selects the kilovoltage and usually the milliamperage, but the equipment regulates the length of the exposure. Automatic timers employ the concept of optimal kilovoltage technique (see under Technique Charts in Chapter 11, Kilovoltage and Quality Control).

When using automatic timing devices, the operator determines when to start the exposure. This is achieved by depressing the exposure button. The exposure ends automatically when a predetermined quantity of radiation is detected. The primary advantage of automatic timing devices is the ability to produce radiographs of uniform density regardless of the size of the patient.

Automatic timing devices are based on four concepts. One concept is for patient size variability to function in the same manner as a variable resistor in an electronic timer. Because automatic timers function on the principle of predetermined radiation measurements, varying patient size changes the rate of radiation absorption (remnant radiation). This regulates the amount of time needed to reach the preset radiation level. The second concept is to employ a device to measure the radiation. The two devices used are ionization chamber or photomultiplier tube. These devices serve as indirect methods of measuring radiation. The third concept is to design the system so that the current is proportional to the radiation measurement. Lastly, a method must exist to terminate the exposure when the quantity of radiation needed to obtain a preset density is reached.

The two types of automatic timers are the ionization chamber and the photomultiplier tube. Often, both types are erroneously referred to as phototimers. The photomultiplier tube and the ionization chamber perform the same function (automatically terminate the exposure). However, the manner in which they achieve the regulation of exposure differs.

IONIZATION CHAMBER

Most ionization chambers are entrance type. That is, they are placed between the patient and the film. To avoid producing a visible image on the radiograph, the ionization chamber has low radiation absorption properties.

An ionization chamber consists of two electrodes separated by an air gap. A direct current is placed on the electrodes. During the x-ray exposure, the remnant radiation enters the chamber and ionizes the air. The positive ions move toward the negative electrode; the negative ions migrate to the positive electrode. This causes a current to flow to the thyratron. The thyratron, in turn, sends a signal to a switch, terminating the exposure (Figure 9–4).

Ionization chambers have three areas for detecting the radiation. These fields usually contain the same surface area but differ in shape. On an upright automatically timed chest unit, the location of the chambers is marked on the surface of the chest holder (Figure 9–5). For routine table work with a source-image distance (SID) of 40 inches, outlines of the detectors may be painted on a plastic plate (similar to a filter). The plate is attached to the bottom of the collimator. Thus, when the collimator light is turned on, the shadow of the detectors is projected onto the patient. This enables the technologist to position the respective detector over the area of interest.

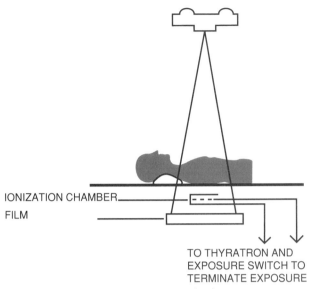

IONIZATION CHAMBER

FILM

TO THYRATRON AND
EXPOSURE SWITCH TO
TERMINATE EXPOSURE

Figure 9–4. Ionization chamber.

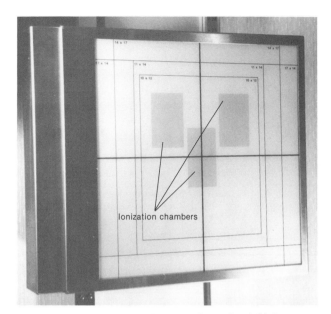

Ionization chambers

Figure 9–5. Ionization detector markings (chest holder).

PHOTOMULTIPLIER TUBE

The photomultiplier tube is an exit type of automatic timer. That is, the photomultiplier tube is located after the film. Often the Bucky tray has a large hole (about 6 inches) in the center, allowing the exiting radiation to strike the photomultiplier tube. A photomultiplier tube is one of many components used for automatic timing. Others are detectors, a light gate, a capacitor, a thyratron and a switch. Before an explanation of the function of these components, a discussion of a photomultiplier tube is in order.

A photomultiplier tube multiplies electrons. This is achieved through the use of a photosensitive cathode, dynodes and an anode. The cathode and the anode contain negative and positive charges, respectively. Figure 9–6 represents the manner in which a photomultiplier tube functions. It can be seen from Figure 9–6 that light strikes the photosensitive cathode and electrons are emitted. The electrons are attracted to the first dynode. A dynode is an electrode. In the photomultiplier tube, the first dynode is less negative (more positive) than the cathode; thus, there is a flow of electrons. The succeeding dynodes become less negative (more positive). There may be as many as 10 dynodes in a photomultiplier tube. When a dynode is hit by electrons, it emits electrons. The number of elec-

trons emitted per electron striking the dynode is a specific multiple factor, e.g., 10 times. The electrons from the first dynode are attracted to the second dynode. Again, there is an increase (by a specific multiple factor) in exiting electrons. This process of multiplying electrons continues until they reach the anode. At the anode, the electrons become current flow.

Figure 9–7 demonstrates the function of an automatic timer using a photomultiplier tube. Located above the photomultiplier tube are the detectors. The ionization type of marking system is used to identify detector location (see above). The three

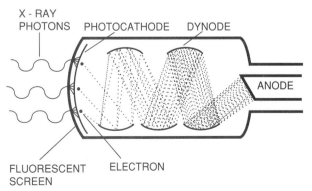

X - RAY
PHOTONS   PHOTOCATHODE   DYNODE

ANODE

FLUORESCENT
SCREEN   ELECTRON

Figure 9–6. Photomultiplier tube.

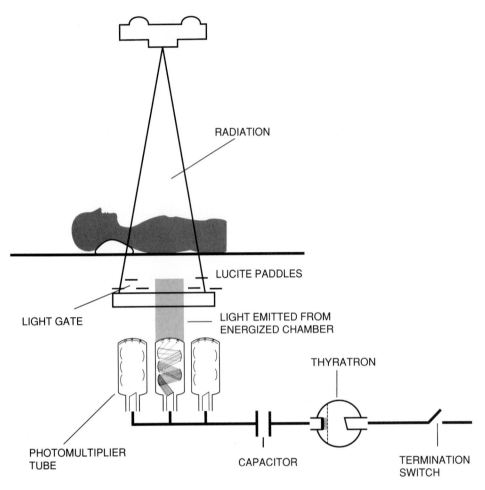

Figure 9–7. Automatic timer using a photomultiplier tube.

detectors are made of several sheets of Lucite (Lucite paddles). Lucite can transmit light as a fiber-optic bundle.

When irradiated, the Lucite emits a light (in proportion to the x-ray intensity) and transmits the light to light gates (located below each detector). The light gates direct the light to the photomultiplier tube. There may be one photomultiplier tube for all three light gates or one photomultiplier tube per gate (for a total of three tubes). The photomultiplier tube changes the light to electrons and multiplies them in a specific ratio. As the electrons strike the anode of the photomultiplier tube, a current flows, charging a capacitor. After it is fully charged, the capacitor conducts a current to the thyratron, which energizes the termination switch, ending the exposure.

BACK-UP TIMER

It is possible to have kilovoltage (kV), milliamperage (mA) and patient size combinations that necessitate a long, e.g., 2–3 seconds, exposure time. This may create a heat unit value exceeding the x-ray tube maximum. The U.S. Department of Health and Human Services (1988) lists a maximum of 600 milliampere-seconds (mAs) for exposures of 50 kV or greater. The maximum is 2000 mAs for exposures of less than 50 kV. Consequently, to protect the x-ray tube and maintain federal standards, a back-up timer is placed in automatic timing devices to terminate the exposure at a preset value. Some units provide a means of selecting different maximum time exposures.

In the overwhelming majority of patients, the

exposure time is well within the back-up time value. However, it is possible that the back-up timer may terminate the exposure before the automatic timing device, ending the exposure. For example, if the back-up timer is set for 0.5 second and a patient requires a 0.8 second exposure, the back-up timer stops the exposure 0.3 second before the needed time (0.8 − 0.5 = 0.3). Consequently, the radiograph is lighter than normal.

In these instances, there are at least three ways to adjust technical factors to obtain a diagnostic radiograph. One method is to increase the milliampere station while maintaining the same kilovoltage. The second method is to increase the kilovoltage and keep the milliamperage the same. Lastly, it is possible to increase both milliamperage and kilovoltage. All these methods increase the amount of remnant radiation entering the detector and decrease the amount of exposure time. Care needs to be taken to use factors that are within the tube limit. If a certain amount of contrast is required for the examination, it is better to maintain the same kilovoltage and alter the milliamperage.

MINIMUM EXPOSURE TIME

A minimum amount of time is needed for automatic timers to respond or react. This is often referred to as minimum reaction time. It is possible to have a minimum reaction time as long as 0.033 (1/30) second. Radiography of objects that are extremely thin may require exposure times shorter than the minimum reaction time. For example, if a minimum exposure time of 0.017 (1/60) second is necessary and the minimum reaction time is 0.033 second, the exposure is twice as long as necessary, resulting in an overexposed radiograph (0.033 − 0.017 = 0.016). To obtain a diagnostic film, the technologist must adjust the factors to increase the time to no less than the minimum reaction time. This may be achieved by decreasing the kilovoltage, the milliamperage or both.

AUTOMATIC TIMER CONTROL PANEL

X-ray generators with automatic timing devices provide the operator with a choice between auto-

matic and manual timed exposures. This is particularly important for table top radiography, e.g., of extremities, because the automatic timer has no effect on these types of procedures. Selecting the automatic button allows the technologist to operate different control panel items than when the manual timing device is energized. This section discusses the control panel items energized with automatic timing devices.

Simple automatic timing devices allow the technologist to select the kilovoltage, the milliamperage, detector chamber, back-up timer (see above) and density. Kilovoltage and milliamperage are selected in the usual manner for optimum kilovoltage technique.

Recall that the duration of the exposure time is determined by the quantity of remnant radiation. The more remnant radiation entering the automatic exposure detector, the less time (exposure) is needed to reach the preset radiation value. Higher kilovoltage or milliamperage settings and smaller patient size increase the remnant radiation (assuming all other factors remain the same). Figure 9–8 shows the effect of these factors on exposure time.

Automatic timers usually have three detectors: one in the center and one located on either side of the center detector. Buttons on the x-ray generator may be depressed to energize the detector. It is possible to energize one, two or three detectors. The design of the equipment determines how many detectors may be energized at one time. The technologist selects the detector(s) located over the area of interest (for more information, see under Precautions).

A control panel item often located on an automatic timer is the density. This control provides a means of increasing and decreasing the radiographic density. The usual range is −4 to +4, with 0 representing normal. The level of density change is usually 25% from the adjacent factor. For example, a setting of +2 is 25% darker than a selection of +1. It should be noted that unlike the case with manually set technique, increasing the kilovoltage or the milliamperage does not change the density. These factors regulate the duration of the exposure. Thus, density is regulated by using the density control.

An alternative to the simple control panel is the computer programmed system (Figure 9–9). These

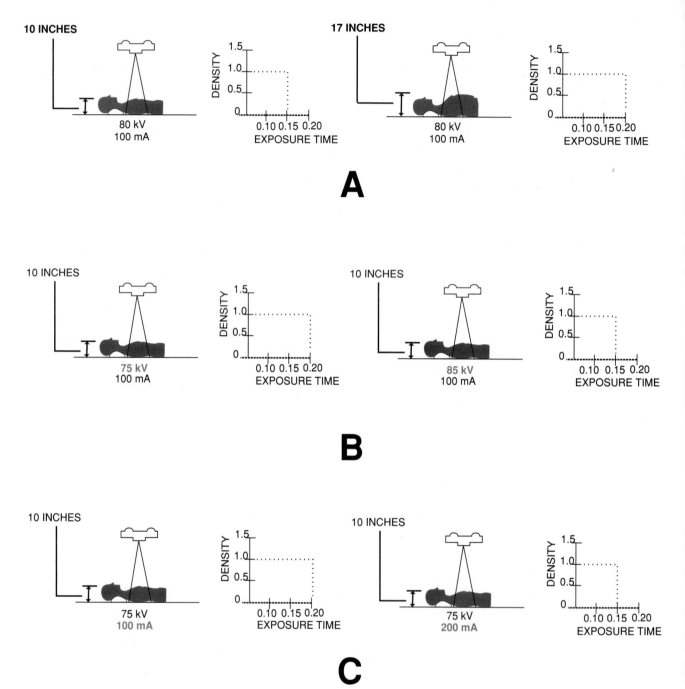

Figure 9–8. Factors affecting automatic exposure time. *A*, Patient size; *B*, kilovoltage; *C*, milliamperage.

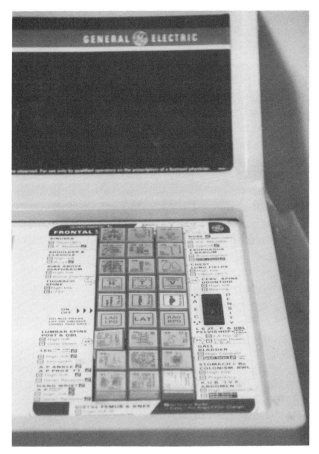

Figure 9–9. Control panel demonstrating the various types of program selections available.

systems provide a variety of control panel choices. Common control panel items enable the technologist to select patient size and position, length of exposure and anatomical part being irradiated.

PRECAUTIONS

Four items may adversely affect the density of a radiograph taken with an automatic exposure timing device:
1. Intensifying screen and film combination
2. Positioning
3. Detector field
4. Collimation.

Automatic exposure timing devices are preset to obtain a specific density for a specific intensifying screen speed and film combination. For example,

photomultiplier tubes require cassettes with little or no lead backing. Using a lead lined cassette with a photomultiplier timing device results in an overexposed film. Thus, it is important that the correct screens and film be used. To maintain the same density when using different intensifying screen speeds, some manufacturers provide a button that changes the sensitivity of the timing device. Unfortunately, technologists sometimes use this button as a means of altering the time to increase the density of a film. Any change in density is best regulated by changing the density knob.

Patient positioning is much more critical with automatic timing devices than with manual timing mechanisms. The appropriate density of the desired area is obtained when the area of interest is over the detector.

Recall that the detector is used to help determine the amount of radiation reaching the film. The technologist selects which detector(s) to use before exposing the film. To obtain the correct density, it is important that the detector field selected is over the area of interest. For example, the lateral (side) detector is energized for a posterior-anterior chest x-ray film. This results in the correct density over the lung field. If the center detector is energized, the density is regulated by the thoracic spine (which is located over the center detector). Thus, the density to visualize the thoracic spine is fine, but the lung field is too dark.

As in all radiographic procedures, it is important to achieve collimation with the area of interest. Any increase in collimation increases the scatter radiation. The scatter radiation is picked up by the detectors, terminating the exposure prematurely.

QUALITY CONTROL

The length of exposure helps determine the amount of radiation absorption by the patient and influences the radiographic quality. Consequently, a properly operating timer is essential.

Many modern x-ray timers operate on electronic impulses. The number of impulses used during a timed exposure is a function of
1. The type of rectification
2. The type of timer employed
3. The type of current (single or three phase) entering the machine.

There are at least three noninvasive instruments used to test timer accuracy. They are (1) the spinning top (for single phase equipment), (2) a synchronous motor driven disc with a small slit (for single and three phase testing) and (3) a digital x-ray exposure timer (for single and three phase units). There is one invasive method used to assess x-ray timer accuracy, the oscilloscope. This text discusses the noninvasive methods of evaluating timer accuracy.

SPINNING TOP TEST

Of the three noninvasive tests, the spinning top test is the simplest. This test is only performed on single phase x-ray units. The synchronous motor or digital x-ray test is required to assess three phase equipment timers.

A spinning top consists of a radiopaque metallic disc. The disc contains a small hole near its periphery, which permits passage of x-rays during exposure. (The hole is imaged as a rectangle. For simplicity, the rectangle is referred to as a dot.) The top spins on a shaft set in a base (Figure 9–10).

To perform a spinning top test, a cassette is placed on the x-ray table and the spinning top is positioned in a corner of the cassette. A minimum of four exposures are made of the spinning top. Thus, the spinning top is placed in one-fourth of the cassette (corner) and the remaining three-fourths is covered with lead. Multiple exposures are used to test the consistency of the timer. A technique setting to obtain at least a 1.5 density is used. Timer settings from 0.07 (1/15) second to 0.1 (1/10) second are recommended for half wave or

self-wave units. A range of 0.04 (1/24) second to 0.05 (1/20) second is preferred for full wave rectified equipment. These ranges limit the number of dots imaged to a sufficient quantity for assessment and decrease the possibility of the dots' overlapping during the spinning of the top.

To obtain an image, the top is rotated on its base at a constant and relatively fast speed so that the top spins for several seconds. A fast speed elongates the dots, facilitating the assessment of their density. While the top is turning, an exposure is made (care should be taken to ensure that the individual who began the top spinning is protected from the radiation during the exposure). This process is repeated for the remaining three exposures. The only change among exposures is to reposition the spinning top over an unexposed one-quarter section of the cassette while protecting the other three-quarters with lead. The same technique is used for all four exposures. After the entire cassette is exposed, the film is developed.

The resulting radiograph reveals a series of dots (Figure 9–11), each dot representing a single pulse of x-ray photons. The number of dots produced in a radiograph is determined by the exposure time setting, the current frequency and the number of useful pulses per cycle (determined by the type of rectification). A half wave or self-wave rectified unit produces one useful impulse, whereas a full wave rectified unit produces two useful impulses (see Chapter 8, Rectification, for more details). One dot is imaged per pulse. To determine the number of dots, the exposure time is multiplied by the current frequency and the number of useful impulses. For example, how many dots are imaged in a radiograph of a spinning top exposed using a half wave rectified, 60 cps x-ray unit and an exposure time of 0.15 second? 0.15 (second) × 60 (cps) × 1 (useful impulse/cycle) = 9 (dots). The test is considered successful if the number of dots is one greater or one less than the expected number.

The density of the dot is evaluated in addition to the correct number of dots. The density of the dot is a function of the x-ray tube current. The darkest part of the dot represents the peak of the current's sine wave (Figure 9–12). An improperly operating timer may not start at zero of the sine wave. This is demonstrated in an unequal distribution of densities within the dots.

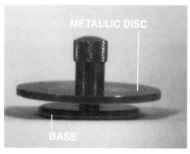

METALLIC DISC

BASE

Figure 9–10. Spinning top.

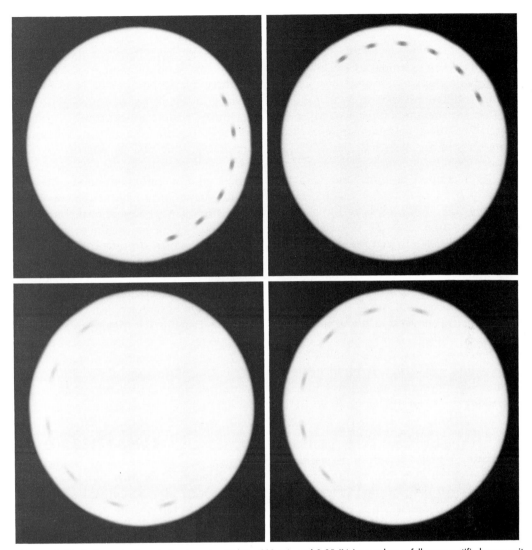

Figure 9–11. Radiograph of a spinning top using 52 kVp, 200 mA, and 0.05 (¹⁄₂₀) second on a full wave rectified x-ray unit.

Figure 9–12. Relationship of the density of a spinning top dot to the sine wave. A = zero, B = peak, C = zero.

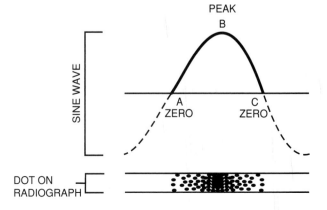

SYNCHRONOUS MOTOR DRIVEN DISC

The synchronous motor is similar to the spinning top in that the synchronous motor employs a brass disc. The primary difference is that the synchronous motor's disc rotates at 1 revolution per second (rps). Some commercially made synchronous motors also contain a penetrometer for assessing the milliamperage (see under Quality Control Tests for Ampere in Chapter 12, Milliampere-seconds and Quality Control).

As stated above, the disc rotates at 1 rps. The disc contains two narrow slits 180 degrees apart and may have a small hole drilled below the slit. To use the synchronous motor, the instrument is plugged into a wall socket and then positioned over one-third of an 8 × 10 inch cassette. An exposure employing a time between 0.033 and 1 second is made. The instrument is moved to the center one-third of the cassette and a second exposure using the same milliampere-seconds but different milliampere and time settings is used. A third and last exposure is made over the remaining one-third of the cassette. Again the same milliampere-seconds

setting is employed, but a milliampere and time setting different from those for the other two exposures is used.

The image on the radiograph consists of two arcs if three phase equipment is used or several slit images if single phase equipment is used (Figure 9–13). Also, dots appear below the slit if the instrument is constructed with a hole below the slit. The accuracy of the timer is checked by measuring the arc or counting the slit images (or dots). For three phase equipment or continuous pulse, single phase units, a special protractor (Figure 9–14) is used to measure the arc. Commercial companies provide a protractor with some times already marked. To determine the arc for times other than those marked on the protractor, multiply the exposure time by 360 degrees. For example, an exposure to 0.2 second has a 72 degree angle (0.2 × 360 = 72). The slit is a three dimensional object and has width. Thus, adding 1 to the calculated degree provides a corrected angle (compensation for the width of the slit). In the previous example, the corrected angle for 0.2 second is 73, or 72 + 1 = 73. Any angle within 10% of the calculated angle is acceptable. Assessment for single phase units employs the

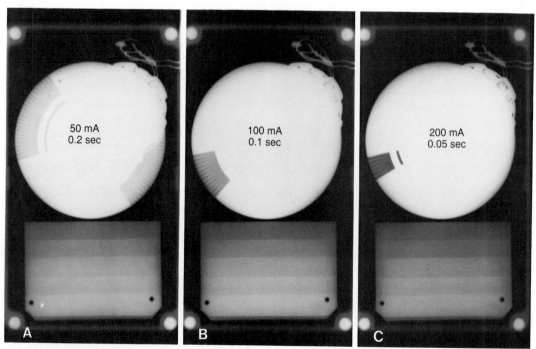

Figure 9–13. Radiographic image produced by a synchronous motor for a full wave rectified x-ray unit.

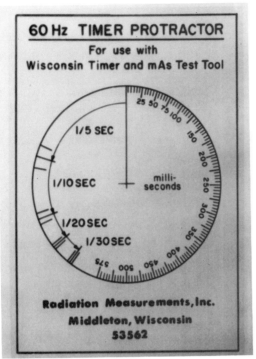

Figure 9–14. Protractor used to measure arc on radiograph of synchronous motor.

number of dots visualized on the radiograph. Refer to discussion under Spinning Top Test for a method to determine the correct number of dots.

DIGITAL METER

Digital meters are computer operated for timer assessment. The digital x-ray exposure timer testing tool is designed to measure the x-ray on time during radiographic exposure. The time indicator, a digital readout, is in pulses for single phase x-ray units and actual exposure time (seconds) for three phase or constant potential x-ray machines. The operator selects the appropriate type of readout before the exposure.

The first step in the operation of the digital meter is to position the device under the x-ray tube. The instrument is turned on. Next the appropriate type of readout is selected, pulse for single phase imaging units and milliseconds or seconds mode for three phase or continuous x-ray machines. Milliseconds are used to time exposures of 0.5 second or

less. Seconds are best used to measure exposures of 1 second or longer.

A 40 inch SID is used for three phase units and 30 inch SID for single phase equipment. The central ray is placed over the designated area on the device and an exposure using the technique settings of 100 mA, 0.1 second 65 kVp is recommended for 30 inch SID. (Note: Some type of system is used to identify if the technique is incorrect. One method uses a red light emitting diode [LED] to indicate an x-ray intensity over range and an amber LED for time over range. Should these LEDs illuminate, technique variables are adjusted appropriately.) After exposure, the time or pulse (depending on the setting) is displayed in a digital readout.

LABORATORY EXPERIENCE

Exposure time and milliamperage are often used to express x-ray intensity. Consequently, tests for assessing one value, e.g., time, often are used to evaluate the other factor, e.g., milliamperage. Thus, it is recommended that Laboratory Experience in Chapter 12, Milliampere-seconds and Quality Control, be reviewed.

Concepts in Medical Radiographic Imaging: Laboratory Manual has two laboratories dedicated to the evaluation of timers. They are Laboratories 13, Timer Test, and 15, Automatic Timers.

The Timer Test laboratory entails assessment of both single phase and three phase equipment. The spinning top, synchronous motor or digital meter instrument may be used to assess single phase units. Three phase assessment is limited to the synchronous motor or digital meter.

Demonstration of the effect of kilovoltage on time for automatic timers is located in Laboratory 15. The researcher performs several exposures at varying kilovoltages and records the time used by the automatic exposure device.

Bibliography

Bushong, SC. Radiologic science for technologists (4th edition). St. Louis: Mosby, 1988.

Carroll, QB. Fuchs's principles of radiographic exposure, processing and quality control (3rd edition). Springfield, IL: Thomas, 1985.

Chesney, DN and Chesney, MO. X-ray equipment for student radiographers (3rd edition). Boston: Blackwell Scientific Publications, 1984.

Cullinan, JE and Cullinan, AM. Illustrated guide to x-ray technics (2nd edition). New York: Lippincott, 1980.

Curry, TS, Dowdey, JE and Murry, RC. Christensen's introduction to the physics of diagnostic radiology (3rd edition). Philadelphia: Lea & Febiger, 1984.

Curry, TS, Dowdey, JE and Murry, RC. Christensen's physics of diagnostic radiology (4th edition). Philadelphia: Lea & Febiger, 1990.

Graham, BJ and Thomas, WN. An introduction to physics for radiologic technologists. Philadelphia: Saunders, 1975.

Gray, JE, et al. Quality control in diagnostic imaging. Baltimore: University Park Press, 1983.

Hendee, WR, Chaney, EL and Rossi, RP. Radiologic physics, equipment and quality control. Chicago: Year Book Medical, 1976.

Hiss, SS. Understanding radiography. Springfield, IL: Thomas, 1980.

McLemore, J. Quality assurance in diagnostic radiology. Chicago: Year Book Medical, 1981.

Selman, J. The fundamentals of x-ray and radium physics (7th edition). Springfield, IL: Thomas, 1985.

Thompson, TT. Cahoon's formulating x-ray techniques (9th edition). Durham, NC: Duke University Press, 1979.

United States Department of Health and Human Resources. Regulations for the administration and enforcement of the radiation control for health and safety act of 1968 (supersedes HEW publication FDA 90–8035). Rockville, MD: U.S. Government Printing Office, April 1988, FDA 88-8035.

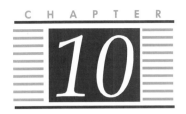

PRODUCTION OF

X-RAYS

INTRODUCTION

Wilhelm Conrad Roentgen, a German physicist, discovered x-rays in 1895. He saw a faint greenish illumination on a fluorescent screen. When placing objects of different densities between the tube and the screen, he noticed that the rays could penetrate some objects with ease and the more dense objects, e.g., lead, were almost opaque. Because he did not know what caused this phenomenon, Roentgen used the symbol x, which represents an unknown in mathematics, to describe the rays. Thus, the term x-rays evolved. In an effort to properly recognize Roentgen for his discovery, the scientific community renamed x-rays Roentgen rays. Unfortunately, this new name is not widely used and the term x-rays continues to be used to most often describe Roentgen's discovery.

Since Roentgen's time, science has been able to improve the methods of x-ray production. The x-ray tubes and accessory equipment, e.g., grids, are much more efficient than the original equipment built in the early 1900s. Experience has also revealed the side effects of x-rays. The hazards of radiation, e.g., cancer, have resulted in the development of protective devices and equipment.

This chapter briefly describes the x-ray circuit. It also includes an in-depth discussion of the x-ray tube. References to the effects of radiation are beyond the scope of this text.

X-RAY CIRCUIT

There are many parts to the x-ray circuit. It is often easier to explain the x-ray circuit and production of x-rays by considering the circuit's components. A common method of dividing the circuit is to refer to the low voltage portion (primary circuit), the high voltage area (secondary circuit) and the filament circuit (Figure 10–1). The low voltage circuit consists of the components located from the main power supply to the primary side of the high tension transformer. The high voltage portion begins at the secondary side of the high tension transformer and ends at the x-ray tube. The filament circuit originates at the tap from the autotransformer and terminates at the filament of the x-ray tube.

LOW VOLTAGE CIRCUIT

The basic function of the low voltage circuit is to direct the incoming voltage to the primary side of the high tension transformer. The primary components of the low voltage circuit are main switch, autotransformer, prereading kilovolt meter, timer and primary coil of the high tension transformer.

The main switch is usually located near the x-ray generator. It is easily recognized, as it is a big metal box attached to the wall. The electricity entering

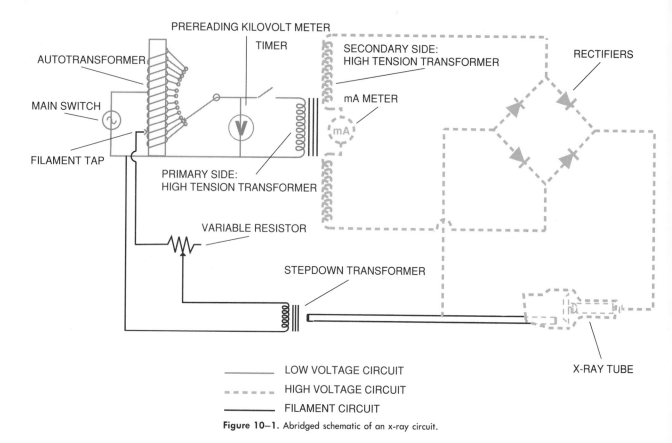

Figure 10–1. Abridged schematic of an x-ray circuit.

the main switch originates from a transformer near the outside of the building. Incoming line conduits carry the electricity from the outside to the main switch box. Located inside the box are large fuses. The fuses serve as a protective mechanism in case the current exceeds its safe range. When the electrical conditions are unsafe, the fuses open the circuit.

When the on/off switch of the x-ray generator is closed (turned on), current passes from the main switch to the primary side of the autotransformer (refer to Chapter 7, Transformers, for more specific information on transformers). The autotransformer regulates the amount of kilovoltage used. This is achieved by moving the tap (Figure 10–1), which is located on the secondary side of the autotransformer. To move the tap, the operator adjusts the kilovoltage knob on the generator. Besides the kilovoltage tap, two other taps are also located on the autotransformer: one for the filament current and the other for the line voltage regulator.

The tap for the filament current is considered

part of the filament circuit and is discussed under Filament Circuit. The line voltage regulator allows the user to adjust the incoming voltage. The peak value of the incoming voltage is affected by all the devices connected to the incoming electrical circuit. If other items are using electricity at the same time, the available voltage is decreased. The line voltage regulator is used to compensate for any voltage fluctuations.

Attached to the secondary side of the autotransformer is the prereading kilovolt meter. This meter measures the amount of voltage at the secondary side of the autotransformer. Recall that the high tension transformer has a fixed ratio. By knowing the ratio of the high tension transformer, it is possible to calibrate the voltmeter to read in terms of kilovoltage. This is the transformer ratio (see Chapter 7). For example, if the fixed ratio of the high tension transformer is 1:1000 and the secondary side of the autotransformer measures 70 V, it is possible to calibrate the meter to read 70,000 V (70 kVp), or 70 × 1000 = 70,000.

Current passes to the primary side of the high tension transformer when the exposure switch is depressed. The duration of the exposure is regulated by the timer (refer to Chapter 9, X-ray Timers and Quality Control, for more specific information on switches and timers). The timer is located in the low voltage side of the x-ray circuit between the secondary side of the autotransformer and the primary side of the high tension transformer.

HIGH VOLTAGE CIRCUIT

Components of the high voltage circuit consist of the secondary side of the high tension transformer, milliammeter, milliampere-seconds meter, rectifiers and x-ray tube. These components and their functions are briefly discussed here. The x-ray tube is discussed under X-ray Tube.

When the current reaches the primary side of the high tension transformer, it travels to the secondary side by mutual induction (refer to Chapter 7, Transformers). The function of the high tension transformer is to step up the voltage from low, 200 V or less, to the thousands of volts.

Connected to the secondary side of the high tension transformer are the meters to read current. One meter is used to measure the larger (exposure times greater than 0.1 [1/10] second) milliampere-seconds values. A special meter, the milliampere-seconds meter, is needed to measure short exposure times.

The production of x-rays requires direct current. Because the incoming voltage is alternating current, there is a need to change it to direct current. This is achieved by rectification (see Chapter 8, Rectification). Several methods are used to rectify a circuit: self-rectification, half wave rectification and full wave rectification. Figure 10–1 represents a single phase, full wave rectified x-ray circuit.

The function of the x-ray tube is to produce x-rays. The manner in which it performs this function is complex (see under X-ray Tube).

FILAMENT CIRCUIT

The filament circuit consists of a tap from the autotransformer, a step-down transformer and a variable resistor. The autotransformer tap provides low voltage (6–12 V) and appropriate amperage (3–5 A) to the filament of the x-ray tube. The step-down transformer is employed to decrease the voltage from the autotransformer. The amount of current to the x-ray filament is regulated by a variable resistor. Recall that, according to Ohm's law (refer to Chapter 5, Electrodynamics), for a constant voltage any increase in resistance decreases the current. The converse is also true. The current exiting the step-down transformer is used for thermionic emission at the x-ray tube.

Thermionic emission is the emission of electrons (created by the heat of the filament current) from the x-ray tube filament (thermionic emission is discussed under X-ray Tube). It is required to produce x-rays. The more current there is at the x-ray filament, the more heat is produced and the greater is the number of electrons emitted.

PRODUCTION OF X-RAYS

Before discussion of the x-ray tube, a brief summary regarding the method of x-ray production is in order. The production of x-rays occurs when high speed electrons are suddenly decelerated or interact with matter. Most of the energy generated during the production of x-rays is heat. Some energy is in the form of light and about 1% is radiation.

The x-ray tube provides all the conditions necessary to produce radiation. The high speed of electrons occurs when a high potential is applied to the electrodes of the x-ray tube. The speed of the electrons approaches one-half of the speed of light. Electron deceleration and interaction with matter results when the electrons strike the target of the anode. Specifics regarding the components of the x-ray tube and their function are discussed below.

X-RAY TUBE

The basic components of the x-ray tube are the electrodes, the vacuum glass envelope and the tube assembly (Figure 10–2). The electrodes consist of the anode and the cathode. The tube assembly, or tube housing, includes the metal shield surrounding the glass envelope and the oil located between the glass and the metal shield.

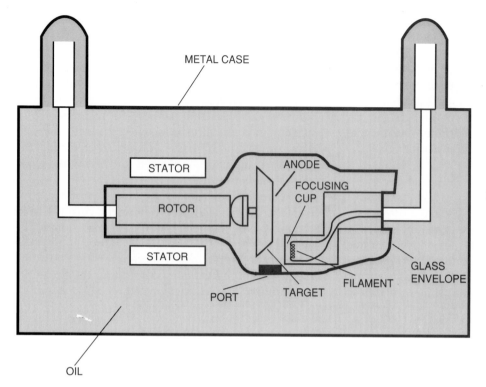

Figure 10-2. X-ray tube.

CATHODE

The cathode of the x-ray tube is the negatively charged electrode. It consists of the filament and the focusing cup (Figure 10–3). Both are negatively charged. The function of the cathode is to serve as the source of electrons needed to produce x-rays.

Filament

The filament is a small coiled wire made of tungsten. Tungsten is used as the metal because it has a high melting point (3370° C), does not evaporate easily and has a high atomic number (74). A high melting point and high evaporation level are necessary because of the large amount of heat (sometimes 3000° C) produced in the tube. Elements with high atomic numbers are needed to provide a good electron source. Sometimes thorium is added to the tungsten to increase the efficiency and prolong the life of the filament.

The true or actual dimensions of the filament are as follows: filament length range is usually 8–15 mm; the diameter range is about 1.5–2.0 mm. The size and shape of the filament help determine the size and shape of the focal spot (the area where the electrons strike the anode). Reference to the focal spot size usually relates to the effective focal spot size. The effective focal spot size represents the dimensions of the focal spot as it appears to the image receptor. Actual filament size differs from the effective focal spot size (see under Anode).

Most modern x-ray tubes contain two filaments

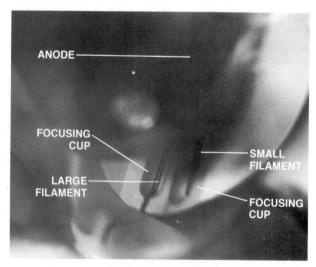

Figure 10-3. Cathode.

of different sizes. The smaller filament is used when a sharp image is required (refer to Chapter 26, Geometric Image Quality). However, small filaments are unable to withstand as much heat as the large filament. Thus, the large filament is employed when the technique results in more heat than the small filament can withstand and when image sharpness is not critical. The specific filament energized is determined when the operator selects the milliamperage.

The filament evaporates with age and use. The evaporation process is slow. Filament evaporation causes the diameter of the filament to decrease (it gets thinner). This increases the possibility for the filament to break, necessitating tube replacement. Filament evaporation also results in the deposition of tungsten on the glass envelope. The deposit acts as additional filtration. It also increases the possibility of arcing. If arcing does occur, it can break the glass and the tube must be replaced.

Thermionic Emission

As mentioned above, the cathode is the source of electrons. This is achieved by a process called thermionic emission. In thermionic emission, the filament circuit (see under Filament Circuit) supplies a current (3–5 A) to the filament. This current heats the filament. The heat causes loosely bound electrons to be removed (boiled off) from their atoms. The electrons released are called thermions. The electrons form a cloud near the filament, which is often referred to as a space charge. When the electrons leave the filament, the filament becomes positively charged. This causes some electrons in the space charge to be attracted back to the filament. In practice, the number of electrons being emitted and the number of electrons returning to the filament are constant. Thus, a state of equilibrium exists. Only a certain number of electrons are emitted (a space charge limit exists).

The thermions remain near the filament as long as no kilovoltage is applied to the electrodes. On application of kilovoltage, the anode becomes positive and the cathode becomes negative. This causes the thermions to move from the cathode to the anode. The greater the kilovoltage applied to the tube is, the faster the electrons travel to the anode, hitting the target at a higher velocity. This results in a beam with more penetrating power than a low voltage beam.

Because the constant application of heat destroys the filament, during ideal times (when no exposure is being made) the amount of current flowing to the filament is lowered to about 5 mA. This lowering of the filament current is called standby. The current is returned to its useful level while the anode is reaching its proper speed (in revolutions per minute) just before exposure.

Focusing Cup

The focusing cup is made of molybdenum and carries the same negative charge as the filament. Tubes with more than one filament have a focusing cup surrounding each filament. The effectiveness of the focusing cup depends on the size and shape of the cup, the amount of charge on the cup, the filament dimensions and the location of the filament within the cup. The function of the focusing cup is to concentrate (focus) the thermions in a narrow path. This is achieved by employing the concept that like charges repel. Thus, the negative charges of the electrons and the focusing cup repel each other. Unfortunately, the negative charges of the electrons also cause the electrons to repel each other. Thus, the highest concentration of electrons is on the outer edge of the path. To make a more uniform intensity of the electron path, the focusing cup charge may be increased (50–100 V) so that it is greater than the filament charge.

ANODE

The anode of the x-ray tube is the positively charged electrode. It is located opposite the cathode at a distance of about 2.5 cm (1 inch). The function of the anode is to stop the electrons and produce x-rays.

Most radiographic x-ray tube anodes are angled. The range of anode angle is 10–20 degrees. The angle of the anode provides a means to have a large actual focal spot size and a small effective focal spot size (Figure 10–4). This phenomena is known as the line focus principle. The mathematical calculation of the size of the effective focal spot is

$$EFS = AFSS \times \sin \Theta \text{ of anode}$$

where EFS is the effective focal spot size, AFSS represents the actual focal spot size, and $\sin \Theta$

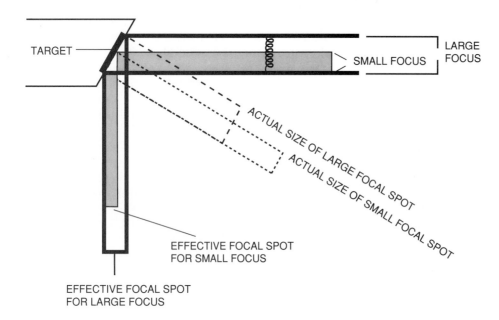

Figure 10–4. According to the line focus principle, the effective focal spot size on a dual focus x-ray tube is smaller than the actual focal spot size.

means the sine of the angle (in this case, the sine of the angle of the anode).

The smaller the effective focal spot size, the better the geometric image quality (refer to Chapter 26, Geometric Image Quality). Effective focal spot size is decreased by decreasing the anode angle. Unfortunately, as the anode angle gets smaller, the heel effect becomes more significant.

The heel effect is an uneven distribution of radiation intensity. In general, the intensity toward the anode side of the image receptor ranges from 75 to 87% and at the cathode side from 105 to 120%. Thus, the heel effect results in the emission of more radiation toward the cathode. The amount of uneven distribution depends on the angle of the anode, the field size and the source-image distance (SID). The heel effect is more prevalent when one employs a short SID, a small anode angle or a large field size. The converse is also true.

The area of the anode where radiation is produced is called the target (where the electrons interact with matter), or focal spot. The target may be mounted on a stationary or a rotating anode.

Stationary Anode

The stationary anode has a tungsten target embedded in copper (Figure 10–5). The target is made of tungsten because of its high melting point and high atomic number. Some targets also have

rhenium mixed with the tungsten. Rhenium is advantageous because it diminishes the target's tendency to become rough or pitted with electron interaction. The copper is useful because it is a good conductor of heat. Thus, it helps dissipate the heat generated when the electrons interact with the target.

Rotating Anode

A rotating anode consists of a 3–5 inch disc mounted on a stem (Figure 10–6). The outer end of the disc is beveled (to obtain an angle) and is where the target is located. The anode uses an induction motor consisting of a rotor and stator to rotate (spin) the disc. Most rotating anode tubes identify the rate of anode rotation as 3300 revolutions per

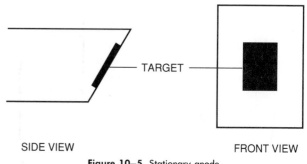

Figure 10–5. Stationary anode.

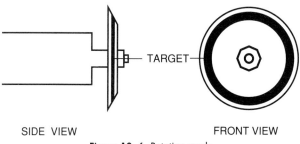

SIDE VIEW   FRONT VIEW

Figure 10-6. Rotating anode.

minute (rpm). However, there is some slippage in the motor, so in practice an anode rotates at between 3000 and 3300 rpm. Special rotating x-ray tubes have a rating of 10,000 rpm.

The rotating anode spins, causing the electrons striking the target to be spread over a large area called the target track. The target track length depends on the speed at which the anode rotates. The more revolutions per minute, the longer the target track is. Long target tracks dissipate the heat over a greater area. This enables the operator to use a higher kilovolt peak, higher milliamperage, or a longer time of operation with anodes having long target tracks.

The amount of load on the focal spot depends on the dimensions of the filament and the diameter of the disc. The smaller the filament is, the more load is on the focal spot. Increasing the diameter of the anode disc increases the circumference. Large diameter discs have longer circumferences, decreasing the load on the focal spot.

Recall that the disc is attached to the motor by a stem. The stem should be short to avoid putting a strain on the motor. The stem is made of molybdenum, which has a high melting point and low thermal conductivity. This is desirable because it limits the amount of heat conducted by the stem to the rotor. This decrease in heat protects the motor and bearings from being burned out.

TUBE ASSEMBLY

As mentioned above, most of the energy generated during the production of x-rays is in the form of heat. Too much heat can destroy the x-ray tube. The oil in the tube assembly helps to cool the x-ray tube. It also helps to protect against spark over,

which may occur when high voltages are applied to the anode and cathode.

When high speed electrons strike the target of the anode, radiation is produced in all directions. The metal tube shield is useful in absorbing stray radiation from the target.

VACUUM GLASS

The anode and cathode are sealed in a vacuum glass envelope. The glass is designed to withstand high temperatures. The vacuum is necessary to allow the electrons to travel from the cathode to the anode uninterrupted. If particles are located in the tube, the electrons interact with them, decreasing the efficiency and life of the tube.

TYPES OF RADIATION PRODUCED AT THE ANODE

Two types of radiation are produced at the anode: Bremsstrahlung and characteristic. Bremsstrahlung is often referred to as braking radiation (from the German translation). Bremsstrahlung radiation occurs when an electron traveling from the cathode enters an atom of the target. The nucleus of the atom attracts the incoming electron and slows (decelerates, or brakes) it. The slowing of the electron produces energy in the form of radiation. One electron usually interacts with several different atoms. Each time the electron interacts, it loses some energy. This results in the production of radiation of different energy levels (a heterogeneous beam).

Characteristic radiation occurs when the electron traveling from the cathode hits and dislodges an inner shell electron (usually an electron in the K or the L shell). The process of characteristic radiation begins with the removal of an inner electron from a target atom, creating a hole, or vacancy, in the shell level where the electron was removed. This hole causes the atom to become unstable (the atom is ionized). To stabilize the atom, an electron from an outer shell moves to fill the hole created by the missing electron. Consequently, another hole is created in the shell from which the electron moved. The new hole is filled by an electron from another shell. This process of filling holes continues until all holes are filled and the atom becomes stable. Every time an electron moves, energy is converted to radiation. The sum of the energy from all electron movement represents the characteristic radiation. The quality of radiation energy emitted from an element is specific to that element and is measured in electron volts. The characteristic radiation of tungsten is about 70 kV. Characteristic radiation is useful when the K shell electron is removed. Electrons removed in shells other than the K shell are too weak to be useful.

HEAT UNITS

About 1% of the energy at the anode is radiation. The remaining 99% is primarily heat. Although the anode is constructed of material with a high melting point, there is a limit as to the amount of heat the anode can experience before it begins to deteriorate.

Knowing the amount of heat produced at the anode is important. Too much heat can create a variety of problems. Common problems caused by excessive heat are melting the target (Figure 10–7B and D), pitting the target (Figure 10–7C), both melting and pitting the target (Figure 10–7E) overheating the bearings or eroding the rotor and anode. A normal target appears as a smooth band (Figure 10–7A).

To prevent overheating that damages the anode, the manufacturer's recommendations regarding preheating the anode should be followed. The preheating process is often referred to as warming up the x-ray tube. It generally involves taking three exposures at 5–10 second intervals at relatively low technique variables, e.g., 200 mA, 2 seconds, 70 kVp.

The heat at the anode is measured in heat units (HU). It is possible to calculate the amount of heat units per single exposure. On single phase machines, this is achieved by multiplying the kilovoltage and milliampere-seconds. Mathematically this is

$$HU = kVp \times mA \times s$$

In six pulse, three phase equipment, the heat units are calculated by multiplying the kilovoltage by the milliampere-seconds and a factor of 1.35, or

$$HU = kVp \times mA \times s \times 1.35$$

The heat unit value for 12 pulse, three phase equipment is kilovoltage times milliampere-seconds and a factor of 1.41, or

$$HU = kVp \times mA \times s \times 1.41$$

On the basis of the previous formulas it can be demonstrated that, relative to heat units, it is better to use a higher kilovoltage than milliamperage. For example, a technique setting of 200 mA, 0.10 second and 85 kVp produces 1700 HU. Using the 15% rule (increase the kilovoltage by 15% and cut the milliampere-seconds by 50%), comparable technique variables are 98 kVp, 100 mA and 0.10 second for a heat unit value of 980 HU. Both techniques produce diagnostic quality film, however, the latter technique results in less heat units to the anode.

METHODS OF PLOTTING HEAT PRODUCTION

X-ray tube manufacturers provide charts to demonstrate the relationship of heat to the x-ray tube.

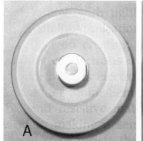 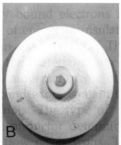 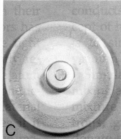 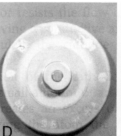 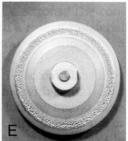

Figure 10–7. Heat damage to anode. *A*, Normal anode; *B*, stationary melt; *C*, surface etching (heavy load); *D*, slow running or multiple melt; *E*, melt over etching with continued overload.

These charts differ from one x-ray tube to another. The basic factors determining the heat rating are type of rectification, waveform (single or three phase), focal spot size and exposure time. In general, heat units are increased with more sophisticated rectification, three phase equipment, a small focal spot size and long exposure times. Three types of charts illustrate the amount of heat produced:
1. Single exposure tube rating chart
2. Multiple exposure tube rating chart
3. Anode heat storage capacity chart.

The single exposure chart is useful for any type of radiography. The multiple exposure graph is most useful for rapid serial filming, e.g., angiography. The anode storage capacity chart is used for long exposures, e.g., fluoroscopy.

SINGLE EXPOSURE TUBE RATING CHART

The single exposure tube rating chart, often referred to as the tube rating chart, is used to determine the amount of heat units generated for a single exposure. The chart plots milliamperage, exposure time and kilovoltage. Two methods are used to plot these factors. One method is to design the chart so that the x axis (horizontal line) represents the exposure time, the y axis (vertical line) is the kilovoltage and the plotted value is the milliamperage (Figure 10–8A). In the second method, the

chart has the exposure time on the x axis, the milliamperage on the y axis and the plotted value is the kilovoltage (Figure 10–8B). Both chart designs are able to determine safe exposure factors. Regardless of the chart design, the process for using the chart is the same.

Two common ways to use the tube rating chart are determining the maximum technical factor values and checking if the set technique is safe. In the former method, the user must know the milliamperage and kilovoltage to be used and set the exposure time according to the chart. The second method allows the operator to set all technique values and check the tube rating chart to make sure the values are safe.

In the first method, determining the maximum safe exposure level, two perpendicular lines are drawn on the graph. To determine the location of the first line, the y axis factor (kilovoltage or milliamperage depending on the chart design) to be used is located. A horizontal line 90 degrees to the y axis is extended to the plotted value on the chart (kilovoltage or milliamperage depending on the chart design). Then a perpendicular line is extended downward to the x axis; this is the exposure time (Figure 10–9). Exposure factors of lower value than the time identified by the line intersecting the x axis are safe.

To determine if a given technique is safe, again two lines are drawn on the chart. To determine the location of the first line, the y axis factor (kilovoltage

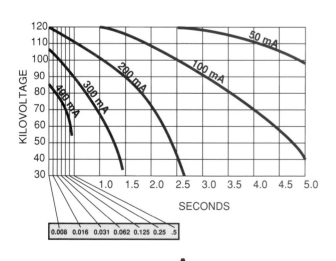

A

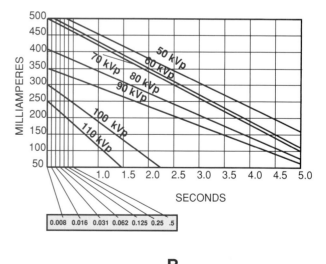

B

Figure 10–8. Single exposure tube rating charts. A, Plotted value is milliamperage. B, Plotted value is kilovoltage.

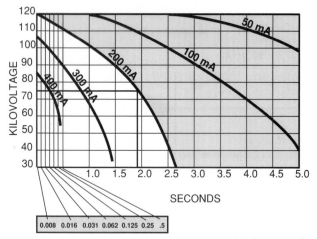

Figure 10–9. Determining maximum exposure value. Any factor outside the computed lines (shaded area) is unsafe.

or milliamperage depending on the chart design) to be used is located. A horizontal line 90 degrees to the *y* axis is extended to the point on the chart representing the plotted value to be used (kilovoltage or milliamperage depending on the chart design). Then a perpendicular line is extended downward to the *x* axis; this is the exposure time (Figure 10–10). If the time set is greater than the computed time, the technique is unsafe and must be adjusted.

MULTIPLE EXPOSURE CHART

Multiple exposures build up heat faster than the tube can dissipate it (cool). Consequently, there is a limit as to how many multiple exposures can be performed. The multiple exposure chart (Figure 10–11) is used to determine the safe number of exposures. Multiple exposures are most often used in any type of serial filming, e.g., cine radiography.

The multiple exposure chart plots heat units (usually on the *y* axis), number of exposures per second (curve on the graph) and the total number of exposures (*x* axis). To determine the maximum number of exposures, the technique variables for each exposure and number of exposures per second must be known. The technical factors per exposure are used to calculate heat units (see under Heat Units). For example, if the technical factors of a three phase, six pulse machine are 85 kVp, 800 mA and 0.05 second, the heat units measurement is 4590 HU, or $85 \times 800 \times 0.05 \times 1.35 = 4590$.

To determine the maximum number of exposures at a rate of three films per second for the previous example of 4590 HU, locate the heat units on the *y* axis. Draw a perpendicular line to the curve representing three films per second. To locate the maximum number of safe exposures, extend a line to the *x* axis from the curve (Figure 10–12).

TECHNIQUE: 70 kVp, 300 mA, 0.5 sec.

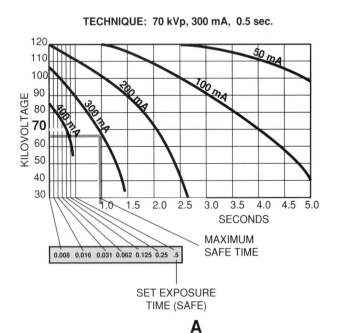

A

TECHNIQUE: 70 kVp, 300 mA, 1.5 sec.

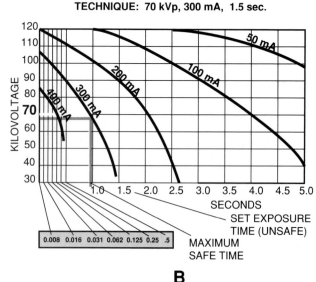

B

Figure 10–10. Determining if a given technique is safe. A, Graph of safe technique. B, Unsafe technique because the exposure time selected is greater than the maximum exposure time allowed.

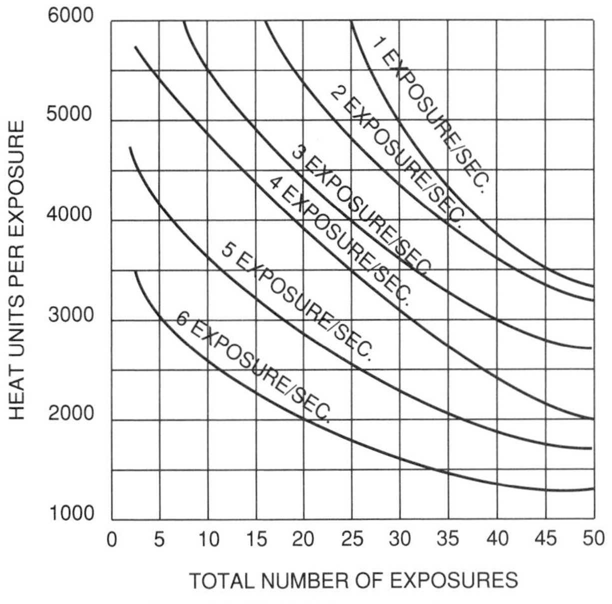

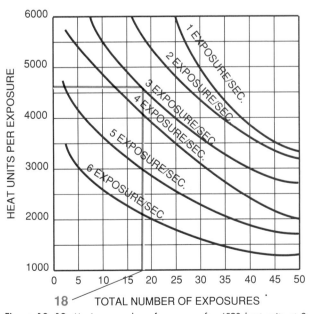

Figure 10–11. Multiple exposure chart.

The multiple exposure chart refers to only the maximum number of safe exposures. It does not address the safety of the individual exposure. To ensure that the technique values are safe for the individual exposure, the operator must also refer to the single exposure chart.

Figure 10–12. Maximum number of exposures for 4590 heat units at 3 exposures per second.

ANODE HEAT STORAGE CAPACITY CHART

The anode heat storage capacity chart (Figure 10–13) demonstrates the storage capacity of the anode and its cooling time. Chart factors include the anode capacity measured in heat units (y axis), time in minutes (x axis), the plotted values relative to the length of time for the anode to cool and the input (exposure) heat units per second plotted values. The anode heat storage chart is useful in determining the anode limits with long exposures, e.g., fluoroscopy.

To determine the input heat units, the kilovoltage, milliamperage and numerical factor, when applicable, are multiplied. For example, the input heat units of fluoroscopy performed at 3 mA, 90 kV on a three phase, six pulse machine is approximately 365 HU. The heat capacity of the anode is deter-

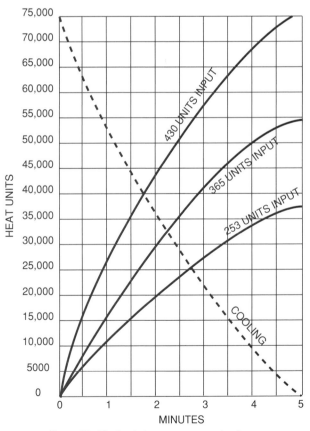

Figure 10–13. Anode heat storage capacity chart.

mined by correlating the time with the input heat units (y axis). This is achieved by drawing a perpendicular line from the time to the input heat units curve and extending another perpendicular line to the y axis. Where the line intersects the y axis is the anode heat storage capacity. For example, if the rate of the previous technique is 4 minutes, the anode chart indicates that the anode heat storage capacity is approximately 50,000 HU (Figure 10–14). In this example, if spot films, millimeter films, cineradiographic films, etc. were taken during the 4 minutes, the heat units for all exposures (kilovolts times milliampere-seconds times numerical factor) are added to the 50,000 anode heat units obtained during fluoroscopy. In Figure 10–14, the maximum anode heat capacity is 75,000 HU. Thus, the maximum heat unit amount reserved for filming, in the previous example is 25,000 HU, or 75,000 − 50,000 = 25,000.

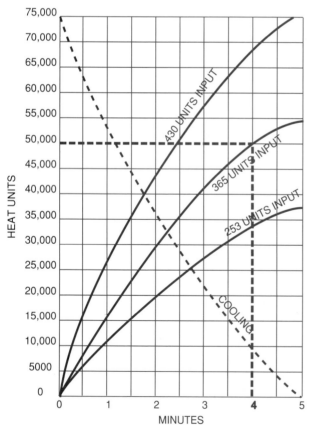

Figure 10–14. Anode heat units for 4 minutes of fluoroscopy at an input of 365 heat units.

FILTERS

The x-ray tube produces radiation in all directions. Much of the radiation is of low energy. This low energy radiation is harmful to humans because it is readily absorbed by the body. Filters are used to decrease the amount of low energy radiation. In diagnostic radiology, filtration is usually measured in equivalent millimeter thickness of aluminum.

There are two ways low level radiation is filtered: inherent filtration and added filtration. As the name indicates, inherent filtration is intrinsic to the x-ray tube. It is built into the tube during manufacturing. The glass envelope, oil, port and tube housing account for the amount of inherent radiation. Generally, inherent radiation is equivalent to 0.5 mm of aluminum.

Added filtration is the filtration added by the operator. Added filtration is usually attached to the end of the collimator located below the port of the x-ray tube. It is used to protect the patient from low level radiation and increase the beam quality (the beam becomes "harder" because of more high energy photons). The amount of added filtration depends on the quality of radiation. Table 10–1 represents the U.S. Department of Health and Human Services recommendation for aluminum filtration for various kilovoltages.

The total amount of filtration is the sum of the inherent and added filtration. For example, if the inherent filtration is 0.5 mm of aluminum and the added is 1.5 mm of aluminum, the total filtration is 2.0 mm of aluminum, or 0.5 + 1.5 = 2.

Filters are constructed in different shapes. Most diagnostic filters are thin flat sheets of aluminum

Table 10–1. U.S. DEPARTMENT OF HEALTH AND HUMAN SERVICES FILTRATION RECOMMENDATION

Kilovoltage	Al Thickness (mm)
40	0.4
50	1.2
60	1.3
70	1.5
80	2.3
90	2.5
100	2.7
110	3.0
120	3.2

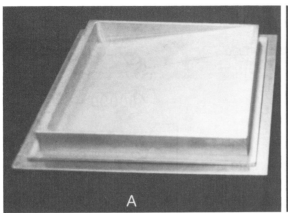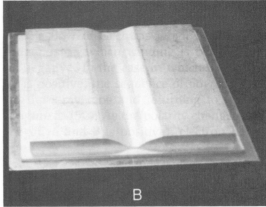

Figure 10–15. *A*, Wedge filter. *B*, Trough filter.

or plastic made to specific aluminum equivalent absorption levels. Two other, less common types of added filters are the wedge and the trough (Figure 10–15). The objective of these filters is to produce a more uniform photographic image.

The wedge filter is thick at one end and thin at the opposite end. It is used for body parts that increase in thickness, e.g., the foot. The thick part of the filter is placed over the thin portion of the anatomical part. For example, if the wedge filter is used for the foot, the thick portion of the filter is placed over the toes.

The trough filter is constructed so the sides or edges of the filter are thicker than the center. It is used for body parts where the center absorbs more radiation than the sides, e.g., the chest. The center of the filter is positioned over the area that absorbs the most radiation. For example, for the chest, the center part of the filter is located over the spine.

LABORATORY EXPERIENCE

Concepts in Medical Radiographic Imaging: Laboratory Manual has two laboratories related to this chapter: Laboratories 16, Focal Spot Size, and 17, Heel Effect.

The Focal Spot Size laboratory allows the investigator to determine the size and shape of the effective focal spot size. The laboratory provides the experimenter with the choice of using a commercial product to test for focal spot size, e.g., pinhole camera and test star pattern, or a simple inexpensive homemade pinhole.

The Heel Effect laboratory is designed to demonstrate the intensity difference of the x-ray beam. This laboratory is performed at two different SIDs to illustrate the decreasing influence of the heel effect at longer SIDs.

Bibliography

Ball, JL and Moore, AD. Essential physics for radiographers (2nd edition). Boston: Blackwell Scientific Publications, 1986.

Bushong, SC. Radiologic science for technologists (4th edition). St. Louis: Mosby, 1988.

Chesney, DN and Chesney, MO. X-ray equipment for student radiographers (3rd edition). Boston: Blackwell Scientific Publications, 1984.

Cullinan, JE and Cullinan, AM. Illustrated guide to x-ray technics (2nd edition). New York: Lippincott, 1980.

Curry, TS, Dowdey, JE and Murry, RC. Christensen's introduction to the physics of diagnostic radiology (3rd edition). Philadelphia: Lea & Febiger, 1984.

Curry, TS, Dowdey, JE and Murry, RC. Christensen's physics of diagnostic radiology (4th edition). Philadelphia: Lea & Febiger, 1990.

Dietz, K. The x-ray tube in diagnostic applications. West Germany: Siemens. (Order number MR A 5/1242.121.)

Eastman Kodak Company. Fundamentals of radiography (11th edition). Rochester, NY: Eastman Kodak Company, 1968.

Eastman Kodak Company. Fundamentals of radiography (12th edition). Rochester, NY: Eastman Kodak Company, 1980. (Publication number M1–18.)

Graham, BJ and Thomas, WN. An introduction to physics for radiologic technologists. Philadelphia: Saunders, 1975.

Hendee, WR, Chaney, EL and Rossi, RP. Radiologic physics, equipment and quality control. Chicago: Year Book Medical, 1976.

Hiss, SS. Understanding radiography. Springfield, IL: Thomas, 1980.

Kelsey, CA. Essentials of radiology physics. St. Louis: Warren H. Green, 1985.

Oman, RM. An introduction to radiologic science. New York: McGraw-Hill, 1975.

Selman, J. The fundamentals of x-ray and radium physics (7th edition). Springfield, IL: Thomas, 1985.

Sprawls, P. Principles of radiography for technologists. Rockville, MD: Aspen, 1990.

United States Department of Health and Human Resources. Regulations for the administration and enforcement of the radiation control for health and safety act of 1968 FDA 88-8035 (supersedes HEW publication FDA 90–8035). Rockville, MD: U.S. Government Printing Office, April 1988.

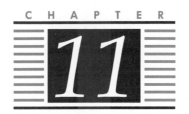

CHAPTER

11

KILOVOLTAGE AND

QUALITY CONTROL

INTRODUCTION

Recall that one factor needed to produce electricity is voltage (see Chapter 5, Electrodynamics). A volt (V) is the amount of force needed to move 1 ampere (A) of current through 1 ohm (Ω) of resistance. In the x-ray circuit, high voltage is used to produce the current flow needed for the production of x-rays (refer to Chapter 10, Production of X-rays). The technologist determines the amount of voltage used during an exposure by adjusting the kilovoltage selector. This positions a tap on the autotransformer to obtain the desired kilovoltage.

This chapter discusses the effects of kilovoltage on the x-ray beam, the patient and the film. Also presented is a summary of quality control tests that may be performed to check kilovoltage output. Before reading this chapter, a review of Chapters 5 and 10 is recommended.

PEAK AND EFFECTIVE KILOVOLTAGES

Electricity entering the x-ray unit travels in a sine wave pattern (see Chapter 5, Electrodynamics). A sine wave may be graphed by plotting the sine of the angle a conductor makes with the magnetic field to the kilovoltage produced (Figure 11–1). The horizontal axis of the graph represents the conductor angle and the vertical axis is kilovoltage. As can be seen in Figure 11–1, the peak, or maximum, voltage

occurs when the angle of the conductor is at 90 and 270 degrees. Because the amount of voltage produced between 0 and 360 degrees varies significantly, to determine the effective value of the kilovoltage, the root-mean-square (RMS) value (the mathematical process used to derive the RMS is beyond the scope of this text) is used. To obtain the effective value, the RMS is multiplied by the peak kilovoltage. For a single phase x-ray machine, the RMS is approximately 0.707. Thus, the RMS for 100 kV is about 70 kV, or 0.707 × 100 = 70. This means that if a technologist selects a 100 kV setting, the effective value of the kilovoltage produced is about 70 kV.

X-RAY BEAM QUALITY

The energy of the x-ray photons depends on the force with which the electrons strike the target. The

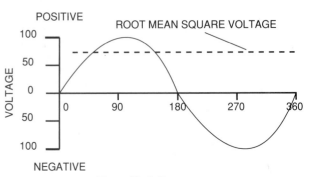

Figure 11–1. Sine wave.

faster the electrons move from the cathode to the anode, the greater is the electron force striking the target. The primary factor regulating the speed of electrons is kilovoltage. As kilovoltage increases, electron speed and photon energy increase.

During an exposure, the kilovoltage value varies relative to the sine wave. Consequently, an x-ray beam contains a variety of photon energies. An x-ray beam consisting of several photon energies is called heterogeneous. Conversely, an x-ray beam containing photons of the same energy is called homogeneous. To illustrate the effect of photon energy on the quality of the x-ray beam, the following discussion refers to a homogeneous x-ray beam.

The quality of an x-ray beam is its ability to penetrate an object. The better the x-ray beam's ability to penetrate an object, the better is the beam quality. The beam's ability to penetrate an object is determined primarily by photon energy. High energy photons have greater penetration than low energy photons. Photon energy is expressed mathematically as $E = h\nu$, where E is the photon energy, h is Planck's constant and ν is the frequency of x-rays measured in hertz (cycles per second). Because h is a constant, in the formula energy is directly proportional to the frequency. In other words, as the frequency increases (becomes higher), there is a corresponding increase in the energy of the photon or beam quality.

The relationship of frequency and x-ray wavelength may also be expressed mathematically. The formula used to express the relationship is $c = \lambda\nu$, where c is the speed of x-rays, λ is the wavelength and ν is the frequency. The speed of x-rays is a constant at 186,000 miles per second, or 3×10^{-10} cm per second (3×10^{-8} m per second). Because the speed of x-rays is constant, the relationship of the wavelength and frequency is inversely proportional, or as the frequency increases, the wavelength decreases (becomes shorter).

In summary,
1. The higher the frequency, the higher the photon energy.
2. The greater the energy, the better the penetration ability and beam quality.
3. The higher the frequency, the shorter the wavelength.

As mentioned above, kilovoltage regulates photon energy. Consequently, the relationship of kilovoltage to frequency and wavelength is the same as the relationship of photon energy to frequency

and wavelength. Thus, as kilovoltage increases, the x-ray beam frequency increases and the wavelength becomes shorter. High frequency, short wavelength x-ray photons have more penetrating power than low frequency, long wavelengths (Figure 11–2). High frequency, short wavelength x-ray photons are produced with high kilovoltage. Thus, high kilovoltage has more penetrating power than low kilovoltage.

HALF-VALUE LAYER

The penetrating power of an x-ray beam is commonly expressed in terms of half-value layer (HVL).

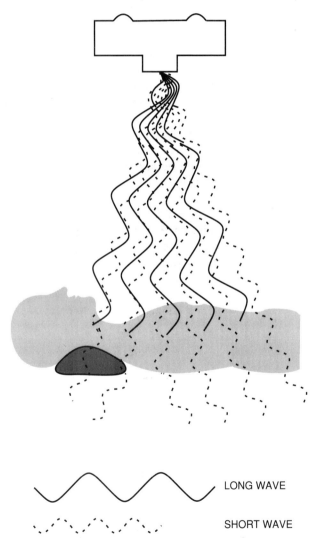

LONG WAVE

SHORT WAVE

Figure 11–2. High frequency, short wavelength photons have more penetrating power than low frequency, long wavelength photons.

The HVL is the amount of thickness of an absorbing material (in diagnostic radiology, the material is aluminum) needed to reduce the x-ray beam intensity to one-half of its original value.

In conventional radiography, knowing the HVL provides information about the absorption rate in the body. This is because the rate at which aluminum and calcium absorb x-rays (absorption coefficient) is almost equal. Thus, if a beam had an HVL of 8 mm of aluminum, an 8 mm bone has the same effect (absorption rate) on the beam as the aluminum. Also, because the ratio of tissue to bone is roughly 5:1, to obtain a similar absorption in tissue and bone necessitates five times the amount of tissue.

CONTRAST

Contrast is the difference between two densities on a radiograph. There are at least three kinds of contrast in radiology (Chapter 27, Photographic Image Quality contains more specific information on contrast). They are subject, film and radiographic. Subject contrast refers to the ability of an object to absorb radiation. Film contrast is inherent in the film and is expressed by the sensitometric curve (refer to Chapter 21, Sensitometry and Processor Quality Control). Radiographic contrast refers to the variety of densities found in the image and is influenced by both subject and film contrast. Kilovoltage is most influential on subject contrast.

A penetrometer (stepwedge) is often used to demonstrate contrast. A penetrometer is usually made of aluminum and is constructed in varying thicknesses (steps). The penetrometer is thin at one end and increases in thickness as one moves to the opposite end (Figure 11–3A). As an x-ray beam enters the penetrometer, the least amount of radiation is absorbed at the thin end. The rate of absorption increases as the thickness of the penetrometer increases. The resulting radiographic penetrometer image is darkest under the thinnest part of the penetrometer and becomes lighter as the thickness of the penetrometer increases (Figure 11–3B). The number of steps visualized on the radiograph de-

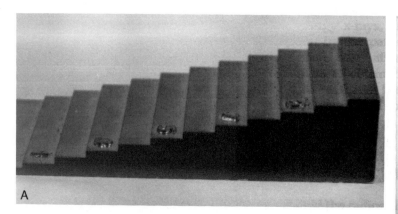

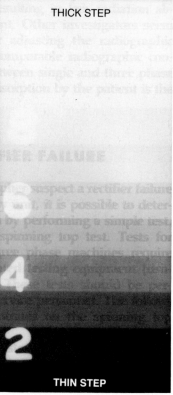

Figure 11–3. A, Aluminum penetrometer. B, Resulting radiograph.

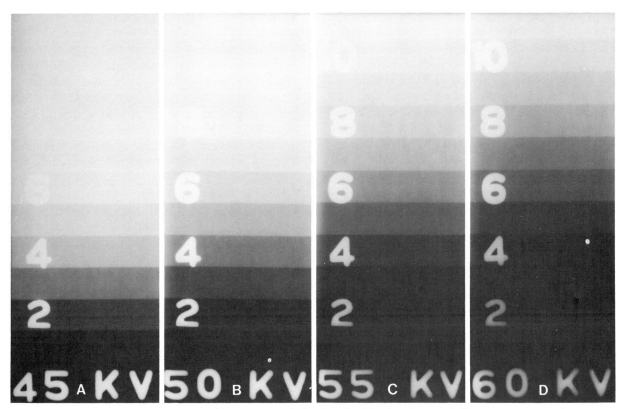

Figure 11–4. In A through D, contrast decreases (more shades of gray) as kilovoltage increases (milliamperage was constant).

pends on the energy of the x-ray beam. The higher the energy is, the more steps penetrated. The steps imaged are often referred to as a scale.

Short scale contrast has few penetrometer steps imaged (few shades of gray). Conversely, long scale contrast has many steps visualized (many shades of gray). Short scale contrast is obtained using low kilovoltage, whereas a long scale is obtained with high kilovoltage. A short scale is referred to as high contrast. Long scale contrast is said to be low contrast. High kilovoltage creates low contrast (Figure 11–4). A decrease in contrast (going from a short scale of contrast to long scale) is demonstrated by an image with less density difference between steps (more grays). Conversely, low kilovoltage results in high contrast (there is a greater difference between densities, less grays).

The terms high contrast and low contrast are relative to what is compared. For example, suppose two sets of radiographs are taken. In each set, all factors are constant except kilovoltage. In set A, radiograph 1 is taken at 60 kV and radiograph 2 is exposed at 80 kV. In set B, radiograph 1 is exposed at 80 kV and radiograph 2 is taken at 100 kV. In set A, radiograph 2 (80 kV) has low contrast when compared with that of radiograph 1 (60 kV). However, in set B, radiograph 1 (80 kV) contains a high contrast when compared with that of radiograph 2 (100 kV). Although contrast is relative, it is generally agreed that radiographs taken below 70 kV are considered high contrast. Low contrast radiographs are usually reserved for exposures greater than 95 kV. Table 11–1 is a summary of the relationship of kilovoltage and contrast.

Table 11–1. RELATIONSHIP OF KILOVOLTAGE AND CONTRAST

Kilovoltage	Scale	Contrast	Gray Shades
Low (≤70)	Short	High	Few
High (≥95)	Long	Low	Many

In practice, high contrast radiographs are usually preferred. Low contrast radiographs often contain too many shades of gray, which interferes with the ability to distinguish one object from another. However, the object being imaged must be considered when determining the level of contrast desired. For example, it is most desirable to use low kilovoltage on a plain radiograph of the abdomen. This results in a high contrast film. However, if the abdomen is imaged with barium in the colon, a high kilovoltage (low contrast film) is needed to image the interior aspect of the colon. The use of high or low kilovoltage is best learned during the practical experience of the technologist.

EXPOSURE LATITUDE

Exposure latitude refers to the range of technical factors that may be employed to obtain a diagnostic radiograph. A diagnostic radiograph contains the correct amount of penetration, density and contrast to demonstrate the object(s) of interest. Kilovoltage is one of the technical factors employed in attaining a diagnostic radiograph. Assuming that all other factors remain the same, a range of kilovoltages may be employed to obtain an acceptable radiograph.

The minimum to maximum (latitude) kilovoltage range is small with low kilovoltage (70 kV or less) and large when high kilovoltage is employed. The amount of kilovoltage latitude is related to contrast. Latitude and contrast are reciprocal values, i.e., as contrast increases (short scale), latitude decreases. For example, radiographs obtained using low kilovoltages have high contrast (few shades of gray). Consequently, any change in kilovoltage has a substantial effect on the amount of images produced on the radiograph. Conversely, high kilovoltage has many shades of gray. Thus, a significant change in kilovoltage is needed for an observable image change on the radiograph. The actual range limits vary with the kilovoltage quantity selected by the technologist. The lower the kilovoltage setting, the less the minimum to maximum limit (latitude). It is generally agreed that kilovoltages below 70 kV have a range of about plus or minus 5 kV. A change of at least 10 kV is needed to have an observable change when employing 100 kV or more.

SCATTER AND PATIENT DOSE

Scatter radiation is the secondary radiation created when the x-ray beam interacts with matter. There are several forms of scatter radiation. In diagnostic radiology, the two forms of radiation interaction of concern are photoelectric and Compton effects. An in-depth discussion of these interactions is beyond the scope of this text. However, a brief summary is appropriate to help understand scatter.

Chapter 10, Production of X-rays, discusses characteristic radiation. Recall that characteristic radiation occurs at the anode and is an interaction between electrons traveling from the cathode and atoms in the target (refer to Chapter 10). The photoelectric effect is the same as characteristic radiation. The difference between characteristic and photoelectric radiation is in the type of energy interacting with the target atom. In the x-ray tube, electrons interact with the target atoms. The photoelectron effect uses photons to interact with matter.

The photoelectric effect occurs when an incoming (incident) x-ray photon hits and dislodges an inner shell electron (usually an electron in the K or the L shell). The result is an absorption of the photon energy, an emission of energy from the atom in the form of a photoelectron and the emission of radiation (Figure 11–5A). The incident photon energy is used (absorbed) to remove the electron. When the electron is removed from the atom, there is a hole, or vacancy, in the shell level where the electron was removed. This hole causes the atom to become unstable (the atom is ionized). To stabilize the atom, an electron from an outer shell moves to fill the hole created by the missing electron. Consequently, another hole is created in the shell from which the electron moved. The new hole is filled by an electron from another shell. This process of filling holes continues until all holes are filled and the atom becomes stable. The movement of electrons results in energy change in the form of radiation (scatter radiation). If an electron from the K shell is emitted, the radiation energy emitted has a wavelength that is characteristic of that atom. The photoelectric effect is prevalent in the x-ray beam at kilovoltages of 70 kV or less. It is also more likely to occur in atoms of low atomic number, e.g., in soft tissue.

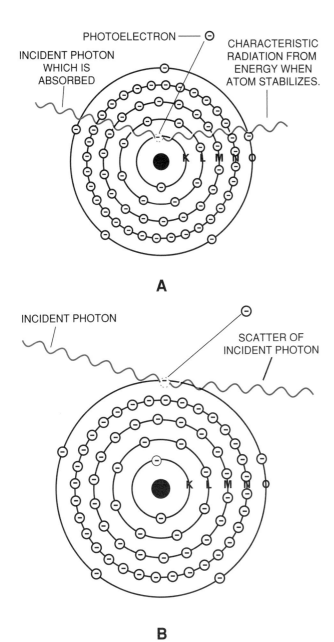

Figure 11–5. A, Photoelectric effect. B, Compton interaction.

Compton interaction occurs when an incident photon dislodges an electron in the outer shell of an atom. The incident photon loses some energy when dislodging the electron and is scattered in a different direction (Figure 11–5B). The scatter of the incident photon is called scatter radiation. The radiation occurring when the electron hole is filled is extremely low and is negligible relative to effects experienced in conventional radiology. In diagnostic radiology, at 80 kV and above, Compton interaction occurs at a greater percentage than does photoelectric interaction. At approximately 180 kV, Compton becomes the predominant type of radiation interaction.

As stated above, the photoelectric effect occurs at the lower kilovoltage range. Recall that low kilovoltage results in less penetration of an object than high kilovoltage. Consequently, the scatter created by the photoelectric effect is usually absorbed in the body. Conversely, the Compton effect occurs at a higher percentage than does the photoelectric effect at 80 kV and above. Because higher kilovoltage is more penetrating, the scatter radiation created by Compton interaction is more apt to strike the film. The scatter exposing the film is called fog. All radiographs contain some amount of scatter. However, if there is more scatter radiation than primary remnant radiation exposing the film, the fog becomes significant and may interfere in the film's diagnostic usefulness.

The decision to employ a high or low kilovoltage has a trade off effect. For example, using high kilovoltage reduces the amount of radiation dosage to the patient but increases the amount of fog on the film and decreases contrast. Conversely, low kilovoltage increases the amount of radiation dosage to the patient but limits fog and increases contrast. Consequently, when determining what kilovoltage to use, one must determine if the need for a high quality radiograph exceeds the effect on patient dose.

TECHNIQUE CHARTS

It is important for a technologist to obtain a diagnostic film on the first exposure. Repeated filming increases the amount of radiation absorption by the patient. One method to limit repeated filming is for the technologist to use a technique chart.

A technique chart allows the technologist to determine the exposure values for a specific examination. The chart contains information on the milliamperage, time, kilovoltage and patient thickness (Figure 11–6). The two types of technique charts available are the variable kilovoltage method and the fixed kilovoltage technique chart.

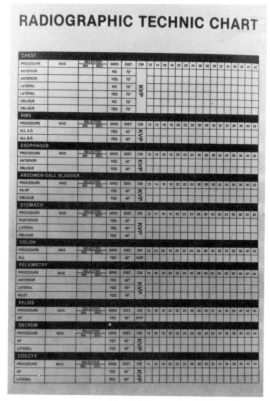

Figure 11-6. An example of a variable technique chart.

In the variable kilovoltage chart, the milliampere-seconds remain constant while the kilovoltage increases 2 kV for every 1 cm increase in object thickness. The kilovoltage is usually determined by multiplying the size of the object by 2 and adding 30 kV (20 kV is added for three phase equipment). For example, if an adult abdomen measures 20 cm, the kilovoltage is 70 kV, or 20 (2) + 30 = 70. A change of 2 kV occurs for each respective 1 cm change in object thickness. In other words, in the previous example of the abdomen, if the patient measured 19 cm, the kilovoltage employed would be 68 kV, or 70 − 2 = 68. An increased abdomen thickness of 1 cm results in a 72 kV exposure, or 70 + 2 = 72.

The second type of technique chart uses fixed kilovoltage. In this method, the kilovoltage remains constant and the milliampere-seconds are altered. The optimum kilovoltage is determined by the formula described for variable kilovoltage and by the radiologist's preference. In deciding the kilovoltage, the radiologist first determines the starting kilovolt-

age from the formula and then assesses the effect of the calculated kilovoltage, e.g., on contrast and patient dose. The kilovoltage is changed if the radiologist decides that there is a need to produce an image of different quality, e.g., contrast, or alter the radiation dose to the patient.

The variable kilovoltage method tends to use lower kilovoltages than the fixed chart. Consequently, the corresponding radiograph has a higher contrast than those obtained using values from the fixed kilovoltage chart. Unfortunately, the variable chart tends to result in an increase in the amount of radiation absorption by the patient. Conversely, the fixed chart usually has a lower patient dose and a lower contrast film.

The use of technique charts is not without problems. One problem is ensuring that the technologist is aware of the patient's condition and adjusts the technique accordingly, e.g., reduces the exposure values when obtaining a chest x-ray film for a person with emphysema. Another problem is that to obtain radiographs of a consistent quality, all technologists must measure body parts in the same location, e.g., measure the chest at midsternum. Unfortunately, technologists tend to be inconsistent where body parts are measured. The most troublesome problem is that, as technologists gain experience in performing the same examinations, they tend to set the exposure values without referring to the technique chart. The more success technologists have in predicting the correct technique, the less apt they are to measure a patient and employ a technique chart. All the problems mentioned introduce the potential for an increase in repeated radiographs. To help eliminate repeated filming, most imaging departments use automatic exposure timers.

The use of automatic timers eliminates the need for technique charts. Most automatic timers are designed to operate on the fixed kilovoltage method. Refer to Chapter 9, X-ray Timers and Quality Control, for a more in-depth discussion of automatic timing devices.

TECHNIQUE COMPENSATION

A diagnostic radiograph of an object may be produced using any one of several different exposure settings. The primary difference among the various techniques is in the amount of radiation absorption by the patient and in the level of contrast or density imaged.

In practice, situations arise (e.g., a patient is unable to hold his/her breath) when it is not practical to employ the technique requested by the radiology department administration. Thus, the technologist must alter the exposure values according to the circumstances. If the decision is to adjust the kilovoltage, a need exists to determine the new milliampere-seconds setting to employ (assuming all other factors, e.g., source-object distance, remain the same). This may be accomplished by using the 13% and 15% rules.

The 13% rule states that, to maintain a diagnostic radiograph, it is possible to decrease the kilovoltage by 13% and double the milliampere-seconds. When increasing the kilovoltage, the 15% rule is applied. This rule states that, to obtain a radiograph of diagnostic quality, kilovoltage is increased by 15% and the milliampere-seconds are halved. The following are examples of the 13% and 15% rules, respectively. In the first example, 80 mAs at 70 kV is employed for an original radiograph. To obtain roughly the same diagnostic quality using a lower kilovoltage, decrease the kilovoltage by 13% and double the milliampere-seconds. This results in a technique setting of approximately 61 kV and 160 mAs, or the kilovoltage calculation is

$$70 \ (0.13) = 9.1$$

$$70 - 9 = 61 \ kv$$

and the milliampere-seconds calculation is

$$80 \ (2) = 160 \ mAs$$

For the second example, assume the original technique is 61 kV at 160 mAs. The radiograph is repeated at a higher kilovoltage. Approximately the same diagnostic quality is obtained by increasing the kilovoltage by 15% and decreasing the milliampere-seconds by one-half. Thus, the resulting technique setting is 70 kV at 80 mAs, or the kilovoltage calculation is

$$61 \ (0.15) = 9.1$$

$$61 + 9 = 70 \ kV$$

and the milliampere-seconds calculation is

$$160/2 = 80 \ mAs$$

Notice that the resulting technique variables in the second example are the same as those in the original technique in the first example.

QUALITY CONTROL TESTS

A variety of instruments test kilovoltage accuracy. They may be divided into two groups: the invasive method and the noninvasive procedures. The invasive method of checking kilovoltage output involves internal measurements of the equipment and requires a qualified service person. This type of testing is not something a technologist is apt to perform and is beyond the scope of this text. However, noninvasive procedures employ instruments that a technologist can easily operate and interpret results from. Thus, this text discusses three types of noninvasive testing devices for kilovoltage. They are a penetrometer, a Wisconsin cassette and a digital kilovoltage meter.

PENETROMETER TEST

Of the three types of tests, the penetrometer procedure is the least accurate. This test consists of checking the reliability of kilovoltage. Reliability refers to how consistent the kilovoltage output is with multiple exposures, using a fixed kilovoltage for given milliampere-seconds (with different milliampere and time stations). To perform the test, the kilovoltage level to be assessed is selected. Then several exposures (the number of exposures depends on the equipment design) are made using the same kilovoltage and milliampere-seconds, but varying the milliampere and time factors. A sufficient amount of radiation is employed to penetrate at least half of the penetrometer steps. The resulting radiograph is a series of penetrometer steps (Figure 11–7), which are compared for density or contrast differences. A machine with a reliable kilovoltage output demonstrates approximately equal densities and contrast. It should be noted that a test result with equal densities and contrast suggests that the kilovoltage is consistent at different milliampere and

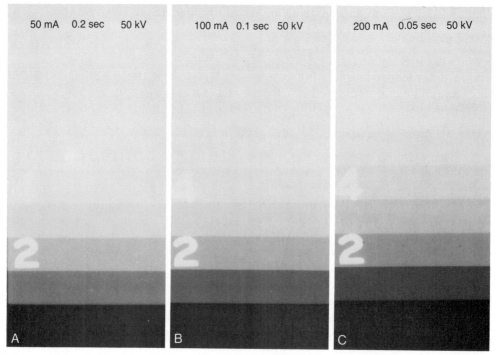

Figure 11—7. Penetrometer test for kilovoltage reliability. Milliamperage and time varied, but kilovoltage and milliampere-seconds were constant.

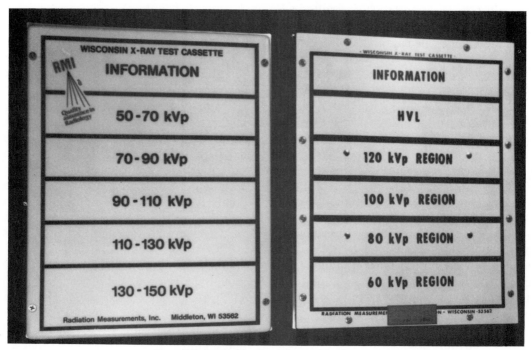

Figure 11—8. Tube side of two Wisconsin cassettes.

time settings. However, this does *not* address the specific kilovoltage output value. For example, if 60 kV is set and the penetrometer images are equal, it is implied that the kilovoltage remained the same from exposure to exposure. However, it is possible the actual kilovoltage output value was 67 kV rather than 60 kV for each exposure.

WISCONSIN CASSETTE

One of the more reliable noninvasive test instruments is the Wisconsin kilovoltage peak test cassette (Radiation Measurements, Inc.) The cassette is designed to measure the peak kilovoltage and HVL. The cassette operates using the concept of x-ray and light attenuation. The construction of the cassette differs radically from that of the conventional cassette (described in Chapter 23, Film Holders and Intensifying Screens). To facilitate comprehension of how the Wisconsin cassette functions, a description of the cassette follows.

The Wisconsin cassette is easily distinguished from a conventional cassette by appearance. The Wisconsin cassette is much thicker and heavier than a conventional cassette. Also, the tube side of the Wisconsin cassette is sectioned and labeled with various kilovoltage ranges, HVL and information (Figure 11–8). The outer portion of the cassette is constructed in three layers. They are (from tube side to back of the cassette): 1/16 inch copper plate, copper stepwedges (or penetrometer) and a lead mask with holes (Figure 11–9). The inner part of the cassette contains one intensifying screen, below which is an optical attenuator (Figure 11–9).

The copper plate on the outer part of the cassette covers all sections of the cassette except the one labeled HVL and information portion. The purpose of the copper plate is to absorb the long wavelengths or low energy photons. This provides a beam with a copper attenuation coefficient that is almost linear. This linear relationship helps to provide a mathematical base used to plot the radiographic density to determine the kilovoltage peak output for a single or three phase x-ray unit.

Below the copper plate are five copper penetrometers, each having 10 steps. The penetrometers are located under the left half of each kilovoltage range and the HVL sections along the long axis of the cassette. The penetrometers vary in thickness relative to the section of the cassette it overlies (kilo-

voltage range or HVL). The thickness of the penetrometers increases as the kilovoltage becomes higher. When the radiation passes through the copper penetrometer, the x-ray beam absorption increases with step thickness. The amount of remnant radiation striking the film varies according to the x-ray absorption. The more x-ray absorption occurs, the less remnant radiation strikes the film.

The last layer of the outer portion of the Wisconsin cassette is a lead mask. The lead mask contains 10 columns of holes arranged in sets of 5 pairs (each pair having 2 columns). Every column consists of 10 holes. The holes of the lead mask permit the passage of radiation, while the lead is used to absorb scatter radiation. Radiation passing through the left column of each pair of holes must first penetrate the copper plate and the copper penetrometer before penetrating the lead plate, whereas the radiation entering the right column of each pair of holes only passes through the copper plate before penetrating the lead shield. This results in density variations of the circles imaged in the left column of each pair of holes. The circles under the right column (reference column) are of relatively equal density.

Beneath the lead mask and located in the inner part of the cassette is an intensifying screen. The

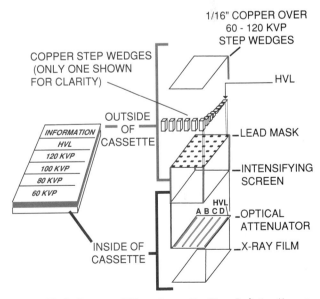

Figure 11–9. Diagram of Wisconsin cassette. (From Radiation Measurements, Inc.)

purpose of the intensifying screen is to convert the x-ray energy to light.

Located under the intensifying screen is an optical attenuator. The optical attenuator is located below the right side of each pair of holes. The objective of the optical attenuator is to filter the light emitted by the screen and striking the film.

The Wisconsin cassette uses the concept of attenuation. In this theory, the radiation under the copper penetrometer (left column) and the light emitted by the intensifying screen beneath the reference column (right side) are attenuated. This produces one circle located in the left column (x-ray attenuated) of an equal density to that in the reference column. Determining the penetrometer step level of the circle with an equal density in the left column and in the reference column results in a linear function of kilovoltage. The step level is used with a calibration curve (supplied by the cassette manufacturer) to determine the peak kilovoltage (Figure 11–10).

The cassette is loaded with the film most often employed in the radiology department. The cassette is position on the x-ray table so that the long axis of the cassette is parallel to the anode and cathode. This limits the influence of the heel effect on the image. Lead numbers or letters may be used to label the x-ray room and test date over the information section of the cassette. Exposures are made individually over each kilovoltage range and the HVL sections. Before making an exposure, the line voltage regulator is adjusted so that it is at its correct location. The kilovoltage employed is equivalent to the voltage labeled on the respective section of the cassette. A milliampere-seconds value capable of providing a density between 0.5 and 2 (with 1 as optimum) in the reference column (right column) is employed. After the film is completely exposed, it is developed.

To determine the peak kilovoltage, the image in the left column that matches one in the reference column is located. The matching image may be located visually or by use of a densitometer. A more accurate match is obtained with a densitometer. After the matching image is determined, the step level of the matching circle is recorded by using the step scale located on the side of the film. It is possible that a density match is between circles or steps, if this occurs the correct step must be extrapolated. This is achieved by using an extrapolation

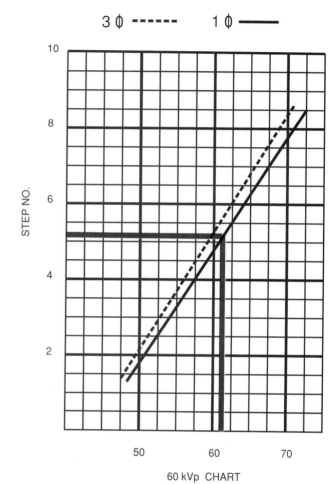

Figure 11–10. Results of the Wisconsin cassette test for a 60 kVp exposure on a single phase x-ray machine. (From Radiation Measurements, Inc.)

formula located in the Wisconsin cassette instruction manual. Finally, the matching step is located on the respective calibration curve to determine the peak kilovoltage (Figure 11–10) or HVL.

The Wisconsin cassette is more accurate at low kilovoltage than high kilovoltage. This is especially true with cassettes manufactured before 1982. Also, because the cassette measures peak kilovoltage and electrical variations influence the kilovoltage value, the Wisconsin cassette is more accurate when a three phase x-ray unit is employed. Although either blue sensitive or green sensitive film may be employed with the cassette, there are minor variations in results. Thus, it is recommended that the cassette be calibrated to coincide with the film most often used in the radiology department. To maximize the results, it is also recommended that the cassette be calibrated every 2 years. Cassettes may be calibrated by sending them to the National Bureau of Standards in Washington, DC, or the University of Wisconsin Radiation Calibration Service (UWRCS) in Madison, WI.

DIGITAL KILOVOLT METER

The digital kilovolt meter is an electronic method of determining the kilovoltage output. The meter senses the intensity of the x-ray beam and adjusts the equipment to measure a wide exposure range. It is able to digitally display the kilovoltage output or, if an oscilloscope is attached, the meter can provide a visual graphic display of the kilovoltage waveform. The information provided by the meter is similar to that from the Wisconsin cassette. However, the meter is easier to use than the Wisconsin cassette and does not require the use of film or a processing room. Unlike the cassette, the meter may vary slightly with changes in the x-ray tube filtration. Corrections can be made for variations by adjusting the HVL or filtration according to a chart provided by the manufacturer.

One common type of digital kilovolt meter is distributed by Radiation Measurement, Inc. (RMI) of Wisconsin (Figure 11–11). To operate the RMI meter, the unit must be turned on. If radiographic kilovoltage is being tested, the rad setting is selected. For measuring fluoroscopic kilovoltage, the fluoro setting is selected. The difference between the rad and fluoro selections is in the time delay

between the beginning of the x-ray exposure and the start of the kilovoltage measurement. The delay is longer for fluoroscopy to ensure time for cable charging and kilovoltage stabilization during fluoroscopy. After the appropriate kilovoltage setting is selected, the meter is positioned so the top of the unit is facing the respective x-ray tube. The x-ray beam is centered over the cross mark located on the meter. The single or three phase button (on the far left) is selected to coincide with the type of x-ray unit employed. A warm-up exposure is made at about 200 mAs and 100 kV. After the warm-up exposure is complete, the kilovoltage and milliamperage to be used are set. A time of 200 ms or longer is selected. After the desired technique variables are set, an exposure is made. The kilovoltage output is displayed immediately after the exposure.

If the kilovoltage range is below or above the measurable range, a "lo" or "hi" display is illuminated on the meter, respectively. If the range is too low, decrease the source-image distance or increase the milliamperage. An increase in source-image distance or a decrease in milliamperage is suggested if the kilovoltage is above the measurable range.

LABORATORY EXPERIENCE

Four practical laboratories in *Concepts in Medical Radiograph Imaging: Laboratory Manual* provide additional learning for the reader. Laboratory 18, Kilovoltage Compensation, allows the experimenter to test the 13% and 15% kilovoltage compensation rules. Laboratory 21, Effect of Kilovoltage on Contrast, provides the experimenter with the opportunity to compare several kilovoltage values relative to contrast. Laboratories 19, Kilovoltage Check, and 20, Half-value Layer, are quality control tests.

The Kilovoltage Compensation laboratory enables the experimenter to obtain four diagnostic radiographs of the same object using four different technical factors. After the radiographs are developed, they are compared for diagnostic quality and differences in density and contrast.

A penetrometer is used in the Effect of Kilovoltage on Contrast laboratory. In this procedure, several radiographs are taken at different kilovoltage values (all other factors remain the same). The radiographs are compared for differences in the number of steps visualized on the penetrometer (contrast).

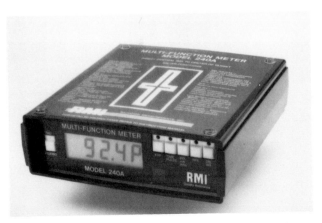

Figure 11–11. Multi-function meter used to test radiographic technique for kilovoltage, time, milliamperage linearity and relative film exposure. (From Radiation Measurements, Inc.)

The Kilovoltage Check laboratory is designed to enable the experimenter to assess the kilovoltage output. Instructions are provided for a kilovoltage reliability check (penetrometer test), as well as tests using the Wisconsin cassette and the digital meter. The accuracy of the measured kilovoltage output depends on the type of test instrument employed.

The Half-value Layer laboratory enables the experimenter the opportunity to assess the HVL. The experimenter may use the Wisconsin cassette or record the exposure rate of several exposures taken at different filtration levels. Both methods require the experimenter to determine the HVL by graphic means.

Bibliography

Bushong, SC. Radiologic science for technologists (4th edition). St. Louis: Mosby, 1988.

Carroll, QB. Fuchs's Principles of radiographic exposure, processing and quality control (3rd edition). Springfield, IL: Thomas, 1985.

Chesney, DN and Chesney, MO. Radiographic imaging (4th edition). Boston: Blackwell Scientific Publications, 1981.

Cullinan, JE and Cullinan, AM. Illustrated guide to x-ray technics (2nd edition). New York: Lippincott, 1980.

Curry, TS, Dowdey, JE and Murry, RC. Christensen's introduction to the physics of diagnostic radiology (3rd edition). Philadelphia: Lea & Febiger, 1984.

Curry, TS, Dowdey, JE and Murry, RC. Christensen's physics of diagnostic radiology (4th edition). Philadelphia: Lea & Febiger, 1990.

DeWerd, LA, and Ranallo, FN. kVp cassette measurements, (editorial). Radiologic Technology, *61* (2):145–146, November/December 1989.

Donohue, DP. An analysis of radiographic quality (2nd printing). Baltimore: University Park Press, 1982.

Eastman Kodak Company. Fundamentals of radiography (12th edition). Rochester, NY: Eastman Kodak Company, 1980.

Hazen, ME. Experiencing electricity and electronics, electron flow version. Philadelphia: Saunders, 1989.

Hiss, SS. Understanding radiography. Springfield, IL: Thomas, 1980.

Hananel, JI. Solving radiographic technique problems. Los Angeles: American Education Review and Advisory Company (AMERAC), 1979.

Lam, RW and Price, SC. The influence of film-screen color sensitivity and type of measurement device on kVp measurements. Radiologic Technology, *60* (4):319–321, March/April 1989.

Lam, RW, and Price, SC. In response—more on kVp measurements (editorial). Radiologic Technology, *61* (2):146, November/December 1989.

McLemore, J. Quality assurance in diagnostic radiology. Chicago: Year Book Medical, 1981.

Radiation Measurements, Inc. Digital kV meter ("Electronic kVp cassette") model 230 (instruction manual). Radiation Measurements, Inc.

Radiation Measurements, Inc. Wisconsin kVp test cassette model 101 (instruction manual). Radiation Measurements, Inc.

Radiation Measurements, Inc. Wisconsin kVp test cassette model 105 (instruction manual). Radiation Measurements, Inc.

Ranallo, FN, et al. Calibration and use of the Wisconsin kVp test cassette. Medical Physics, *15* (5):768–772, September/October 1988.

Selman, J. The fundamentals of x-ray and radium physics (7th edition). Springfield, IL: Thomas, 1985.

Simpkin DJ: The Wisconsin kVp test cassette with orthochromatic film. Medical Physics, *9* (1):110–111, January/February 1982.

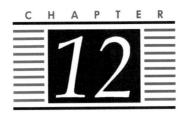

MILLIAMPERE-SECONDS AND QUALITY CONTROL

INTRODUCTION

Electrical current is a flow of electrons. An ampere is the unit used to measure current flow (see Chapter 5, Electrodynamics). One ampere is equivalent to 1 C (a coulomb is a quantity of charge equal to 6.25×10^{18} electrons) per second. In the x-ray circuit, the current is measured in a fraction of an ampere called a milliampere (1 mA = 0.001 [1/1000] A).

Milliamperage represents the x-ray intensity or exposure rate of the x-ray beam. The duration of the exposure rate is determined by the exposure timer. The amount of the exposure rate and the length of time the exposure rate occurs represent the quantity of the x-ray beam (number of x-rays produced). The quantity of the x-ray beam is determined by multiplying the exposure time (usually in seconds) by the milliamperes (mA × s = mAs).

The amount of milliampere-seconds used during a x-ray exposure is determined when the technologist sets the milliampere and time selectors. The milliampere selector regulates the amount of heat (and subsequent number of electrons produced in the electron cloud) needed for thermionic emission. The milliampere setting also determines which filament is energized in x-ray tubes with two filaments. The timer setting selects the length of time the current flows from the cathode to the anode.

This chapter discusses the effects of milliampereseconds on the x-ray beam, the patient and the film. Also presented is a summary of quality control tests that may be performed to check milliampere and time outputs. A review of Chapter 5, Electrodynamics; Chapter 9, X-ray Timers and Quality Control; and Chapter 10, Production of X-rays, is recommended.

LAW OF RECIPROCITY

As mentioned above, the quantity of the x-ray beam is measured in milliampere-seconds. Recall that milliampere-second is obtained by multiplying the milliamperes by the time in seconds. The law of reciprocity, as it relates to imaging, states that different milliampere and time factors may be used to obtain the same milliampere-second value. For example, 10 mAs may be obtained by using 100 mA at 0.1 second (100 × 0.1 = 10) or 200 mA for 0.05 second (200 × 0.05 = 10). Thus, theoretically, an infinite number of milliampere and time combinations can be employed to obtain the same milliampere-second value. However, the number of combinations available is limited by the milliampere and time increments on the x-ray machine. Also, notice that the relationship of milliamperage and time is inversely proportional when different combinations are used for the same milliampere-seconds. In other words, as milliamperage increases, time decreases and vice versa.

The law of reciprocity is consistent when milliampere-second exposures are made using direct film holders. However, there is a reciprocity failure when milliampere-seconds are used with intensifying screens. This failure occurs because the film in the intensifying screen is exposed by light instead of by radiation. If a film is exposed using a high intensity of light for a short time or a low intensity of light for a long time, a decrease in the expected film density results. It should be noted that this reciprocity failure exists at milliampere and time settings that are at the extreme ends of the exposure range. Also, modern electrical designs, intensifying screen construction and film composition have made the reciprocity law failure essential negligible.

MILLIAMPERE-SECONDS AND DENSITY

Milliampere-seconds represent the quantity of x-rays. As the milliampere-second value doubles, the quantity of radiation also doubles. The quantity of radiation is directly proportional to the density on a film. Thus, the milliampere-seconds value has a linear or direct relationship to density; changing the milliampere-seconds alters the amount of film density. However, the human eye is limited in its ability to detect density changes. In general, a 15% density change must occur before the human eye is able to detect a difference. A densitometer is used to measure minor changes in density that elude the human eye. Minor density changes are significant in some cases, e.g., sensitometry (see Chapter 21, Sensitometry and Processor Quality Control) and insignificant in other instances, e.g., conventional diagnostic film reading.

INVERSE SQUARE LAW

Recall that x-rays originate from a point and emerge in a fanlike configuration from the x-ray tube. Thus, as the distance from the source of the

x-rays (tube) increases, the irradiated area becomes larger (Figure 12–1). Consequently, the same amount of radiation must spread over a larger area, or is thinner. This phenomenon is represented by the inverse square law, which states that the intensity is inversely proportional to the square of the distance. The mathematical expression of the inverse square law is $I = 1/d^2$, where I is the intensity and d is the distance.

In conventional radiography, the inverse square law is used to determine milliampere-seconds compensation (assuming that all other factors remain the same) associated with source-image distance (SID) changes. The formula used to calculate changes in milliampere-seconds is $mAs_2/mAs_1 = (SID_2)^2/(SID_1)^2$, where mAs_2 is the new milliampere-

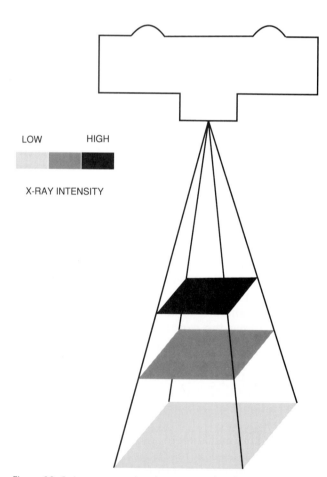

LOW   HIGH

X-RAY INTENSITY

Figure 12–1. Inverse square law demonstrating that the x-ray beam from the tube originates at a point and fans outward. As the distance from the origin (tube) increases, intensity decreases inversely in proportion to the square of the distance from the source to the area irradiated.

second value, mAs_1 is the old milliampere-second value, SID_2 is the new SID and SID_1 is the old SID. For example, if a radiograph is taken at 100 mAs and 72 inch SID, what is the milliampere-second value if the radiograph is repeated using a SID of 40 inches? (See the following calculations for the answer.)

$$X/100 = (40)^2/(72)^2$$
$$X/100 = 1600/5184$$
$$5184X = 1600 \,(100)$$
$$5184X = 160,000$$
$$X = 160,000/5184$$
$$X = 30.86 \text{ mAs}$$

MILLIAMPERE-SECONDS AND THE PATIENT

The milliampere-second value determines the number of x-rays produced. Radiation absorption by the patient is partly determined by the amount of radiation the patient receives. In general, the more radiation, the more the patient absorbs (assuming the penetration or kilovoltage value of the x-ray is unchanged). Because the milliampere-second value has a direct effect on the amount of radiation, any change in milliampere-seconds has a corresponding change in the radiation absorption by the patient. Thus, exposures of high milliampere-seconds should be avoided whenever possible. Unfortunately, some procedures, e.g., mammography, normally require high milliampere-second exposures. It is essential that, in procedures requiring high milliampere-seconds, extra care be taken to avoid repeated filming.

QUALITY CONTROL TESTS FOR TIMERS

Chapter 9, X-ray Timers and Quality Control, contains information about timers. The reader is referred to Chapter 9, which contains a detailed discussion of timer quality control, for information regarding quality control tests for timers.

QUALITY CONTROL TESTS FOR MILLIAMPERE

Two instruments are commonly used to check the milliampere output. They are the penetrometer and an ionizing chamber (usually a dosimeter). A penetrometer infers milliampere output through density measurements. Dose measurements are used to infer milliampere output when using a dosimeter.

Test results are dependent on other factors besides milliamperage. Thus, regardless of the instrument employed, milliampere tests are performed if the following four conditions exist:
1. The processor is operating properly.
2. The timer is accurate.
3. Techniques and equipment that have no reciprocity law failure are employed.
4. The kilovoltage output is accurate.

Of the two instruments available for testing the milliampere output, the dosimeter is more accurate than the penetrometer. This is a result of a reduced number of variables (the processor, the film or the screen) that might influence the outcome of the test.

The penetrometer or the dosimeter is used to examine three milliampere principles. One is to assess consistency of a given milliampere-seconds output regardless of the milliampere or time setting used. The second principle evaluates the accuracy of the linear relationship among milliampere stations. The last principle examines the ability of a given milliampere station to produce the same output from one exposure to the next.

The process to test the consistency of a given milliampere-seconds output is performed by making several exposures using the same milliampere-second setting but different milliampere and time stations (all other factors remain the same). For example, 20 mAs is the same if an exposure is made at 200 mA for 0.1 (1/10) second or 400 mA at 0.05 (1/20) second. Test results should demonstrate similar outputs for each exposure. If the penetrometer is employed as the test instrument, accurate milliampere stations image equal densities of each respective step for all exposures (Figure 12–2). Using the dosimeter as the test instrument demonstrates equivalent dose readings.

To test the linear relationship of the milliampere stations, exposures are taken using several different milliampere-second values (altering milliamperes while all other factors remain constant). For example, because milliamperage is linear, 200 mA should produce twice the intensity of 100 mA. Thus, an exposure at 200 mA for 0.5 (1/2) second has twice the density (100% more) than an exposure at 100 mA for 0.5 second. Penetrometer tests demonstrate

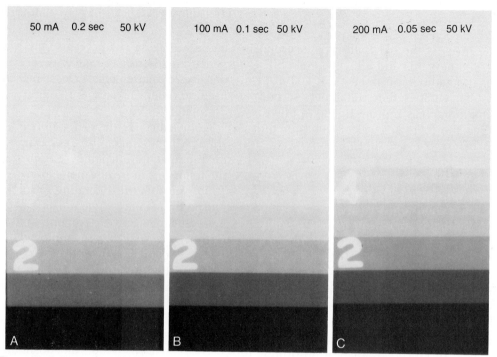

Figure 12–2. Penetrometer test results using the same milliampere-seconds but different milliamperage and time stations.

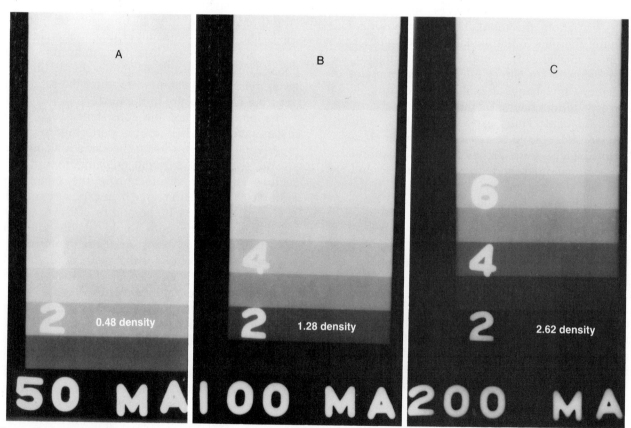

Figure 12–3. Penetrometer test results for linear relationship of milliamperes using 59 kVp, 0.2 second and varied milliampere values as indicated on radiograph. As the milliampere value doubled from *A* to *B*, there is a 167% increase in density (67% more than expected). When the milliampere value doubled from *B* to *C*, there is a 104% increase in density (within normal limits).

density differences of the respective steps equivalent to the respective linear function among the exposures (Figure 12–3). Dosimeter test results reveal dose rates equivalent to the linear function among the exposures. Results that are plus or minus 10% are considered acceptable.

The last principle is evaluated by making several exposures using the same milliampere and time settings. Multiple exposures using the same milliampere and time settings should produce similar outputs. If the penetrometer is employed as the test instrument, the image has equal densities of each respective step for all exposures (Figure 12–4). Using the dosimeter as the test instrument demonstrates equivalent dose readings for all exposures. Results of plus or minus 5% are considered acceptable.

LABORATORY EXPERIENCE

Four laboratory procedures are associated with this chapter. They are Laboratories 24, Effect of Milliampere-seconds on Density; 23, Law of Reciprocity; 13, Timer Test; and 22, Milliampere Check. The Timer Test laboratory is also related to Chapter 9, X-ray Timers and Quality Control; thus, the experimenter may already be familiar with this laboratory.

The Effect of Milliampere-seconds on Density laboratory enables the investigator to demonstrate the relationship between milliampere-seconds and density. In this laboratory, six exposures are made of a penetrometer at increasing milliampere-second values. The six penetrometer images are compared for density changes.

The Law of Reciprocity laboratory allows the experimenter to determine the validity of the law of reciprocity. In this laboratory, three exposures are made at the same milliampere-second setting but different milliampere and time settings. The densities of each exposure are measured and compared.

The following information on the Timer Test laboratory is for individuals who did not perform this laboratory while studying Chapter 9. Laboratory 13 allows the experimenter to assess the accu-

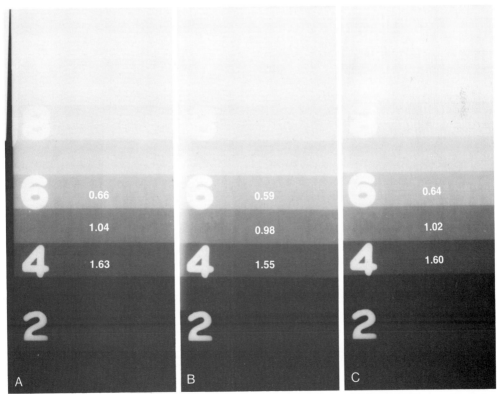

Figure 12–4. Penetrometer test results for multiple exposures of same technique (50 kVp, 100 mA and 0.2 second), demonstrating similar densities of three steps, respectively.

racy of the timer on single or three phase equipment. The spinning top instrument is used for single phase equipment testing. The experimenter may use one of two instruments to test three phase equipment. They are the synchronous motor and a digital meter. More specific information about the use of these instruments is located under Quality Control in Chapter 9.

The Milliampere Check laboratory contains three experiments. One checks the consistency of a given milliampere-seconds output regardless of the milliampere or time setting used. The second experiment evaluates the accuracy of the linear relationship of one milliampere station to another. The last experiment examines the ability of a given milliampere station to produce the same output from one exposure to the next. All experiments allow the researcher to choose a penetrometer or a dosimeter to check the milliamperage.

Bibliography

Bushong, SC. Radiologic science for technologists (4th edition). St. Louis: Mosby, 1988.

Carroll, QB. Fuchs's Principles of radiographic exposure, processing and quality control (3rd edition). Springfield, IL: Thomas, 1985.

Chesney, DN and Chesney, MO. Radiographic imaging (4th edition). Boston: Blackwell Scientific Publications, 1981.

Chesney, DN and Chesney, MO. X-ray equipment for student radiographers (3rd edition). Boston: Blackwell Scientific Publications, 1984.

Cullinan, JE and Cullinan, AM. Illustrated guide to x-ray technics (2nd edition). New York: Lippincott, 1980.

Donohue, DP. An analysis of radiographic quality (2nd printing). Baltimore: University Park Press, 1982.

Eastman Kodak Company. Fundamentals of radiography (12th edition). Rochester, NY: Eastman Kodak Company, 1980.

Hendee, WR, Chaney, EL and Rossi, RP. Radiologic physics, equipment and quality control. Chicago: Year Book Medical, 1976.

McLemore, J. Quality assurance in diagnostic radiology. Chicago: Year Book Medical, 1981.

Selman, J. The fundamentals of x-ray and radium physics (7th edition). Springfield, IL: Thomas, 1985.

IMAGE INTENSIFICATION AND ACCESSORY EQUIPMENT

INTRODUCTION

Conventional radiography produces still images or pictures of the human body. This type of imaging records the condition of the part as it appeared at the time of x-ray exposure. However, some organs within the body, e.g., the heart, are constantly moving. Often the movement is so fast that a routine radiograph is unable to record the information needed to make a proper diagnosis. Also, sometimes it is desirable to watch the organ's movement to assess its function. The imaging modality of choice to capture organ movement is fluoroscopy. Accessory equipment may be attached to the fluoroscopic unit to record the image (make a permanent copy) for further study.

This chapter addresses the equipment aspect of fluoroscopy. Among the topics are equipment needs, the basic function of the equipment and the various types of accessory equipment (attachments) associated with fluoroscopy.

CHARACTERISTICS OF THE HUMAN EYE

Before a discussion of fluoroscopy, a brief review of the characteristics of the human eye is in order. Because there are many parts to the human eye, this discussion is limited to the portions of the eye that relate to fluoroscopy: the cones and the rods.

Cones are sensitive to color and are used for daylight vision. Cone vision is often referred to as photopic vision. Many cones are located on the retina in the center of the eye (the fovea). The large number of cones contributes to good visual acuity (ability to distinguish objects).

The rods are sensitive to shades of gray and function best in dim light. Vision using the rods is called scotopic vision. Rods are located outside the fovea of the retina, making the visual acuity with the rods poor. It takes several minutes for the rods to adapt (function) to changes from bright light to dim light. Visual acuity in dim light may be improved by looking at an object using peripheral vision (utilizing the location of the rods). Also, visual acuity is increased by moving the eye rather than staring at an object. The rods are sensitive to a blue-green light. Thus, original fluoroscopy screens were constructed of phosphor, which emitted a greenish light.

DIRECT FLUOROSCOPY

The earliest form of fluoroscopy employed a system in which the operator viewed the image directly (thus the name direct fluoroscopy). In its simplest form, fluoroscopic equipment consists of an x-ray tube and a fluorescent screen (Figure 13–1). The x-ray tube and the fluorescent screen are located opposite each other and are connected by a metallic rod. The attachment of the tube to the screen provides a means for them to move simultaneously while maintaining their position opposite one another. The screen also has the ability to move up or down the metallic rod attachment. The closer the screen is to the object, the sharper the image. The

direct fluoroscopic screen is coated with zinc cadmium sulfide phosphor. This phosphor emits light photons when stimulated by x-rays. The back of the screen is lead lined to protect the operator from radiation.

The basic principle of operation of a direct fluoroscopic unit is for the remnant radiation to strike the fluoroscopic screen, emitting light. The intensity of the light is directly proportional to the amount of x-ray energy striking the phosphor. The higher the x-ray energy, the brighter the light illumination of the screen.

Direct fluoroscopy has three major disadvantages: only one person is able to view the image, the room needs to be completely dark for fluoroscopic viewing, and the patient dose is high. Because only one person can observe the anatomy, it is not possible for an attending physician, intern or radiology resident to view the image simultaneously with the operator. The need to perform fluoroscopy in a completely dark room requires the operator to allow his/her eyes to adapt to the dark before entering the room. Fluoroscopic operators constantly move from a dark room to a white-lit room. This means the eyes are continually changing to adapt from use of the cones to use of the rods. However, the constant adaption and readaption is eliminated by wearing red goggles when in white light. The red color of the goggles acts as a filter of wavelengths, helping to maintain the scotopic vision. The poor efficiency of the fluorescent screen requires a lot of remnant radiation to achieve the appropriate brightness. Consequently, there is a high radiation dose to the patient.

IMAGE INTENSIFICATION

In the early 1950s, a system of fluoroscopy was developed that is still in use. This system employs an image intensification tube. The function of the image intensification tube is to increase (intensify) the brightness of the light produced from a fluoroscopic screen. One advantage of increasing the brightness is that it eliminates the need to perform fluoroscopy in a completely darkened room. Accessory equipment can be added to the image intensifier to provide a means of recording the image and to enable the viewing of the image by several people simultaneously. Some accessory items include tele-

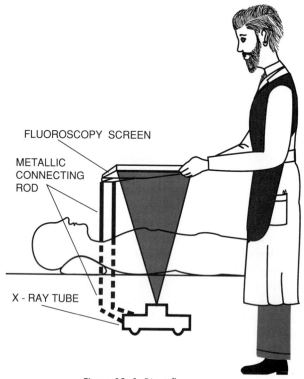

FLUOROSCOPY SCREEN

METALLIC CONNECTING ROD

X - RAY TUBE

Figure 13–1. Direct fluoroscopy.

vision, spot filming equipment and cineradiographic equipment (see below).

As in direct fluoroscopy, in image intensification the x-ray tube is connected to the fluorescent screen (image intensifier). Some units have the intensifier located under the table and the x-ray tube above the table. This allows the tube to be used for conventional filming as well as fluoroscopy. However, most fluoroscopy units have the intensifier above the table and the tube below the table. Thus, if conventional radiography is to be performed, a second x-ray tube must be installed. Some modern intensifier and x-ray tube attachments (C-arm) allow for angled (transverse) as well as horizontal and vertical movements.

The U.S. Center for Devices and Radiological Health identifies the safety features associated with fluoroscopic equipment. Some of the more important safety features of which a technologist should be aware are the following: a minimum of 18 inches from the x-ray tube to skin must be maintained, the radiation emitted can not exceed 10 roentgens (R) per minute, a drape (usually leaded rubber) must be attached to above-table image intensifiers, and the exposure must be attached to a 5-minute alarmed timer. Of these features, the 5-minute timer is most apt to be misused or abused. The timer should always be allowed to expire (run down).

When the timer expires, an alarm or buzzer should sound. This advises the operator that the patient received 5 minutes of fluoroscopy. Unfortunately, sometimes the technologist resets the timer before it expires. This practice never allows the operator to hear the alarm. Thus, the amount of patient exposure is unknown.

IMAGE INTENSIFICATION TUBE COMPONENTS AND FUNCTION

Figure 13–2 diagrams the basic components of an image intensification tube. An image intensification tube consists of an input phosphor, a photocathode, a focusing lens, an anode and an output phosphor. These components are enclosed in a vacuum glass. The vacuum glass is surrounded by a casing protecting it from damage and shielding the operator from scatter radiation.

The following is a brief summary of image intensification tube function. Remnant radiation strikes

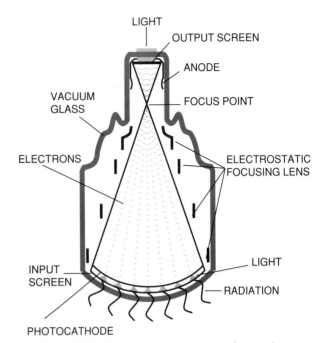

Figure 13–2. Components of an image intensification tube.

the input screen, producing light. The light from the input screen hits a photocathode, emitting electrons. The electrons accelerate to the output screen as a result of the potential difference between the photocathode (negative charge) and the anode (positive charge). As the electrons travel to the anode, they are shaped or focused by the electrostatic lens. The electrons strike the output screen, which changes the electron energy to light. Because the electron quantity is proportional to the original x-ray intensity (direct proportion), the light image is the same as the image produced at the input screen. The difference is that the image at the output screen is smaller and inverted.

INPUT PHOSPHOR

As stated above, the original input phosphor was made of zinc cadmium sulfide. Currently, input phosphor is constructed of cesium iodide. This material is more desirable because it absorbs more photons (has a greater quantum detection efficiency) than zinc cadmium sulfide. Because cesium iodide has a better quantum detection, it is possible to use less of the phosphor and smaller crystals to obtain a sufficient amount of brightness. This results in a thinner input phosphor layer than is possible with zinc cadmium sulfide. The thinner layer increases the resolution (sharpness) of the image. Also, the higher quantum detection efficiency means less radiation is needed to obtain the desired brightness. Consequently, the radiation dose to the patient is reduced.

Image sharpness is also improved by constructing the crystals on the input phosphor so that the ends are pointed (Figure 13–3). The pointed end limits the amount of diffusion of light, increasing the image sharpness. Another factor affecting the sharpness of the image is the distance from the input phosphor to the photocathode.

As shown in Figure 13–2, the input phosphor is located close to the photocathode. The closer they are, the less diffusion of light and the better the image definition. However, the input phosphor and the photocathode should never touch; if they come in contact with one another, a chemical reaction can occur, destroying the phosphor. Consequently, a thin transparent layer attaches the input phosphor to the photocathode. The layer's thinness allows the input phosphor and the photocathode to be close to one another, and its transparency provides a means for light transmission from the input screen to the photocathode.

The diameter of the input screen is determined during manufacturing. Common diameters are 6 and 9 inches. However, the diameter may be as large as 12 or 14 inches.

PHOTOCATHODE

The photocathode is usually made of antimony and cesium compounds. When these compounds come in contact with light, they emit photoelectrons (often referred to as electrons). The number of electrons emitted is proportional to the brightness of the input screen. The brighter the screen is, the more electrons are emitted. As is the case for all electrons, they carry a negative charge.

ELECTROSTATIC FOCUSING LENS

The electrostatic focusing lens (electrodes) is positively charged. The lens focuses the electron stream as it travels from the photocathode to the anode. To avoid distortion, the electrons must travel the same distance from any point on the input screen to its opposite position on the output screen. This is achieved by having the input screen curved.

Also, during the focusing process, the electrons cross at a point called the focus point. The crossing of the electrons at the focus point inverts the image on the output screen. The distance from the focus point to the output screen varies according the size of the input screen. The larger the input screen, the shorter the distance between the focus point and the output screen.

ANODE

The anode is located in the neck of the intensifying tube. As with all anodes, it carries a positive charge. The potential difference between the photocathode and the anode is about 25 kVp. This potential difference causes the electrons to move from the photocathode to the anode.

OUTPUT PHOSPHOR

The output phosphor is made of zinc cadmium sulfide. This phosphor is used because it emits a light to which film is sensitive, thus enabling a permanent record to be made of the image. The output screen also has a thin aluminum plate. The aluminum is used to prevent light from returning to the photocathode (retrograde movement) and activating it again.

The image on the output screen is substantially smaller than the image on the input screen. An intensifying tube is often identified by the ratio of the input screen to the output screen. The output screen is usually 1 inch. Thus, a 6-inch input screen

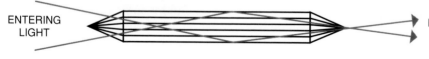

ENTERING LIGHT   EXITING LIGHT

Figure 13–3. Shape of crystal on input screen.

with a 1-inch output screen has a 6:1 ratio. However, because the output screen is often 1 inch, this type of tube is usually referred to as a 6-inch tube (the 1-inch output screen is inferred).

OUTPUT SCREEN ATTACHMENTS

Several items may be attached to the output end of the image intensification tube. Some attachments are a mirror system used to view the image, a television monitor, photospot filming device or a cineradiographic equipment (Figure 13–4). These attachments are discussed in more detail below.

IMAGE INTENSIFICATION TUBE BRIGHTNESS GAIN

Recall that the purpose of an image intensification tube is to increase the brightness of the image on the fluorescent screen (input phosphor). The degree of brightness is measured using one of two methods. The first method is to compare the luminance

of the output screens between the original direct fluoroscopy screen (Patterson type B-2) and the current image intensification output screen for the same exposure value. This method of determining brightness gain is discouraged for two reasons. First, the brightness of the Patterson type B-2 output screen is not standardized and varies from screen to screen. Second, the brightness of the screen deteriorates with age.

The preferred method of identifying the brightness gain is to use the conversion factor. The conversion factor is the ratio of the output luminance to the exposure rate at the input screen. Luminance is measured in a unit called candela (cd). (The explanation of candela is beyond the scope of this text.) The conversion factor formula is

$$\text{Conversion factor} = \frac{cd/m^2}{mR/second}$$

Two factors affect the brightness: the rate at which the electrons strike the output screen (determined by voltage), and the degree of image minification. Thus, brightness gain is identified, in this

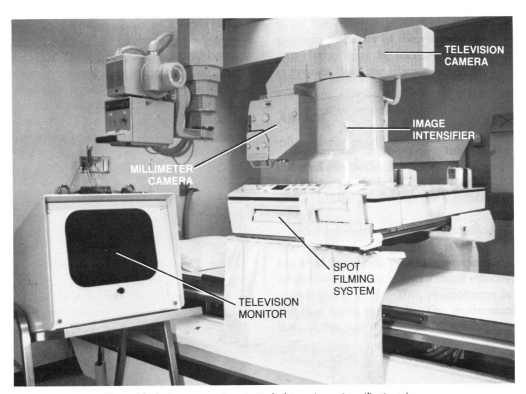

Figure 13–4. Accessory equipment attached to an image intensification tube.

text, as the product of the minification gain and the flux (voltage) gain.

Brightness gain = minification gain × flux gain

Minification gain is created by the reduction in size of the image from the input screen to the output screen. The minification gain depends on the relationship of the area of the input screen to the area of the output screen. The input and output screens are circular. Recall that the area of a circle is pi (π) times the radius squared, or $A = \pi r^2$, where A is the area and r represents the radius. Also, recall that the diameter of a circle has two radii. Thus, a radius is equivalent to one-half a diameter, or D/2, where D is the diameter. Because D/2 is the same as r, it is possible to substitute D/2 for r in the formula for the area of a circle. The new (and equivalent) formula for the area of a circle becomes

$$A = \pi(D/2)^2, \text{ or } \pi(D)^2/2^2, \text{ or } \pi(D)^2/4$$

As stated above, minification gain is the reduction of the area of the input screen to the area of the output screen. If one employs the formula for the area of a circle, the minification gain formula (where D_i is the input screen diameter and D_o is the output diameter)

$$\text{Minification gain} = \frac{\dfrac{\pi}{4}(D_i)^2}{\dfrac{\pi}{4}(D_o)^2}$$
$$= \frac{\pi(D_i)^2}{\pi(D_o)^2}$$
$$= \frac{(D_i)^2}{(D_o)^2}$$

The flux gain is the amount of brightness increase when a light photon strikes the output phosphor. This is usually a factor of at least 50. The total brightness gain range (minification times flux gain) of an image intensification tube is usually 1000 to 6000.

MULTIFOCUS IMAGE INTENSIFICATION TUBE

As mentioned above, image intensification tubes are available in a variety of sizes. It is possible to have a tube with more than one size of input screen.

A tube having two input screen sizes is called a dual focus tube. One with three sizes is identified as trifocus tube. The most common type of multifocus tube is the dual focus tube. These are usually constructed with 6-inch and 9-inch input screens (Figure 13–5). The size of input diameter is regulated by changing the voltage on the focusing lens, which alters the shape of the electron beam.

Recall that the distance from the focus point to the output screen varies with the size of the input diameter. The smaller the diameter is, the farther the focus point is from the output screen. As a result, the image on the output screen is magnified. Consequently, the smaller input diameter of a dual image intensification tube is used for magnification purposes.

When employing the smaller input diameter, the number of electrons striking the output screen is less than with a larger input diameter. Thus, on a dual focus tube, the brightness of the image on the output screen is less with the smaller input screen. To increase the brightness, the amount of radiation is increased. This increases the radiation dose to the patient.

VIGNETTING

Theoretically, the electrons striking the output screen do so such that the image is proportional to

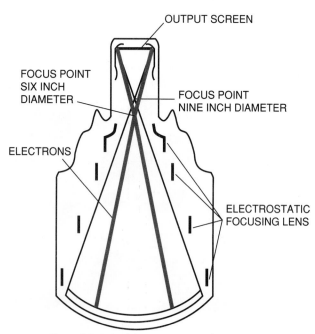

Figure 13–5. Dual focus image intensification tube.

the input screen. However, in practice, the electrons on the peripheral edge of the output screen are angled more than those at the center of the screen. This creates distortion (decreasing sharpness) and reduces the brightness. This decrease in sharpness at the periphery is called vignetting.

VIEWING THE INTENSIFIED IMAGE

MIRROR SYSTEM

The simplest method of viewing the image produced at the output screen of the intensifier is by using mirrors. Briefly, mirrors project the image on the output screen of the image intensifier to the exterior. This is achieved by using several mirrors in series and angling them to project the image where desired (Figure 13–6). The last mirror is mounted on the outside of the image intensifier near the operator's eye level. This system has several disadvantages. The primary disadvantages are that the intensity of the image decreases as it is projected from one mirror to the next, viewing is limited to one person, and the field (image) is small.

TELEVISION SYSTEM

Television has been commercially available to the U.S. public since the 1950s. Most people are familiar with the basic concept in which commercial television is transmitted (telecasted) and viewed. Free television images are transmitted over the air waves, received by an antenna and displayed on a screen. Recently, cable networks (paid television) have evolved. In these systems, the image originates from the network and is transmitted to the individual viewer via cables. (Some transmissions may originate in distant locations, e.g., foreign countries. In these instances, the signal may be sent to the network via a satellite.) Television systems employed with image intensification operate on the same principle as commercial television. The primary difference is that, although the open air and cable transmissions may employ the air waves to send signals, the televisions used in imaging departments are closed circuit. A closed circuit television system transmits the signal through various electrical components via cable connections.

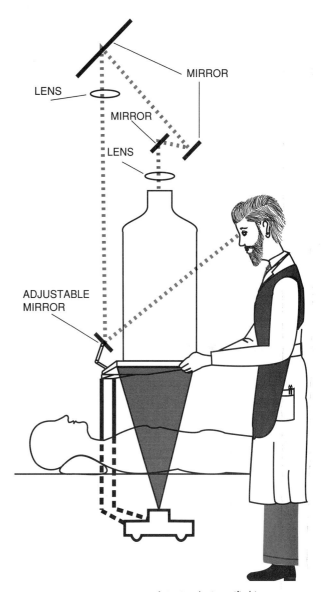

Figure 13–6. Mirror system of viewing the intensified image.

Television technology is complex. Current research in this area is resulting in the development of a high resolution television screen. Also, research is continuing to improve the method of displaying the image. Of particular interest is the continued investigation of replacing the picture tube with a smaller and higher resolution screen. An in-depth consideration of television is beyond the scope of this text. This discussion is designed to briefly summarize the basic operation of the major portions of a closed circuit television system.

Basic Operation

A closed circuit television system attached to an image intensifier consists of a camera, a control unit and a monitor. The basic function of the camera is to receive the light image on the output screen of the image intensification tube, change the light image into an electronic signal and send the signal to the control unit. The control unit is responsible for amplifying the image and synchronizing it with the monitor. The monitor changes the electronic signal to a visible image recognizable by the human eye.

Images are displayed on the monitor as individual still pictures (frames). The speed with which the frames are displayed tricks the human eye into thinking the image is in motion (motion integration). This is achieved because the minimum time the eye needs to see an image is approximately 0.2 second. A rate of 15 frames per second is fast enough for the eye to retain the previous image while displaying the current image. Consequently, the eye sees the various frames as a motion picture.

A second feature of the eye is the time needed to distinguish brightness intensities (brightness integration). Brightness integration is shorter than motion integration. Thus, a rate of 15 frames per second is fast enough to allow the eye to see motion but is too slow to achieve brightness integration. Consequently, at 15 frames per second, the eye sees the image flickering. A rate of at least 25 frames per second is needed to remove flicker. However, the ability to visualize flicker has been recorded with rates as high as 50 frames per second. Ideally, a rate of 50 frames per second eliminates all flicker.

Television Camera

The first component of a closed circuit television system is the television camera or pickup tube. The function of the pickup tube is to convert the light from the output screen of the image intensification tube to an electrical current. Two types of pickup tubes are used in radiography; the Vidicon and Plumbicon. The Plumbicon has a different type of phosphor located on the target. It provides a better contrast and shorter lag time than the Vidicon does. However, the Plumbicon pickup tube has an increased rate of quantum mottle. Both tubes are compact (about 6 inches in diameter and 10 inches in length) and lightweight (less than 10 pounds). The pickup tube is attached to the output section of the image intensification tube (see Figure 13–4).

There are two methods of attaching the pickup tube to the image intensification tube. One method is to use a fiberoptic connection (coupling); the other method uses a lens system. The fiberoptic system connects directly to the image intensifier. It provides better resolution than the lens system. However, the fiberoptic coupling does not provide a means to attach recording devices, such as cineradiographic equipment.

Figure 13–7 is a diagram of a Vidicon pickup tube. The basic components of the pickup tube are

Electron gun
Frontal plates (target plate, signal plate and face plate)
Focusing coils
Deflecting coils
Control grid

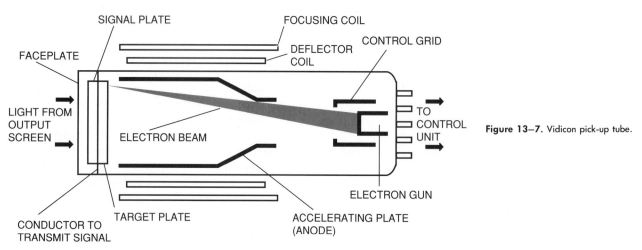

Figure 13–7. Vidicon pick-up tube.

The pickup tube operates when light from the output tube of the image intensifier is transmitted through the glass face plate and signal plate, striking the target plate. The signal plate is thin enough to transmit light and is made of graphite to conduct electricity. The target contains antimony trisulfide crystals. The important characteristic of the target is that the resistance of the crystals changes relative to the light intensity received from the output screen of the image intensifier. The more light received, the less the resistance (more positive charge) of the crystal. Lower resistance crystals produce a greater electrical signal than high resistance crystals. This produces a signal that is a duplicate of the image on the output screen.

The electron gun emits electrons and sends them in a concentrated stream (the control grid helps concentrate the electrons) to the target. The electrons scan the target in a manner similar to a person reading a page in a book. For example, the electrons start in the upper left corner and move to the right side (active trace) of the target. On reaching the right side, they return to the left side at a level slightly lower than that of the first scan and start a new left to right scan. When the electrons are located in the lower right corner of the screen, they return to the upper left corner to repeat the scan process. This method of movement (left to right, up and down) is achieved by varying the charge levels of the electrostatic focusing and deflector lens. One complete scanning process of the screen is called a raster.

As the electrons strike the crystals on the target, they are conducted to the signal plate. Recall that the signal plate transmits the electrical signal to the control unit. The strength of the electrical signal depends on the resistance of the crystals in the target. Low resistance crystals result in a strong electrical signal.

Control Unit

The pickup tube signal is sent to the control unit. The control unit is complex in its operation. A simplified explanation of the unit is that the unit is responsible for amplifying the electrical signal received from the pickup tube, synchronizing the electron movement and pulses between the pickup tube and the television monitor.

Television Monitor

The television monitor is a type of cathode ray tube. It is also known as a kinescope. The most common lay term for a television monitor is a picture tube. The major components of a kinescope are electron gun, anode, focusing coils and deflector coils (Figure 13–8). The function of the television monitor is to convert the electronic signal received from the control unit into a visible image.

The monitor is much larger than the pickup tube but is similar in function. As with the pickup tube, the monitor has an electron gun that emits electrons. The electrons emitted are synchronized by the control unit so that they are of the same intensity and location as the electrons generated by the pickup tube. This provides a means of reproducing the image exactly as it appears at the output screen of the image intensifier.

The control grid concentrates the electrons into a beam. The electrons move in the same raster pattern

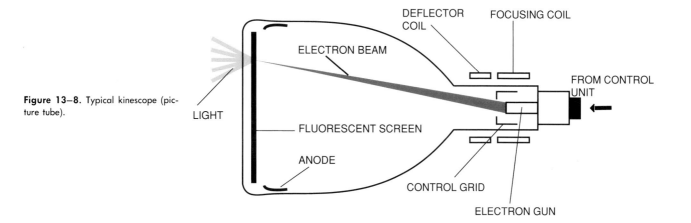

Figure 13–8. Typical kinescope (picture tube).

as those of the pickup tube. As with the pickup tube, the focusing and deflector coils move the electron beam left, right, up and down. The electrons strike the anode of the monitor. The anode consist of small fluorescent crystals, which emit light when stimulated by electrons.

The intensity of the light is directly proportional to the intensity of the electrons. When the screen is viewed from a distance (at least 25 inches), the individual crystals appear as a solid picture. This is analogous to the case with a picture printed in a newspaper. The newspaper picture is made of many small dots. When it is viewed closely, the individual dots are visible; however, from a distance the dots merge and appear as one image.

In the United States, the electron gun of the kinescope makes one complete top to bottom scan of the monitor in 1/60 second (this is equivalent to one electrical cycle). One scan is called a field and contains 262.5 horizontal scan lines. A complete frame consists of two fields, or 525 horizontal scan lines, and takes 1/30 second. To provide an illusion of motion, the frame frequency must be at least 25 frames per second. Because 1 frame takes 1/30 second, there are 30 frames in 1 second. To provide a better image, an interlace method of scanning is used. In the interlace method, the first field scans the even numbered lines on the monitor. The second field scans the odd numbered lines. A new and different image is produced over the entire screen with every field or 1/60 second. Thus, 60 different fields are imaged in 1 second. This field rate is sufficient to meet the brightness integration of the eye so that no flicker is visualized.

VIEWING SYSTEM COMPARISON

The type of viewing system employed is often a matter of space availability and economics. The least expensive system requiring the least amount of space is direct fluoroscopy. However, the quality of the image is so poor and the amount of radiation dose to the patient is so great that this method is essentially nonexistent. Thus, the viewing systems most often used are mirror (second most expensive) and television (most expensive). Sometimes a unit may have both mirror and television attachments. The mirror system limits the number of people able to view the image to one. Also, the brightness of a

mirror unit is lower than that of the television system. The lower illumination also has a higher patient dose and poorer image quality than television. Table 13–1 compares the various viewing systems.

PREINTENSIFIER TUBE (SPOT FILM) IMAGE RECORDING

The earliest recording device used with image intensification tubes is the spot film device. This system is being replaced by the use of photospot (millimeter) filming. Unlike other recording devices, the spot film employs regular conventional sized films and cassettes. The cassette is placed in a film carriage located near the image intensification tube (see Figure 13–4). Before the exposure, the operator selects the area of the film to be exposed (Figure 13–9). There are usually several types of field exposures. For example, it is possible to expose the entire film or only one-fourth of the film. In the former case, the film has one exposure on one film, this is often referred to as a 1:1 (pronounced 1 on 1) setting. The latter example results in four exposures on one film, 4:1 (4 on 1) exposure.

To record an image, the operator energizes the spot filming switch. The switch moves the spot film from its storage place in the carriage to a position located between the patient and the image intensification tube. Because spot film recording requires a much higher milliampere value than fluoroscopy, the switch also changes the milliampere value to 100 mA or greater. This process of moving the film and changing the milliamperage takes time. Consequently, there is a short delay from the time the spot film switch is energized to the time the actual exposure is made.

Table 13–1. VIEWING MODALITY COMPARISON

Item	Direct	Mirror	Television
Quality	Poor	Good	Good
Observers	1	1	Many
Patient dose	High	Medium	Low
Cost	Low	Medium	High
Room space	Small	Average	Large
Brightness	Dim	Bright	Very bright

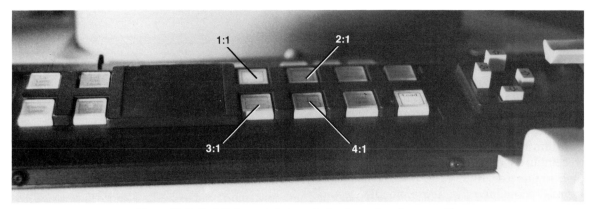

Figure 13–9. Spot filming controls demonstrating the number of exposures/film.

During the delay, the operator is unable to see the image, and the anatomical part is still moving. Consequently, it is possible that the part may be in an anatomical phase, e.g., emptying of the stomach, different from that desired. Also, the filming process is slow. It takes several seconds from one exposure to the next. This also contributes to recording the wrong phase of movement of an anatomical part.

Spot films are advantageous because they produce images of high quality and are easily stored. Two disadvantages of spot filming are the slow filming rate and the high exposure technique (high patient dose).

OUTPUT SCREEN IMAGE RECORDING METHODS

LENS SYSTEM

Common methods used to record the image at the output screen include photospot (millimeter camera) recording, cineradiography and magnetic tape or disc recording. All these methods require that a lens system be positioned after the output screen. Thus, a brief discussion of the lens system is in order.

Located immediately after the output screen is a complex lens system called the collimator or objective lens. This system focuses the light from the output screen into parallel lines (Figure 13–10). The exiting light from the collimator lens enters the next system.

If several recording images are used, the next system is the image distributor or beam splitter. The beam splitter is a partially reflective mirror. It allows the majority of light (usually 80–90%) to be transmitted to the pickup tube of the television system. The remaining light is directed to a recording device, e.g., cineradiographic equipment. Some beam splitter mirrors rotate to change the direction of light from one recording system to another.

The last lens system is the camera lens. This system focuses the parallel light from the collimator lens onto the film. As the name indicates, the camera lens is part of the camera.

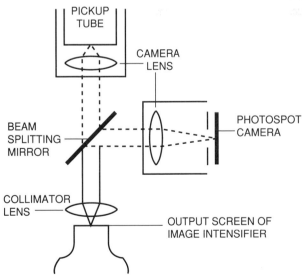

Figure 13–10. Lens systems located at the output screen of the image intensifier.

PHOTOSPOT

Photospot recording uses light to expose the film, thus the name photospot. The film used for photospot recording may be roll or cut type. The photospot system is often referred to as the millimeter camera. The millimeter camera consists of a storage film reel (unexposed film), a pull arm, an aperture, a take-up film reel or magazine (exposed film) and a shutter (Figure 13–11).

The millimeter camera is commonly available in three sizes, 70 mm, 90 mm and 105 mm. The actual size of the image is slightly smaller. This is because the holes on the side of the film used to move the film occupy some area of the film. The larger the film, the better the film quality of the image. However, larger film requires more radiation for exposure, which increases the patient dose. Because the individual frames are small relative to conventional film, a special plastic or self-adhesive holder may be used to store the film (Figure 13–12). Roll film is cut before it can be stored in the plastic container.

Photospot filming is faster than spot filming. The maximum rate of photospot recording is generally 12 exposures (frames) per second. This rate is fast

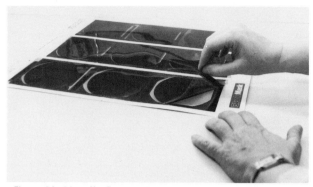

Figure 13–12. Self-adhesive millimeter film holder storage container.

enough to record slowly moving organs, e.g., movement of the esophagus during swallowing.

To record an image, the operator energizes the photospot switch. This opens the shutter of the camera, allowing the light emitted from the beam splitter to enter the aperture of the camera, exposing the film. After exposure, the film is advanced. While the film is advancing, the shutter closes, preventing light from entering the camera. The exposed film is transported to the take-up reel or magazine. This process is synchronized with the x-ray exposure so that radiation is produced only when the shutter is opened. The exposed film is developed in the same processor used for conventional films. Sometimes, a lead film is attached to the millimeter film. This is especially useful for roll film to prevent the natural curl of the film from jamming the processor.

CINERADIOGRAPHY

Cineradiography is similar to photospot recording. Cineradiographic film is available in 16-mm and 35-mm sizes. As with photospot film, the actual size of the image on the film is slightly smaller than the film. Also, the larger film has better image quality and requires more radiation, increasing patient dose. Cineradiography differs from photospot recording in the number of frames that can be exposed per second. Cineradiographic frame rates are much faster than photospot frame frequency. Framing rates for cineradiography are a function of the sine wave. In the United States, where electricity is produced at a 60 cycle per second rate, the cineradiographic frame frequency is a multiple of

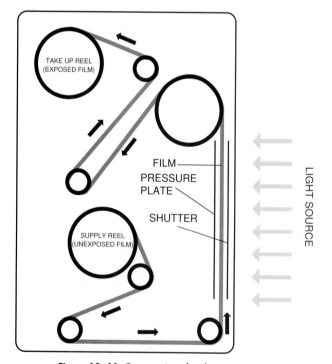

Figure 13–11. Cross section of a photospot camera.

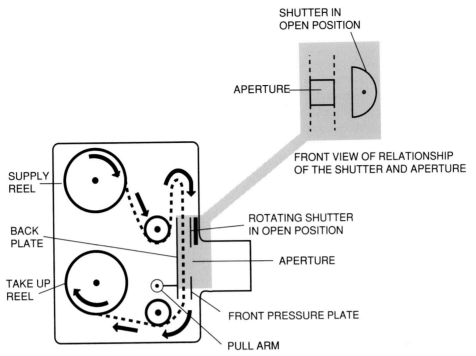

Figure 13–13. Cross section of a cinefluorography camera.

60. Common rates for cine are 7.5, 15, 30 and 60 frames per second. The high framing speed is useful in organs that move rapidly, e.g., the heart.

The cineradiographic camera is similar to a commercial movie camera. The cineradiographic camera consists of shutter, camera lens, aperture, film reels, front pressure plate, pull down arm and back plate (Figure 13–13). Image recording is comparable with that with the photospot camera. An image is recorded on cineradiographic film when the shutter opens and exposes the film. The pull down arm advances the film one frame. The front pressure plate holds the film against the back plate. While the film is advancing, the shutter is closed. This process is synchronized with the x-ray pulse. After exposure, the cineradiographic film is developed in a special processor. It is important that the processor be properly maintained to obtain high quality images.

Recall that both photospot and cineradiographic films are rectangular and the output screen is circular. Thus, it is impossible to expose the film without either overexposing the patient or having some areas of the film unexposed. Exposing a frame of film is called framing. There are several types of framing. The two most common types are exact framing and overframing (Figure 13–14). In exact framing, 100% of the image is recorded on only 60% of the film. Overframing demonstrates 60% of the image on 100% of the film. This method results in a magnified image and increases the patient dose.

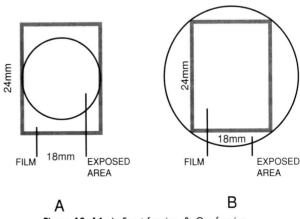

Figure 13–14. A, Exact framing. B, Overframing.

MAGNETIC TAPE OR DISC

Recently, the use of magnetic tape and disc has become a popular means of imaging. Among the U.S. public, the use of magnetic tape or disc to project movies is widespread. Projection of movies is achieved by attaching a videotape recorder (VTR) or videocassette recorder (VCR) to a television monitor. The principles of using VCR and magnetic tape or disc to image a fluoroscopic image are identical. As with a home VCR, fluoroscopic magnetic tape or disc requires a magnetic recorder and television monitor.

Before discussion of the function of a magnetic recorder, a review of electricity and magnetism is appropriate. Recall that a magnetic field surrounds an electrical current. Also, some materials are easily magnetized (ferromagnetic). Thus, it is possible to induce a magnetic field in a ferromagnetic object by placing the object near the magnetic field. This constitutes the basic principle of how an image is recorded on tape or disc. Playing back the image employs the concept of moving a magnetic field (moving tape or disc) through a stationary conductor (wiring of the unit). This process induces an electrical current in the wire. More specific information regarding recording and playback follows.

The magnetic recorder consists of a device to record the image (tape or disc) and a metallic core to record or play back the image (Figure 13–15). The metallic core is often identified as a read/write head. To demonstrate how a magnetic recorder works, the following discussion relates to a magnetic tape system.

The magnetic tape unit is placed between the control unit and the television monitor. Recording

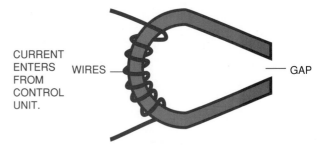

Figure 13–16. Read/write head.

begins when the electronic signal is received from the control unit. The signal enters the magnetic recorder via wires. These wires are attached to the read/write head (Figure 13–16). The current induces a magnetic field in the head. The magnetic field intensity is directly proportional to the intensity and direction of the electrical current. Surrounding the head is a thin tape (usually Mylar) containing magnetic material (generally iron oxide). A magnetic field is induced in the tape when the tape moves past the head gap. The intensity and direction of the magnetic field is directly proportional to the current (Figure 13–17).

Unlike the case with film, no processing is needed to view the image. Rather, to play back the image, the tape is rewound to the appropriate area. After the tape is rewound, the play button is depressed. The tape moves across the head, inducing the identical magnetic field pattern of the tape on the head. The magnetic field induces an electrical current of equal intensity on the wires attached to the head. The current is transmitted to a television monitor, where it is converted to a visible image.

Magnetic discs function in the same manner as tapes. The disc is circular and flat. Its appearance is similar to that of a phonographic record. There are hundreds of individual grooves on the surface of the disc. The grooves are where the image is magnetized. Discs are more advantageous than tape because discs can randomly (immediately) access an image and they provide a higher resolution, especially in the slow/stop frame mode.

RECORDING MODALITY COMPARISON

All recording modalities have advantages and disadvantages. Often, selecting one modality over

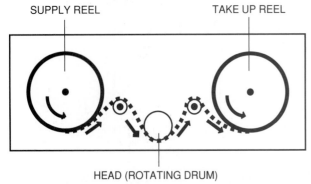

Figure 13–15. Top view of reel to reel magnetic tape recorder.

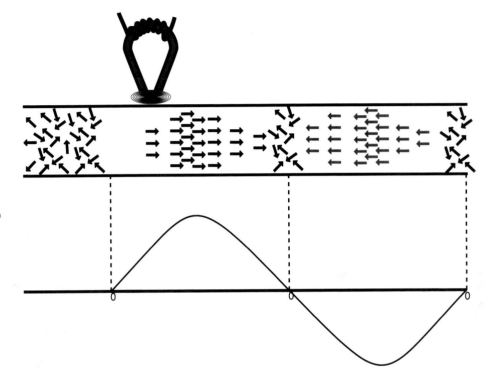

Figure 13–17. Intensity and direction of magnetic field induced on tape.

Table 13–2. RECORDING MODALITY COMPARISON

Item	Spot Film	Photospot	Cineradiography	Magnetic Tape or Disc
Quality	Excellent	Good	Good	Poor
Storage	Sheet	Sheet	Roll	Reel/disc
Patient dose	High	Low	Low	Low
Reusable	No	No	No	Yes
Processor	X-ray	X-ray	Special	None
Frame rate	1/s	12/s	60/s	60 rpm

another requires a compromise of other factors. The spot film provides the best film quality. The films are also easily stored in the patient's record folder. However, spot filming has a high patient dose and is slow. It is not recommended for motion studies. The photospot system is useful in studying limited motion organs. The quality of the image is poorer than that achieved with spot filming. However, there is a significant decrease in patient dose. For extremely fast organ movement, cineradiography is the modality of choice. However, it requires a special processor and the film rolls are cumbersome to store. Magnetic imaging is most useful when a need exists to see the image immediately. It has the advantage of being reusable and does not require a processor. Storing the tapes for future reference is cumbersome. Table 13–2 summarizes recording modality comparison.

Bibliography

Ball, JL and Price, T. Chesney's Radiographic imaging (5th edition). Boston: Blackwell Scientific Publications, 1989.

Bushong, SC. Radiologic science for technologists (4th edition). St. Louis: Mosby, 1988.

Chesney, DN and Chesney, MO. Radiographic imaging (4th edition). Boston: Blackwell Scientific Publications, 1981.

Chesney, DN and Chesney, MO. X-ray equipment for student radiographers (3rd edition). Boston: Blackwell Scientific Publications, 1984.

Cullinan, AM. Producing quality radiographs. New York: Lippincott, 1987.

Cullinan, JE and Cullinan, AM. Illustrated guide to x-ray technics (2nd edition). New York: Lippincott, 1980.

Curry, TS, Dowdey, JE and Murry, RC. Christensen's Introduction to the physics of diagnostic radiology (3rd edition). Philadelphia: Lea & Febiger, 1984.

Curry, TS, Dowdey, JE and Murry, RC. Christensen's Physics of diagnostic radiology (4th edition). Philadelphia: Lea & Febiger, 1990.

Hendee, WR, Chaney, EL and Rossi, RP. Radiologic physics, equipment and quality control. Chicago: Year Book Medical, 1976.

Kelsey, CA. Essentials of radiology physics. St. Louis: Warren H. Green, 1985.

Sprawls, P. Principles of radiography for technologists. Rockville, MD: Aspen, 1990.

United States Department of Health and Human Resources. Regulations for the administration and enforcement of the radiation control for health and safety act of 1968. FDA 88-8035 (supersedes HEW publication FDA 90–8035). Rockville, MD: U.S. Government Printing Office, April 1988.

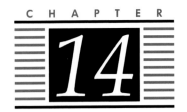

CONVENTIONAL TOMOGRAPHY AND QUALITY CONTROL

INTRODUCTION

The human body is a three dimensional object having length, width and depth. A conventional radiograph of the human body is a two dimensional representation of the organs and is unable to demonstrate depth. This two dimensional portrayal of the organs makes them appear as if they are in the same plane (the organs overlap each other). For example, when viewing a conventional anterior-posterior radiograph of the abdomen, it is impossible to tell if the gallbladder is more anterior or more posterior than the thoracic spine. In the majority of imaging procedures, this organ overlapping is of no consequence and does not interfere with the film's diagnostic utility. However, sometimes there is a need to remove superimposition of organs to obtain a diagnostic radiograph. There are five ways to circumvent the superimposition of organs:
1. Stereoradiography
2. Magnification
3. Rotation of the patient
4. Breathing technique (a form of tomography)
5. Tomography

Stereoradiography is a special technique in which two radiographs are exposed at different tube positions. Chapter 20, Film, Film Processing and Photographic Techniques, provides detailed information about stereoradiography.

An object's magnification is related to the ratio of the object-film distance (OFD) to the source-object distance (SOD), or OFD/SOD (see Chapter 26, Geometric Image Quality). Magnification increases when the SOD is short relative to the OFD. Magnification is useful in demonstrating the structure of interest when objects are anatomically far apart. The part farthest from the film has the greatest magnification and is essentially blurred, leaving the object closest to the film (object of interest) visible. An example is a posterior-anterior mandible radiograph taken at a short source-image distance (SID). In this example, the cervical spine (part farthest from the film) is blurred, leaving the mandible visible.

Sometimes the mere rotation of the human body is enough to move one object away from another. The farther apart the objects are, the less degree of rotation is required to visualize them separately.

The breathing method is also useful in blurring objects obscuring the visibility of other structures. In this method, it is important that only the object needing to be blurred moves. An example is a breathing technique for the lateral thoracic spine. In this example, a long exposure is used while the patient is breathing. The ribs are blurred, facilitating the visibility of the thoracic spine.

Tomography (body section radiography) is a special method of imaging in which the tube and the film move in opposite directions while the patient is stationary. This method is designed to obtain a diagnostic image of an object lying in a specific plane while blurring structures lying above or below (superimposed on) the plane of interest. The principles and methods necessary for this process to occur are presented in this chapter.

NOMENCLATURE

Research and development of tomography occurred in the early 1900s. At that time, there were many individuals in several countries performing experiments relative to tomography. It was common for individual researchers to use different terminology in describing similar processes. This diversity of terms presented communication problems. For example, the terms planigraphy, stratigraphy and laminography are synonyms for tomography. Recognizing the need to standardize terminology, in 1962 a subcommittee of the International Commission on Radiological Units and Measures (ICRU) established the generic term tomography to describe all forms of body section radiography. Even today with the standard terminology, it is not unusual to find that in different geographical locations different terms are used to describe the same item or process. To avoid any semantic problems that may arise, the following is the nomenclature used in this text:

Tomogram–the radiograph produced by a tomographic unit.

Fulcrum–the pivot point about which the tube and the film move.

Fulcrum level–the distance from the fulcrum to the table top.

Objective plane (focal plane)–the plane where the area of the object appears sharp or is in focus.

Exposure angle–the angle formed by x-ray beam movement during exposure.

Amplitude–the tube movement or shift measured in inches or centimeters per second.

Tube shift–the distance the tube travels.

Tube trajectory–the path of the tube during movement.

Blur–the distortion of objects outside the objective plane.

Blur margin–the edge of the blurred object.

TUBE MOVEMENTS

There are six common types of tube movements used in tomography. They are (from simplest to most complex) rectilinear, curvilinear, elliptical, circular, spiral and hypocycloidal (Figure 14–1). These tube trajectories are classified relative to the direction of tube travel. Because rectilinear and curvilinear tube movements are in one direction, they are classified as unidirectional. The remaining tube trajectories move in a variety of directions and are classified as pluridirectional or multidirectional.

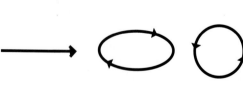 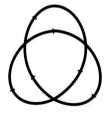

LINEAR   ELLIPTICAL   CIRCULAR   SPIRAL   HYPOCYCLOIDAL

Figure 14–1. Conventional tomographic tube movements.

In all of these movements, the tube is attached to the film and both revolve around a point called the fulcrum. It is important that the tube and the film move in opposite directions.

UNIDIRECTIONAL CONVENTIONAL TOMOGRAPHY

Unidirectional, or linear, tomography is the simplest type of tube movement. Owing to its simplicity, it is a good model for explaining the principles of tomography. Thus, of the various types of tube trajectories, unidirectional is discussed in detail.

The advantage of linear tomography is that the equipment is inexpensive and can be attached to almost any radiographic unit with only minor modifications. The tomographic equipment is easy to assemble and disassemble. Thus, it takes about 10–15 minutes to convert a conventional radiographic room to perform linear tomography and vice versa. The apparatus needed to convert a radiographic room for linear tomography are a metal rod, a fulcrum level attachment and a tomographic control panel.

In linear tomography, a metal rod attaches the tube to the Bucky tray (Figure 14–2). The purpose of the rod is to ensure that the tube and the Bucky tray move in opposite directions during the exposure (Figure 14–3). The movement of the tube over distance is accomplished by energizing a motor, which is usually attached near the tube head or the back of the table.

Connected to the side of the table is the fulcrum level attachment (Figure 14–4). The fulcrum level

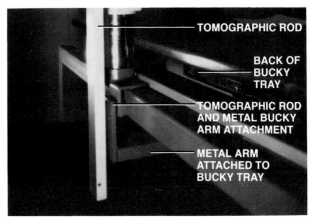

Figure 14–2. Linear tomographic unit.

attachment is used to adjust the height of the fulcrum (relative to the table top) to the area of interest. The height is adjusted by manually turning a knob or pressing an electronic button, which turns a worm gear, moving the fulcrum either up or down.

The length of the exposure is determined by the speed of the x-ray tube travel and the exposure angle. Some linear tomographic units allow the operator to adjust the tube travel speed. This speed is usually measured in inches or centimeters per second (amplitude). As the speed of the tube increases, the exposure time decreases. Another factor determining the length of the exposure time is the exposure angle. Adjusting the exposure angle usually changes the distance between two microswitches. The greater the exposure angle, the greater the distance between the microswitches. As the distance increases, the exposure time increases,

Figure 14–3. Unidirectional tomographic tube movements.

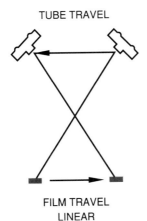

TUBE TRAVEL

FILM TRAVEL
LINEAR

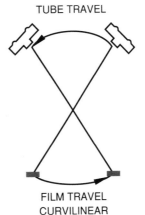

TUBE TRAVEL

FILM TRAVEL
CURVILINEAR

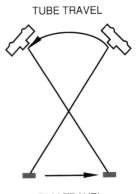

TUBE TRAVEL

FILM TRAVEL
LINEAR WITH CURVILINEAR

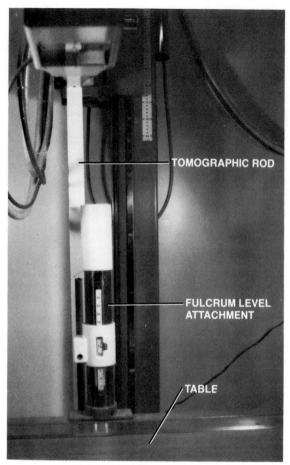

Figure 14–4. Fulcrum level attachment.

Proper equipment setup involves connecting the fulcrum level attachment to the table and connecting the rod to the tube and the Bucky tray. All knobs used to connect the equipment, e.g., the knob used to secure the rod to the tube, must be tight. Because the tube moves along the longitudinal axis of the table, the longitudinal tube lock must be off (open). Also, the lock used to secure the Bucky tray must be off to enable the Bucky tray to move during exposure. The only other lock that needs to be off is the mechanism used to angle the tube. Locks that must be on are the transverse, center and vertical locks. Engaging these locks ensures that the tube is centered and maintains a constant OFD/SOD ratio during the exposure.

In linear tube movement, the tube trajectory is such that the SIDs at the extreme ends of tube travel are longer than those at midtravel (see Figure 14–3). This increased distance decreases the x-ray beam intensity (by the inverse square law). The tomographic film density varies relative to the beam intensity. By visual observation of the movement, it seems that there should also be a variation in magnification. However, the ratio of the OFD to SOD for all points of travel is the same (Figure 14–7). Thus, the magnification is unchanged.

To correct the variation of x-ray beam intensity and maintain uniform tomographic film density, the linear tube movement may be modified to a

assuming that the amplitude is constant. Tomographic units that permit the operator to change speed and exposure angle usually have a chart to determine the exposure time (Figure 14–5).

The tomographic control panel is used to operate the tomographic apparatus (Figure 14–6). This panel is usually a separate unit mounted on the wall near the main control panel or near the x-ray table. The panel contains switches to control the exposure angle, the fulcrum level, the tube speed and the motor that moves the tube. When the tomographic control panel is turned on, the direction of the current is altered so that it bypasses the conventional radiographic control of the tube and engages the tomographic motor needed for tube movement. Before using the control panel to energize the tomographic unit, the operator must properly set up the tomographic equipment.

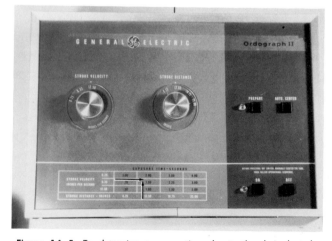

Figure 14–5. To determine exposure time, locate the desired stroke velocity (inches per second), move across the row until the column representing the desired stroke distance (inches) is reached and read the exposure time. In this example, a velocity of 8.33 inches per second and stroke distance of 12.50 inches has an exposure time of 1.50 seconds.

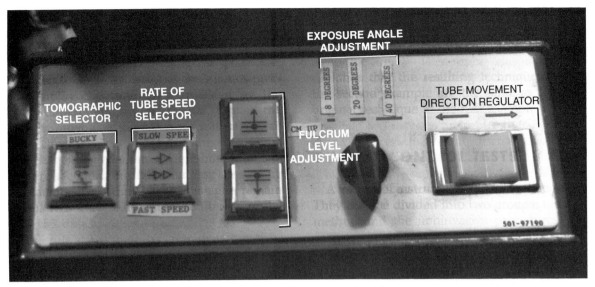

Figure 14–6. Tomographic control panel.

curvilinear trajectory (see Figure 14–3). In a curvilinear trajectory, both the tube and the film move in an arc. This results in a constant SID and uniform beam intensity throughout the entire tube travel.

It is not unusual for imaging departments to utilize a combination of linear and curvilinear movements. In this combination, the tube moves in an arc while the film movement is straight (see Figure 14–3). Consequently, the SID is constant, but the OFD/SOD ratio changes. The fluctuation in the OFD/SOD ratio causes a variation in the degree of magnification. However, in practice, the variation in magnification is too small to be detected by the human eye and does not affect the radiograph's diagnostic quality.

PLURIDIRECTIONAL CONVENTIONAL TOMOGRAPHY

Linear tube movement has the disadvantage of creating streaks on the tomogram, decreasing image sharpness. The streaks are a direct result of the type of tube movement (see under Blur for detailed information on linear streaks). Altering the type of tube trajectory to be multidirectional improves the sharpness of the tomographic image. There are four basic multidirectional tube movements. They are elliptical, circular, spiral and hypocycloidal (see Figure 14–1).

The elliptical movement is a slight variation from linear. Rather than moving in a straight line, the tube travels in an elliptical pattern. This trajectory tends to be limited to only one exposure angle

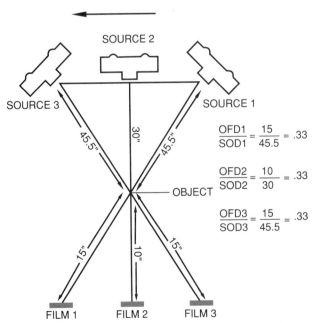

$$\frac{OFD1}{SOD1} = \frac{15}{45.5} = .33$$

$$\frac{OFD2}{SOD2} = \frac{10}{30} = .33$$

$$\frac{OFD3}{SOD3} = \frac{15}{45.5} = .33$$

Figure 14–7. Effect of linear movement on magnification. Note that the ratio of object-film distance (OFD) to source-object distance (SOD) is constant for all tube positions.

selection of 40 degrees. The circular pattern is an improvement over an elliptical one. The exposure angle changes when the radius of the circle is varied. The specific exposure angle is determined by the radii choices provided on the equipment. Spiral travel provides excellent image sharpness. However, it allows only small exposure angles. The most complex and efficient multidirectional movement is hypocycloidal. This movement has a fixed exposure angle of 48 degrees. The large exposure angle creates a thin objective plane (see under Thickness of Objective Plane), limiting the use of hypocycloidal trajectory to small anatomical parts.

In all these movements, it is important that the grid revolve to avoid grid cutoff or the unwanted radiation absorption of the primary beam (Chapter 24, Grids and Quality Control, has an in-depth discussion of grid cutoff). To obtain a sharp image, the film moves opposite the tube while maintaining the same position. In other words, film may be positioned north-south (N-S), and as the film rotates in a circle it maintains a N-S orientation. Figure 14–8 demonstrates the relationship of the film and grid relative to tube movement for a circular trajectory.

FULCRUM

The fulcrum is the pivot point of the rod connecting the tube and the Bucky tray. This pivot point is important because all structures located in the plane of the fulcrum (objective plane) and parallel to the tube movement remain in a constant position on the film during the tube travel (Figure 14–9). Consequently, these structures are well defined (sharp) on the tomogram. Because all objects above or below the objective plane move, they are blurred and are less visible on the tomogram than the stationary structures (see under Blur and Thickness of Objective Plane for the concept of image blurring and clarity). The anatomical part of interest is imaged by adjusting the fulcrum level to coincide

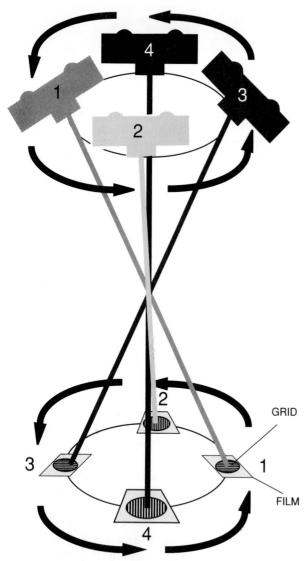

Figure 14–8. Relationship of film and grid to circular trajectory. Film maintains the same position and grid revolves.

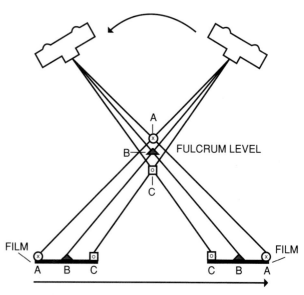

Figure 14–9. Relationship of points in and around the fulcrum level to their position on the film. Points A and C move from one side of the film to the other, whereas point B (fulcrum level) maintains its position.

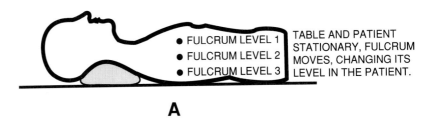

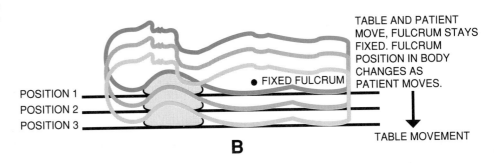

Figure 14–10. In a movable fulcrum (A), the patient and table are stationary while the fulcrum moves. A fixed fulcrum (B) has a stationary fulcrum about which the patient and table move.

with the height of the part. This may be achieved by either adjusting the level of the fulcrum (variable fulcrum) or using a fixed fulcrum and moving the part (Figure 14–10).

CHANGING THE FULCRUM LEVEL

The most common method of changing the fulcrum level for linear tomography is for the fulcrum itself to be movable. In this method, the patient remains at the same level and the height of the fulcrum is moved up or down until the desired plane is reached (Figure 14–10).

A fixed fulcrum is utilized most often with pluridirectional or specialized skull units. Changing the level of the fulcrum requires the object to move up or down (usually by adjusting the height of the table or Bucky tray) until the desired plane and fixed fulcrum are at the same level (Figure 14–10). Care needs to be taken when adjusting the fulcrum level on a unit for skull radiography. In these units, the patient is usually erect and tends to reposition his/her head (misalignment) when the Bucky tray moves. To obtain the proper fulcrum level, the object must be positioned identically for each level. Rotation of the part between levels images a plane other than the area of interest. Patient misalignment

does not tend to be an issue if the patient is recumbent and the entire table moves. In these cases, the patient is lying down, facilitating stability and making it relatively easy for the patient to maintain position as the table moves from one level to the next level (Figure 14–10).

DETERMINING FULCRUM LEVEL

The desired fulcrum level is usually determined by viewing two conventional radiographs of the object (e.g., anterior-posterior and lateral). An anterior-posterior radiograph helps locate the object relative to its lateral (right or left) placement in the body (Figure 14–11). The lateral film is useful in locating the object relative to its anterior-posterior position (Figure 14–11). Both films help determine the location of the object relative to its superior-inferior direction in the body.

The anterior-posterior and lateral measurements are used to obtain a scout tomogram at the middle of the object. Using the measurements of Figure 14–11, a scout tomogram would be taken with a fulcrum level set at 14 cm (assuming the patient is lying supine on the x-ray table). The central ray would be located 15 cm below the patient's shoulder and 10 cm from the patient's right side.

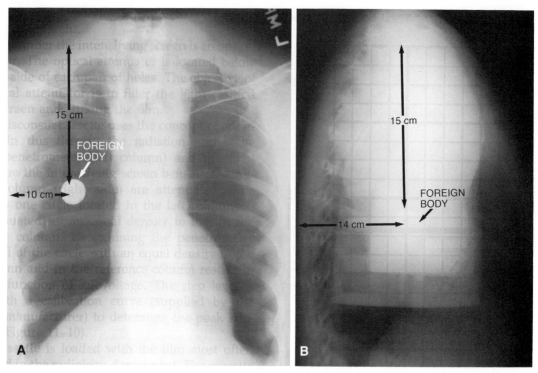

Figure 14—11. Determining fulcrum level. A, Anterior-posterior film is used to assess the lateral position of the object. B, Lateral radiograph helps locate the object relative to its anterior-posterior position in the body. Both films are used to identify the superior-inferior position of the object.

Because conventional radiography demonstrates some magnification, exact measurements are not always possible. Thus, it is not unusual for the initial scout tomogram to be located outside the midline of the object. To help determine a more accurate location of the object, a second scout tomogram may be taken 2 mm (for small objects) or 2 cm (for large objects) above or below the calculated midline of the object. Comparing the two scout tomograms provides a sense of direction as to whether to set additional fulcrum levels higher or lower than the initial scout tomogram. For example, if the first scout tomogram demonstrates a sharp image of the object of interest and the second scout tomogram (set 2 cm posterior to the first scout) shows the object blurred, but a well-defined vertebral spine, it can be assumed the object is anterior to the first fulcrum level. Thus, additional fulcrum levels would be taken at a height greater (more anterior) than the first scout tomogram. Another reason to take scout tomograms is to determine proper technique. A dark scout film necessitates that subsequent tomograms be exposed at lower

kilovoltage on milliampere settings. The converse is true for light scout tomograms.

MULTISECTIONAL CONVENTIONAL TOMOGRAPHY

Multisectional, or multilayer, conventional tomography is the ability to obtain multiple fulcrum levels (objective planes) during one tomographic exposure. The difference between single and multisectional images is in the cassette.

BOOK CASSETTE

Single layer (objective plane) tomography employs the same cassette used in conventional radiography. These cassettes hold a single sheet of film sandwiched between a pair of intensifying screens (Chapter 23, Film Holders and Intensifying Screens, addresses conventional radiographic cassettes in detail). To obtain four different objective planes requires four different exposures, with cassettes and fulcrum levels being changed between exposures.

Multisectional conventional tomography uses a special book cassette. These cassettes are constructed to hold several x-ray films at one time. Each film is sandwiched between a pair of intensifying screens. Each pair of intensifying screens is separated from its adjacent pair of screens by a radiolucent (e.g., polyester foam) spacer. The spacer material allows easy penetration (low absorption) of radiation. The width of the spacer used for book cassettes varies from 0.5 cm to 1 cm. The exception is a plesiotomogram. A plesiotomogram is a tomogram obtained using a special spacerless book cassette. The distance between films is the thickness of the intensifying screens (1 mm).

A specific book cassette contains spacers of the same width, e.g., 1 cm. The maximum number of films contained in a book cassette usually ranges from three to seven. The maximum number of films a specific book cassette can accommodate is determined by the manufacturer during construction of the cassette. The more films a book cassette stores,

the larger the cassette is. Large book cassettes cannot fit in a normal Bucky tray and must be placed in a special tray or drawer located under the Bucky tray.

Book cassettes are able to image several objective planes with one tomographic exposure. The number and distance between the objective planes is a function of the book cassette construction. A book cassette containing three films separated by 1-cm spacers images three different objective planes 1 cm apart (Figure 14–12). For example, assume a radiologist requests that multisectional tomograms be obtained at levels 18, 19, and 20 cm. To achieve these planes, the tomographic fulcrum is set at the highest level desired, in this case 20 cm. The tomographic fulcrum corresponds to the top film of the book cassette. To obtain the three levels simultaneously, a book cassette containing three films with 1-cm spacers is placed in the Bucky tray. The top film (film closest to the table top) represents the *set* fulcrum level of 20 cm. The middle film corresponds to an *effective* fulcrum level (an effective fulcrum level is the point at which the film and the tube pivot) of 19 cm. The last film in the book cassette

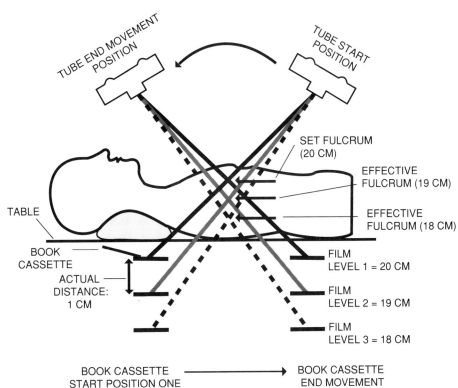

Figure 14–12. Multiple objective planes obtained with a book cassette (cassette size is enlarged for illustration purposes).

is at an effective fulcrum level of 18 cm. These multiple objective planes occur because the ratios of OFD to SOD for all three points are the same.

As x-rays pass from one film to the next, some radiation is absorbed by the spacers, screens and film. To obtain similar densities among the films, the speed of the intensifying screens increases as the distance from the film to the table top increases. The increase in intensifying screen speed helps to compensate for the decrease in radiation intensity.

Because there is a limit as to the fastest speed available for the bottom intensifying screen, the variations of speed among the screens need to be considered as a unit. Basically, the bottom screen establishes the fastest speed. As one moves closer to the top of the book cassette, screen speed is reduced (becomes slower). The top screen has the slowest speed. Consequently, to obtain the density needed for a diagnostic tomogram, the top screen requires a higher exposure value than that for single layer tomography.

DOSE

The amount of radiation dose to the patient is less for multisectional conventional tomography than for single cassette tomography containing the same number of tomograms. It would appear that, when using a five film book cassette, the patient would receive one-fifth the amount of radiation received by a patient exposed using five individual tomograms. However, the absorption of radiation by the book cassette and the varying intensifying screen speeds require a higher exposure value than that for single layer tomography. It is estimated that a patient exposed using a book cassette receives about one-half the amount of radiation received by a patient exposed using a single tomography method. The actual amount of exposure decrease obtained by using a book cassette is a factor of the thickness of the cassette and the specific technical factors employed.

When considering the dose to the patient in both single and multiple conventional tomography, proper radiation protection techniques should be applied. For example, special care must be taken when the cornea of the eye is irradiated. The cornea is sensitive to radiation and should be protected with a lead shield during tomography. Other radia-tion protection techniques for this area include the use of a round cone and rare earth screens.

ADVANTAGES

There are several advantages to multisectional conventional tomography. These include saving time by reducing the number of exposures, extending the life span of the x-ray tube by using fewer heat units, decreasing radiation exposure to the patient and obtaining different objective planes of an organ while it is in the same physiological phase, e.g., respiration.

DISADVANTAGES

The primary disadvantage of multisectional conventional tomography is poor radiation quality. The decreased tomographic detail is a result of the fast speed of the intensifying screens and the scatter radiation produced from the book cassette. A dis-advantage of lesser consequence is the increased costs for special cassettes and possible Bucky equip-ment. The cost is usually incurred in the initial purchase.

BLUR

FACTORS AFFECTING BLUR

The objective of tomography is to remove (blur) images that obscure structures of interest. Images are blurred by having them move from one point on the film to another (see Figure 14–9). The greater the movement is, the more the image is blurred. Images that maintain a constant position on the film appear well defined (sharp). During tomography, structures located in the objective plane maintain a constant position on the film, while objects above and below the objective plane change their location on the film. Four factors affecting the degree of image blurring are the distance the object is from the objective plane, the tube trajectory, the exposure angle and the distance of the object from the film.

The farther an object is from the objective plane, the more it moves, increasing blurring. The mathematical relationship expressing movement of an object is

$$Movement = 2d \tan \theta/2$$

where d is the distance of the object from the fulcrum and θ is the exposure angle. An object 6 cm from the fulcrum moves twice as far as an object 3 cm from the fulcrum (assuming that the exposure angle is constant). This may be illustrated by inserting the appropriate numbers in the movement formula, or

d = 3 cm	d = 6 cm
θ = 30 degrees	θ = 30 degrees
Movement = 2(3) {tan 30/2}	Movement = 2(6) {tan 30/2}
Movement = 6(tan 15)	Movement = 12(tan 15)
Movement = 6(0.2679)	Movement = 12(0.2679)
Movement = 1.6074 cm	Movement = 3.2148 cm

In practice, the relationship of the distance an organ or pathologic feature (object) is from the objective plane is a function of the human body. Thus, although the tomography operator can adjust the objective plane (fulcrum) level, the distance of other organs to the plane of interest is out of the control of the operator.

One factor that affects blurring and is under the operator's control is the type of tube trajectory used. As discussed above, tube movement may be unidirectional or pluridirectional (see under Tube Movements). Maximum blurring of an object occurs when the structure is perpendicular to the direction of the tube movement. Objects parallel to tube movement have a minimum amount of blurring. Figure 14–13 shows tomograms of an object 3 cm above the objective plane; the tomograms demonstrate the degree of blurring of four types of tube trajectories. It can be seen from Figure 14–13 that pluridirectional tube trajectories, e.g., hypocycloidal, have the greatest amount of blurring. The simplest tube movement, linear, demonstrates that it is possible for an object to be outside the objective plane and be unblurred (sharp). Objects parallel to linear tube movement cause streaks (parasite lines) that are readily visible on the tomogram (Figure 14–14). The increased efficiency of the pluridirectional tube trajectories is attributed to the ability of the tube to change directions so that few objects are parallel to the tube movement.

A third factor affecting the amount of blurring is exposure angle. As the exposure angle becomes wider, the amount of blurring increases. Exposure angle is discussed under Thickness of Objective Plane.

The object's distance from the film is the last factor affecting the amount of blurring. Objects farthest from the film are blurred more than objects close to the film (assuming that both objects are the same distance from the fulcrum level).

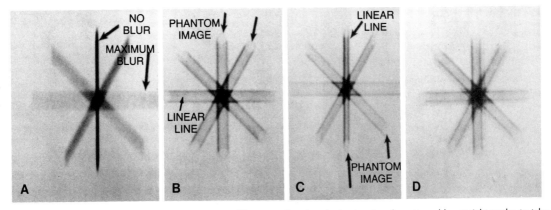

Figure 14–13. Effect of tube trajectory on blurring. A, Linear (no blurring in direction of tube travel and maximum blur at right angles to tube travel). B, Circular (equal blurring around radius. Phantom images and linear lines are present in the object [see arrows]). C, Elliptical (combination of linear and circular blur characteristics). D, Hypocycloidal (maximum blur all over). (From Phillips Medical Systems.)

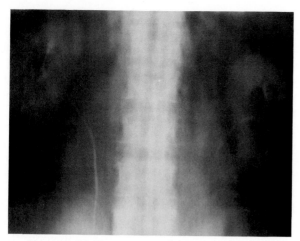

Figure 14–14. Linear tomogram demonstrating blur streaks.

PHANTOM IMAGES

All types of tube movements produce phantom images. Phantom images are pseudoshadows appearing on a tomogram. These shadows do not represent a real object but do give the illusion of being real structures. These shadows may interfere with the film's diagnostic value. Circular, linear and short exposure angle tube trajectories are the most common types of tube movements apt to create phantom images of significance to hinder film interpretation. Phantom images occur by either blur margin overlap or displacement of a blurred image. (It should be noted that parasite lines, or streaks, seen on linear tomography are not classified as phantom images. The streaks are unblurred images of a real object.) In blur margin overlap, the margin from one object overlaps the blur margin of another object (Figure 14–15). Phantom images created by displacement are commonly produced in short exposure angle circular tomography. Often, these images are shadows from dense objects and give the appearance of a less dense (soft tissue) structure located within the focal plane.

THICKNESS OF OBJECTIVE PLANE

As indicated above, the degree of blurring increases as the distance from the fulcrum level increases. Thus, the blurring of images is a gradual

process. Also, the human eye is limited in its ability to perceive blurred images. Consequently, the eye accepts a certain amount of blur as a sharp image. The amount of blur the eye accepts is subjective and varies from one individual to another. The gradual blurring and the limitation of the human eye's ability to recognize blur contribute to the objective plane's having a certain amount of thickness.

Thus, even though in theory a plane represents points without thickness, in practice the objective plane has thickness. This thickness often results in tomography being described as radiography of a slice, or slab, of the human body. The slice, or slab, is often referred to by radiographers as a cut. The radiographer should be extremely cautious to avoid using the term "cut" in the presence of patients. The lack of imaging experience by patients often causes the misinterpretation of the word "cut" to mean surgery. This misinterpretation may not always be communicated verbally to the radiographer. The thought of having or needing surgery

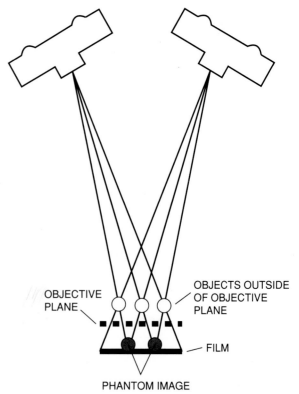

Figure 14–15. Phantom image: blur overlap.

results in unnecessary stress and anxiety to the patient.

The amount of thickness of the objective plane is a function of the exposure angle. Most tomographic machines permit the operator to change the exposure angle. The greater the angle, the thinner the objective plane (Figure 14–16). Section thickness may be determined by using a simplified version of a formula developed by Kieffer (Selman, 1985, p. 448). The formula is

$$h = B/\{\tan \theta/2\}$$

where h is section thickness, B is maximum permissible blur and θ is the exposure angle. For example, if the maximum permissible blur is 0.5 mm, when using an exposure angle of 10 degrees, the section thickness is approximately 5.7 mm, or

$$h = 0.5/\{\tan 10/2\}$$
$$h = 0.5/ \tan 5$$
$$h = 0.5/0.08749$$
$$h = 5.7 \text{ mm}$$

An increase of exposure angle to 40 degrees decreases the thickness of the section to approximately 1.4 mm, or

$$h = 0.5/\{\tan 40/2\}$$
$$h = 0.5/\tan 20$$
$$h = 0.5/0.3640$$
$$h = 1.4 \text{ mm}$$

Tomography employing an exposure angle between 5 and 10 degrees produces a thick objective plane. This type of tomography is called zonography. The film produced by zonography is called a zonogram. The differences between a zonogram and a large exposure angle tomogram are in the thickness of the objective plane and the amount of contrast. Zonograms have a thicker objective plane and a higher contrast (fewer shades of gray) than do tomograms using large exposure angles. Zonography is useful in removing an object from surrounding structures. In zonography, the object tends to be viewed as a unit (one large section). The use of exposure angles greater than 10 degrees is indicated when there is a need to study an object

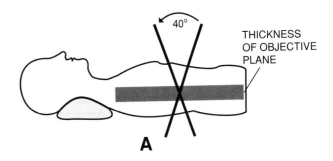

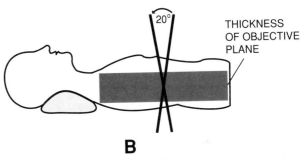

Figure 14–16. Effect of exposure angle on thickness of objective plane. A, Large angle results in a thin section. B, Small angles produce a thick objective plane.

in more detail. This is achieved by examining the object in sections instead of as a unit.

As stated above, some tomographic units use amplitude to describe tube travel. If the tube travel remains constant, any change in SID alters the exposure angle, which affects the thickness of the objective plane (Figure 14–17). For example, a tube moving at a rate of 12 inches per second travels 36 inches for a 3 second exposure. Figure 14–17 demonstrates the exposure angle increase (creating a thinner objective plane) when the same amplitude (12 inches per second) and exposure time (3 seconds) are used at shorter SIDs. Regulating objective plane thickness by amplitude is impractical and is discouraged. Section thickness is best altered by adjusting the exposure angle.

It is advantageous to adjust the thickness of the objective plane to correspond to the part being imaged. Because the sizes of organs vary, large organs, e.g., lung, are better imaged using a thick objective plane. Small organs, e.g., inner ear, are best imaged using a thin objective plane.

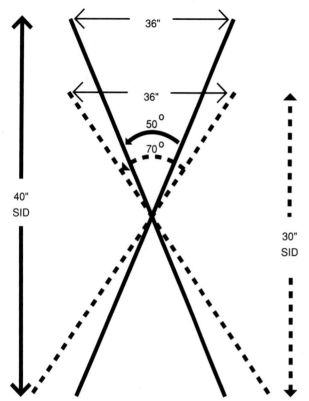

Figure 14–17. As the source-image distance (SID) decreases from 40 inches to 30 inches, the exposure angle increases, assuming the amplitude (12 inches per second) and the exposure time (3 seconds) remain constant.

TOMOGRAPHIC QUALITY CONTROL

When assessing the effectiveness of a tomographic unit, the following 11 areas should be tested:

1. Tube motion (trajectory)
2. Mechanical stability
3. Completeness of exposure
4. Tube travel speed constancy
5. Symmetrical relationship of the exposure angle to the table and itself
6. Exposure angle
7. Thickness of the objective plane
8. Blur margin
9. Blur quality
10. Resolution
11. Focal plane

Many of the assessments may be conducted during one exposure of an appropriate test tool. A simple pinhole test instrument can be employed to

determine tube motion, mechanical stability, completeness of exposure, tube travel constancy, exposure angle and symmetrical relationship. The remaining tests can be achieved by using a composite phantom. This is a type of phantom that contains several items, e.g., wire patterns, wire mesh, bone.

PINHOLE TEST

To conduct a pinhole test, a lead shield with a 2–3 mm hole drilled in the center is needed. The lead shield is placed about 5 inches (12 cm) above the fulcrum level and is exposed with the desired technique and tube movement. The geometric configuration of the tube is readily visible (Figure 14–18) on the tomogram.

Examination of the image for smoothness determines the mechanical stability of the tube movement. Tube trajectories that are unstable (shake or

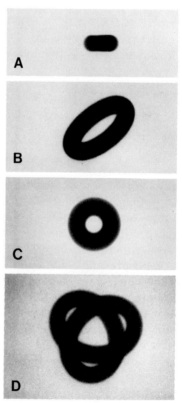

Figure 14–18. Pinhole test demonstrating the geometric configuration of the tube (trajectory). A, Linear; B, elliptical; C, circular; D, hypocycloidal.

vibrate during exposure) demonstrate an uneven image.

Inspecting the image to ensure that it is solid (no unexposed areas) assesses the completeness of the exposure. A solid line (unbroken) image represents a complete exposure.

If any changes in density are observed throughout the image, there is a variation in tube travel speed. The denser areas indicate a higher exposure rate and possible slow tube travel. A properly operating tomographic unit has a constant tube travel rate.

The location of the image relative to the table indicates if tube travel is symmetrical. Also, comparing the center of the image to the outer edges (radii) assesses the symmetry of the image to itself.

To determine the exposure angle, the pinhole is placed at the level of the fulcrum. Two exposures are made while the film is stationary. The first exposure is made with the central ray perpendicular to the film. The second exposure is made as the tube moves through its cycle. The exposure angle is calculated by measuring the distance between the pinhole and the film and measuring the distance between the image of the perpendicular central ray and the edge of the tube movement image (Figure 14–19). The exposure is determined by the formula

$$\text{Tan } \theta = \frac{\text{distance between central ray and image}}{\text{distance between pinhole and film}}$$

COMPOSITE PHANTOM

One type of composite phantom is made by 3M Company in St. Paul, MN. This phantom is designed to perform several tests using one exposure. The fulcrum is set at midphantom level during the exposure.

Section thickness is one of the tests of the composite phantom. Section thickness is determined by viewing the image of two slanted wires and a ruler. One wire is slanted to a 5 cm depth and is used to measure centimeter levels. The second wire has a 1-cm inclined depth and measures millimeters. Observing the areas appearing sharp (well defined) of the wires and comparing them with the appropriate scale on the ruler indicates the thickness of the objective plane. Because the acuity of human eyes differs, the length of the sharpness is subjective.

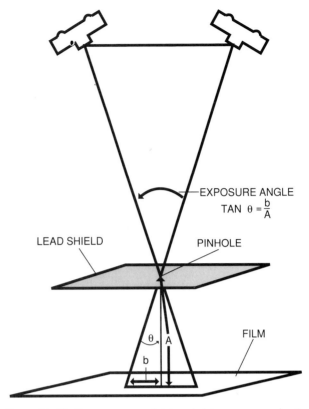

Figure 14–19. Measurements needed to calculate exposure angle. A, Pinhole to film distance; b, central ray to edge of tube movement image distance.

Another test of the composite phantom is assessment of blur quality. The blur quality is obtained by imaging two copper wire patterns. One wire consists of a series of arcs and the other is an eight-pointed star pattern. The arc pattern is exposed 5 mm above the objective plane and the star pattern is at the fulcrum level. By analyzing the images, it is possible to determine the blur quality. The arc pattern demonstrates the blur pattern for objects outside the objective plane. The star pattern, being at the fulcrum level, should be well defined.

Blur margin is tested by using nine wires located in the composite phantom. The center wire is perpendicular, while the remaining wires are inclined at 5 degree increments. A good tomogram demonstrates a circular center wire, with the remaining wires being oval.

To assess resolution, the composite phantom has three wire meshes consisting of differing numbers of lines per inch. The lines per inch of the wire meshes are 20, 30 and 50. An exposure is made with the fulcrum level at the middle of the wire meshes. The tomogram is inspected to determine which wire mesh has the sharpest image. The wire mesh with the sharpest image represents the resolution level. A good tomographic unit is able to resolve (demonstrate) 50 lines per inch.

The last test of the composite phantom is used to assess the focal plane. It consists of taking a tomogram of a bone with a simulated lesion. The lesion is removed and a conventional radiograph is taken. The tomogram and radiograph are compared for focal plane quality.

VARIATIONS OF CONVENTIONAL TOMOGRAPHY

Many techniques evolved from the fundamental principles of conventional tomography. Of these techniques, autotomography, pantomography, skip tomography and computed tomography (CT) are discussed briefly.

AUTOTOMOGRAPHY

Autotomography is a method of blurring unwanted structures. In this technique, the tube and film remain stationary while the patient moves. An example of autotomography is breathing technique for a lateral thoracic spine or sternum film.

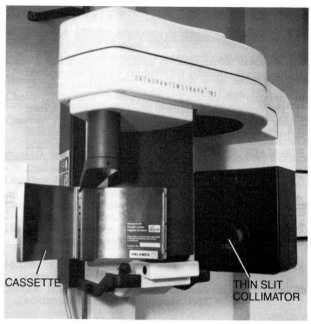

CASSETTE   THIN SLIT COLLIMATOR

Figure 14–20. Pantomograph machine.

PANTOMOGRAPHY

Pantomography is limited to radiography of curved surfaces, usually of the skull area, e.g., mandible. This technique requires the use of a curved cassette. During pantomography, the tube moves, exposing the film using a thin (narrow) slit beam restrictor (Figure 14–20 is an example of a

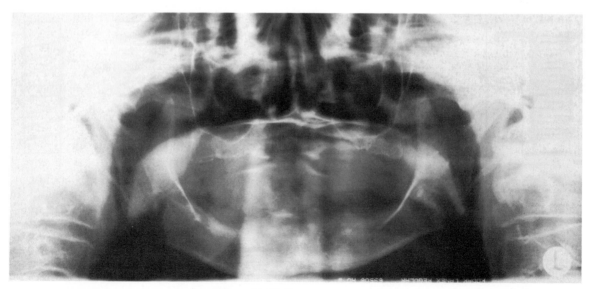

Figure 14–21. Pantomogram.

pantomograph unit). The slit prevents diverging x-rays from striking the film. Thus, only straight rays expose the film. Because divergent rays are responsible for producing penumbra (blurred area) on the film, the image produced appears motionless and sharp. The resulting pantomogram (film) is a flattened image of a curved surface (Figure 14–21).

SKIP TOMOGRAPHY

Skip tomography is a tomographic technique in which the exposure stops during the center of the tube travel (Figure 14–22). The intent is to avoid imaging dense objects that overlay the structures of interest. This technique is best applied when the dense object and structure of interest are located far apart. Also, it is important to use this technique with a large exposure angle to include the distances skipped and those exposed.

COMPUTED TOMOGRAPHY

The use of CT in medicine originated in the United States about 1975. CT is similar to conven-

Figure 14–23. Computed tomographic image. (Courtesy of Mr. Ken Wintch.)

tional tomography in that the tube and detectors (film in conventional tomography) move around a stationary patient. Unlike conventional tomography, CT does not use a film to produce images. Rather, the image is produced when the remnant radiation (the x-rays emitted from the patient) are recorded by a detector and sent to a computer for image construction. The computer analyzes the information received from the detectors and constructs an image. This image may be reproduced on radiographic film (Figure 14–23) for later use. Special equipment is required to produce CT images. The explanation of the principles of CT and its equipment is beyond the scope of this text.

LABORATORY EXPERIENCE

As indicated under Tomographic Quality Control above, numerous procedures may be performed to test tomographic equipment. The experiments in *Concepts in Medical Imaging: Laboratory Manual* concentrate on tomographic principles instead of assessment of equipment efficiency. Laboratories #25, Fulcrum Level, and #26, Thickness of Objective Plane, may be performed on any type of tomographic unit.

The Fulcrum Level laboratory #25 provides the experimenter with the opportunity to locate the fulcrum level and determine its relationship to the clarity of the tomogram. In this laboratory, the individual uses a constant exposure angle and takes five exposures at different fulcrum levels. Each tomogram is assessed to determine the clarity level.

The Thickness of Objective Plane laboratory (#26) allows the experimenter to observe the relationship of the exposure angle to the thickness of the objec-

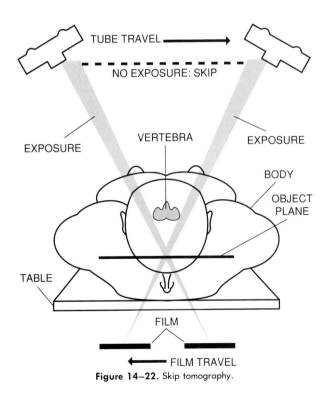

Figure 14–22. Skip tomography.

tive plane. In this laboratory, four tomograms are taken using different exposure angles while a constant fulcrum level is maintained. By comparing the amount of clarity visualized on the tomogram, the experimenter is able to determine the effect of the exposure angle on the thickness of the objective plane.

Bibliography

Ballinger, PW. Merrill's atlas of radiographic positions and radiologic procedures (6th edition). St. Louis: Mosby, 1986.

Berrett, A. Modern thin-section tomography. Springfield, IL: Thomas, 1973.

Bushong, SC. Radiologic science for technologists (4th edition). St. Louis: Mosby, 1988.

Chesney, DN and Chesney, MO. Radiographic imaging (4th edition). Boston: Blackwell Scientific Publications, 1981.

Cullinan, AM. Producing quality radiographs. Philadelphia: Lippincott, 1987.

Cullinan, JE and Cullinan, AM. Illustrated guide to x-ray technics (2nd edition). Philadelphia: Lippincott, 1980.

Curry, TS, Dowdey, JE and Murry, RC. Christensen's introduction to the physics of diagnostic radiology (3rd edition). Philadelphia: Lea & Febiger, 1984.

Curry, TS, Dowdey, JE and Murry, RC. Christensen's physics of diagnostic radiology (4th edition). Philadelphia: Lea & Febiger, 1990.

Gray, JE, et al. Quality control in diagnostic imaging. Baltimore: University Park Press, 1983.

Kodak Company. Fundamentals of radiography (12th edition). Rochester, NY: Eastman Kodak Company, 1980.

Littleton, JT. Conventional tomography in perspective. Radiographics 6 (2):336–339, March 6, 1986.

McLemore, J. Quality assurance in diagnostic radiology. Chicago: Year Book Medical, 1981.

Selman, J. The fundamentals of x-ray and radium physics (7th edition). Springfield, IL: Thomas, 1985.

Swallow, RA and Naylor, E, editors. Clark's positioning in radiography (11th edition) Rockville, MD: Aspen, 1986, pp. 379–391.

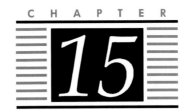

FUNDAMENTALS OF COMPUTER TECHNOLOGY

KEVIN M. McNEILL

INTRODUCTION

Conrad Roentgen discovered x-rays in 1895. The primary medical use of radiation from 1895 to approximately 1975 was for the production of radiographs. In the early 1970s, radiographic imaging underwent a major change. At this time, nuclear medicine imaging (gamma camera) and computed tomographic equipment made use of computers to produce images. Unlike previous equipment, these systems produced computerized images that could be stored on diskettes or magnetic tape. Hard copies of the images were produced on radiographic film. The introduction of these types of equipment began a revolution regarding the manner in which future images would be produced. Currently, computerized imaging has expanded and is commonly employed for conventional radiography, ultrasound, nuclear medicine and magnetic resonance imaging. The advent of the common use of computers in imaging departments resulted in the need for technologists to become familiar with computer technology.

The study of computer technology can be extensive. New advances occur almost daily. The intent of this chapter is to present a basic fundamental background of computer technology. Chapter 16, Digital Imaging Overview, presents fundamental concepts of digital imaging. The information in both these chapters is useful in providing a basic foundation of computer technology, enabling the reader to pursue more advanced concepts.

COMPUTER TERMINOLOGY

As computer technology developed, new terminology also evolved. To assist individuals with little or no background in computers, the following brief definitions of key terms and phrases used throughout this chapter are provided. It is recommended that readers familiarize themselves with the meaning of these terms.

Address–a value specifying the unique location of a stored piece of information in the memory unit.

Arithmetic and logic unit (ALU)–the functional circuitry in the central processing unit that performs arithmetical operations (e.g., add, subtract) and logical operations (e.g., and, or) on data. Computers often contain more than one ALU.

Analog input–a continuous variable electronic signal.

Bit–the smallest unit of information in a digital system. A bit may have a value of either 1 or 0, which may be interpreted in several ways, e.g., true or false, on or off and as the coefficient of a power of 2.

Bus–an electrical data path allowing the parallel exchange of many bits of information between components of a computer system. A typical computer may have several buses, both internal and external.

Byte–a grouping of eight bits as one unit of information. A byte may represent 256 different values.

Central processing unit (CPU, processor)–a group of functional elements that provide fundamental data manipulation and control operations at the heart of the computer system. These functional elements consist of the ALU, the control unit and the main memory.

Control unit–the element in the CPU that supervises the functioning of the computer as a whole, especially decoding instructions to configure the ALU for the appropriate operation.

Digital input–input that is represented by a limited number of discrete or quantized values.

Direct memory access (DMA)–a method of transferring information to/from computer memory that does not require the use of the CPU. Input/output (I/O) controllers with appropriate DMA control circuitry can move data to/from memory directly. The alternative requires the CPU to move data between memory and the input/output device.

Hardware–equipment or physical aspect of the computer. Hardware consists of the CPU and peripheral devices.

Indirect addressing–an instruction format in which the instruction word contains the address of the data to be operated on rather than the data itself. After the instruction is fetched from memory, an additional operation is required to fetch the data.

Input/output devices–devices such as terminals and printers that perform a translation between electronic signals suitable for the computer to "read" (machine language) and symbols (letters or characters) that humans understand.

Interface–circuitry that decodes, interprets and sends signals between the computer and peripheral devices. It also synchronizes the data flow rate between the computer and peripheral devices.

Kernel–the set of programs in an operating system that implement the most primitive functions of the system.

Memory–the components of digital computers that provide the capability for storing information. The hierarchy of storage devices includes registers, random access memories (RAMs), magnetic discs, magnetic tape and optical discs. The main memory associated with the CPU is made up of RAM.

Operand–the data that are the target of an operation specified in a computer instruction. Some instructions may specify multiple operands in source and destination fields. Each operand is specified by a field in the instruction word.

Software–a set of instructions or programs that tell the computer what to do.

Word–a grouping of several bits into one unit of information. The number of bits often varies with different types of computers. Sixteen bit words are common for minicomputers, whereas 64 or more bits are common for supercomputers.

BRIEF HISTORY

The earliest computing machines were mechanical calculators developed in the early seventeenth century. These machines used pegged wheels to add, subtract, divide and multiply. In the early nineteenth century, Charles Babbage developed the analytical engine. Babbage's machine was a mechanical, program controlled, digital computer with punched card I/O, an arithmetical unit, storage and a printing mechanism.

At the end of the nineteenth century, Herman Hollerith developed a code for using punched cards to represent numerical and logical data. His machines for tabulating and sorting the cards were highly successful. In the early twentieth century, Hollerith's company merged with two others to form the company that would become the International Business Machines Corporation (IBM).

During the early twentieth century, many developments and efforts were aimed at building a general purpose electronic computer. The most influential research in this area occurred in the 1940s at the Moore School of Engineering at the University of Pennsylvania by John Mauchly and J. Presper Eckert. Their work led to the development, in 1946, of the first electronic computer called the electronic numeric integrator and calculator (ENIAC). It contained 19,000 vacuum tubes and 1500 relays. Its primary use was the computation of ballistic trajectories but, by the end of its development, it was essentially a general purpose computer. The ENIAC was capable of 5000 additions or subtractions per second. It had 312 words of hard wired program storage and was used for 10 years.

While the ENIAC was still being developed, its inventors, joined by John von Neumann, began planning its successor, the electronic discrete variable computer (EDVAC). The EDVAC was different from its predecessor and basically completed the invention of the modern digital computer. Unlike the ENIAC, which worked with decimal digits, the EDVAC was a binary computer and therefore required substantially fewer tubes. Also, the EDVAC was designed with about 100 times the amount of internal memory capacity of the ENIAC. The designers of the EDVAC realized that the control instructions, as well as the data for the specified computations, could be placed in the machine's memory as a stored program. This change from the previous methods of hard wiring the instructions or placing them on punched tape was the critical development that made the EDVAC essentially a modern computer. Today, any computer utilizing programs stored in memory with the data on which the programs operate is classified as having a von Neumann architecture.

Because the plans for the EDVAC had been widely published, the concepts it contained influenced computer designers to develop other computers with stored programs. In 1949, the electronic delay storage automatic calculator (EDSAC) was built at Cambridge in the United Kingdom. This machine had 1024 words of primary memory and 4600 words of magnetic drum storage. It was the first machine to execute a stored program rather than a hard wired program.

In the 1950s, IBM introduced the 700/7000 series and I/O channels, improving the efficiency of computer communication with the external environment. The development of the universal automatic computer (UNIVAC I), in 1951, introduced a magnetic tape system. The early 1950s also marked the development of high level languages designed to reduce the burden of programing in machine language. FORTRAN (formula translation) was introduced in 1957 and is still the standard language for scientific programing.

The transistor, which replaced vacuum tubes, was introduced to digital computer circuitry in 1958. This advance allowed machines to become smaller and generate less heat than the preceding vacuum tube based machines. IBM introduced its first transistorized system, the 7070, in 1960. It was not successful because it lacked compatibility with earlier IBM machines. There were numerous other computer advances in the 1960s, including

1. Implementation of the first virtual memory system at Manchester University using an ATLAS computer in 1962
2. In 1963, the creation of the first computer (Burroughs B-5000) for high level programing languages
3. Control Data Corporation (CDC) introduced the CDC 6600, which took the leading role in the development of supercomputers.

CDC machines were the first major departure from traditional von Neumann architecture. Supercomputers are generally much faster, have large amounts of memory and are extremely expensive. To gain the increase in speed, the CDC 6600 used multifunction processing in which multiple operations are performed simultaneously.

Also, during the 1960s, large mainframe computers began being replaced by smaller minicomputers. Digital Equipment Corporation (DEC) introduced the first generation of minicomputers with the PDP-1 in 1960. Minicomputers dramatically reduced the cost of computing as well as the size of the machines. The most successful of the PDP series was the PDP-11, which evolved into the VAX family with the release of the VAX-11/780 in 1978. In the mid-1960s, IBM introduced one of its most successful series, the System/360. At the end of the decade CDC introduced the 7600 supercomputer with pipelined processing, the most commercially successful technique for speeding up sequential computers.

The 1970s witnessed the establishment of a new class of computer, the microcomputer. The Intel 4004, 4 bit processor, led the way, followed by the Intel 8080. The Intel line evolved into a highly successful series of processors that were at the heart of the personal computer explosion. Another successful family of microprocessors was developed by Motorola. That company's 68000 family is used widely in real time and industrial control computers.

Currently, advances in parallel processing and multiprocessing are challenging the role of the supercomputer. Although known for many years, parallel computing techniques have only become commercially feasible on a large scale since 1980. Parallel techniques utilize many processors, which may work together or independently. Parallel processors offer a significant price advantage over supercomputers but suffer from a lack of available software. The shortage of software is due to the difficulty of decomposing problems into parts that can be computed in parallel.

DIGITAL LOGIC

Digital computers operate on digital information. Unlike analog information, which is continuous, digital information is discrete or quantized. Analog input functions similarly to a wind watch with a second hand. The time indication on a wind watch, like analog information, is continually in motion (this is evidenced by the constant motion of the second hand). Digital information is displayed in a similar manner to a quartz watch with a digital display. The quartz watch displays time in individual segments, e.g., 7:22.

In a digital computer, information is represented by a limited number of discrete or quantized values. The components making up the computer are binary. That is, only two discrete values are allowed.

Therefore, digital computers use the binary number system in which there are two digits: 0 and 1. A single binary digit is called a bit. A bit may have a value of either 1 or 0, which may be interpreted in several ways, e.g., true or false, on or off and the coefficient of a power of 2.

Because the circuits making up the computer deal with binary information, it is natural for the computer to perform its operations using the base 2 number system. However, people are most familiar with decimal numbers (base 10); also, binary numbers can be quite cumbersome. For example, the value of the binary number 1101011 is not readily recognized by most people. However, the equivalent decimal number, 107, does convey meaning to most people. Figure 15–1 demonstrates binary to decimal conversion.

The computer uses groups of bits to represent information using the base 2 system. For example, 8 bits are grouped together to form a byte, which can represent 256 (2^8, or $2 \times 2 \times 2 \times 2 \times 2 \times 2 \times 2 \times 2 = 256$) different values. Just as with decimal numbers, the bit position in a byte indicates a power of the base by which the bit value is multiplied. Figure 15–1 illustrates the conversion of an 8 bit binary number to its decimal equivalent.

It is convenient to represent binary numbers using octal (base 8) or hexadecimal (base 16) numbers. Each octal digit represents 3 bits (2^3, or $2 \times 2 \times 2 = 8$), whereas each hexadecimal digit represents 4 (2^4, or $2 \times 2 \times 2 \times 2 = 16$) bits of a binary number. Therefore, octal and hexadecimal numbers are more compact and the conversion to and from binary is quite straightforward. Hexadecimal numbers may be confusing when first encountered because they include A, B, C, D, E and F to represent

BINARY VALUE
0 1 0 0 1 1 0 1

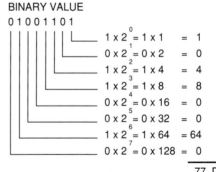

$$1 \times 2^0 = 1 \times 1 = 1$$
$$0 \times 2^1 = 0 \times 2 = 0$$
$$1 \times 2^2 = 1 \times 4 = 4$$
$$1 \times 2^3 = 1 \times 8 = 8$$
$$0 \times 2^4 = 0 \times 16 = 0$$
$$0 \times 2^5 = 0 \times 32 = 0$$
$$1 \times 2^6 = 1 \times 64 = 64$$
$$0 \times 2^7 = 0 \times 128 = 0$$

77 DECIMAL VALUE

Figure 15–1. Binary to decimal conversion.

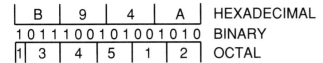

| B | 9 | 4 | A | HEXADECIMAL |

1 0 1 1 1 0 0 1 0 1 0 0 1 0 1 0 BINARY

|1| 3 | 4 | 5 | 1 | 2 | OCTAL

Figure 15–2. Relationship of binary, octal and hexadecimal notations.

10, 11, 12, 13, 14 and 15, respectively. Figure 15–2 shows the relationship between a 16 bit binary number and its octal and hexadecimal representations. Table 15–1 lists several numbers in binary, octal, hexadecimal and decimal forms. The advantage of octal and hexadecimal over decimal systems is the ability to easily determine the status of individual bits in the equivalent binary form.

In the computer, the binary values are represented by electrical signals of different voltages. Generally, each value covers a range of voltages to allow for small variations in the signal. The value 1 may be represented by a signal between 4.5 to 5 V, while 0 is represented by a signal in the range of 0 to 0.5 V. Other voltage levels are not allowed.

GATES, ADDERS AND FLIP-FLOPS

To operate on binary values, digital computers use basic building blocks called gates. Gates take

one or more signals as inputs and produce an output digital value that is a logical function (e.g., and, or, nor) of the inputs. The logical function is based on Boolean algebra. An in-depth explanation of logical functions is beyond the scope of this text. However, Figure 15–3 is an example of a simple logical function.

In Figure 15–3, two switches are connected in series to a light bulb. For the light bulb to illuminate, both switches must be on (closed). In computers, it is possible to represent the on position (closed) with a binary value of 1. Conversely, the switch position of off (open) may be represented by the binary value of 0. Thus, when switches 1 and 2 have a value of 1, the light bulb illuminates. All other value combinations do not illuminate (off) the bulb (see truth table accompanying Figure 15–3).

Logic gates commonly used as building blocks are shown in Figure 15–4, along with a truth table that shows the relationship between the inputs to the gate and its resulting output.

Table 15–1. BINARY, OCTAL AND HEXADECIMAL REPRESENTATION OF SEVERAL DECIMAL NUMBERS			
Decimal	**Binary**	**Octal**	**Hexadecimal**
1	00000001	001	01
2	00000010	002	02
3	00000011	003	03
4	00000100	004	04
5	00000101	005	05
6	00000110	006	06
7	00000111	007	07
8	00001000	010	08
9	00001001	011	09
10	00001010	012	0A
11	00001011	013	0B
12	00001100	014	0C
13	00001101	015	0D
14	00001110	016	0E
15	00001111	017	0F
16	00010000	020	10
32	00100000	040	20
64	01000000	100	40
128	10000000	200	80
255	11111111	377	FF

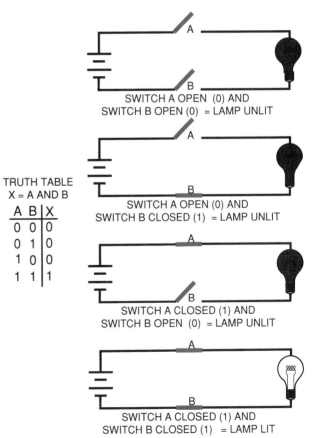

TRUTH TABLE
X = A AND B

A	B	X
0	0	0
0	1	0
1	0	0
1	1	1

SWITCH A OPEN (0) AND
SWITCH B OPEN (0) = LAMP UNLIT

SWITCH A OPEN (0) AND
SWITCH B CLOSED (1) = LAMP UNLIT

SWITCH A CLOSED (1) AND
SWITCH B OPEN (0) = LAMP UNLIT

SWITCH A CLOSED (1) AND
SWITCH B CLOSED (1) = LAMP LIT

Figure 15–3. Effect of the *and* logical function.

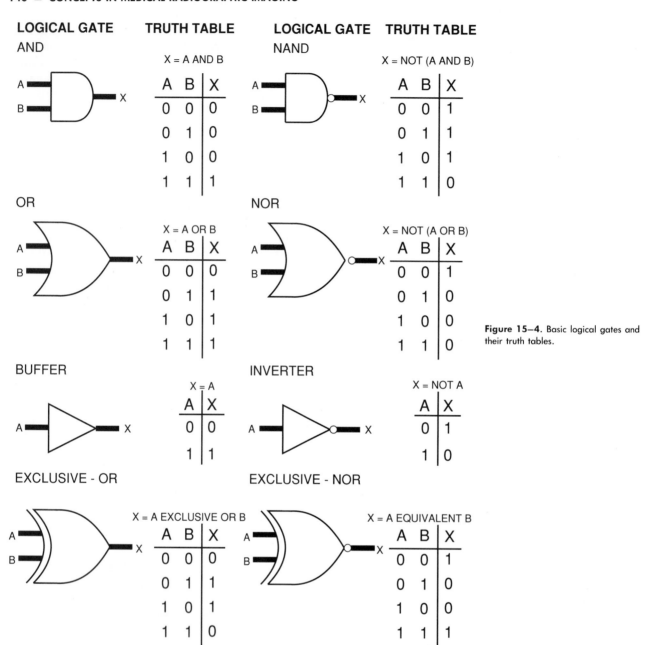

Figure 15–4. Basic logical gates and their truth tables.

The basic gates are combined into larger elements called combinatorial circuits. These elements perform more complicated functions and are often represented by graphic symbols of their own. By giving common combinatorial circuits their own symbol, the design of digital circuits is simplified. Figure 15–5 shows a combinatorial circuit to compute the sum of 3 input bits and return the sum and a carry. This circuit is called a full adder and it is the most basic function for generating arithmetical operations in digital computers.

Gates and adders alone are not enough to build a computer because they lack the capability to store information. Another circuit, called a flip-flop, is a binary cell that can store a single bit. Commonly used flip-flops have two outputs, usually called Q and Q'. The normal output is represented by Q, whereas Q' is its complement. That is, if Q has the

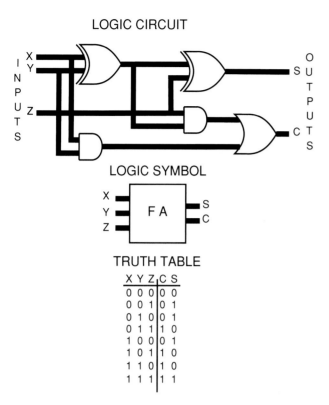

LOGIC CIRCUIT

LOGIC SYMBOL

TRUTH TABLE

X	Y	Z	C	S
0	0	0	0	0
0	0	1	0	1
0	1	0	0	1
0	1	1	1	0
1	0	0	0	1
1	0	1	1	0
1	1	0	1	0
1	1	1	1	1

Figure 15–5. The full adder.

value 1, Q' has the value 0. Conversely, when Q has the value 0, Q' has the value 1. There are several types of flip-flops; however, discussion of one illustrates the basic principles.

An important aspect of many flip-flops is their synchronous nature. The inputs are allowed to change only at discrete intervals. Control of the input signals is provided by the use of a clock-pulse. A clock-pulse is a signal that alternates between 0 and 1 at a regular interval and that is distributed throughout the system. The flip-flop maintains its binary state of 0 or 1 until the next clock-pulse arrives. At that time, the inputs determine the new state of the flip-flop. Figure 15–6 illustrates a clocked RS flip-flop and a characteristic table showing the relationship of the input and output signals.

Gates and flip-flops are interconnected to form sequential circuits. The gates provide the capability to generate outputs, which are a function of the inputs; while the flip-flips store state information. The output of the total sequential circuit is a function of the current state of the circuit, as maintained

by the flip-flops and external inputs. Many common sequential circuits are available as integrated circuits, eliminating the need for designers to build up sequential circuits from the gate level.

REGISTERS

A particularly important type of sequential circuit is a register. A register contains a number of flip-flops and other gates which serve to control the transitions of the flip-flops. A register with N flip-flops is an N bit register and can store any binary number of N bits. Registers are usually capable of parallel loading; a control signal enables loading of data. Figure 15–7 shows an 8 bit register. Digital computers use large numbers of registers. One important register is called the program counter.

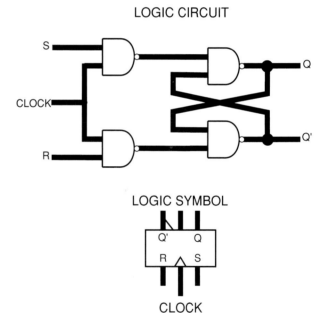

LOGIC CIRCUIT

LOGIC SYMBOL

STATE TABLE

R	S	Q(t+1)	DESCRIPTION
0	0	Q(t)	STATE REMAINS UNCHANGED
1	0	0	RESET (CLEAR) THE FLIP - FLOP
0	1	1	SET THE FLIP - FLOP
1	1	?	ILLEGAL

Figure 15–6. An RS flip-flop.

LOGIC CIRCUIT

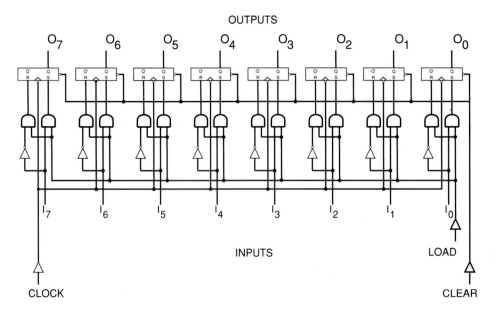

Figure 15–7. An 8 bit register.

LOGIC SYMBOL

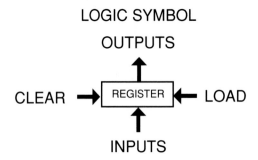

This register keeps track of the location of the next instruction to be executed by the computer and is used to fetch that instruction from memory.

Other important circuits are decoders and multiplexers. Decoders have N inputs and 2^N (i.e., 2 to the Nth power) outputs. For any N bit binary number provided as input, only one of the 2^N outputs is enabled. This function is useful in decoding memory addresses and is discussed further below. Multiplexers allow input from one of 2^N input lines to be sent to a single output line, under the control of N bits, which select the input line.

MEMORY

ORGANIZATION

The computer must have a mechanism to store program instructions and data. This mechanism is provided by a collection of storage registers and control circuitry. This collection is called memory and several types exist, but the basic principles are common for all types. The memory stores binary information in a group of bits, called a memory word, which is accessed as a single unit. A memory word is accessed by a unique address, which encodes its location in the memory unit. Memory that permits accessing of words in any order is called random access memory (RAM). RAM that cannot be updated is referred to as read only memory (ROM). ROM is often used to contain permanent codes, which must not be changed. Some memory systems, such as magnetic tape, scan words in the order they are stored. For example, to access a word in the middle of a magnetic tape, all information preceding the requested word must be scanned.

The bits of the memory word may represent any binary coded information, such as numbers, alphanumerical characters and program instructions. The way that individual bits are stored depends on the type of memory and may be based on flip-flops, magnetic core, magnetic bubbles or magnetic domains.

Memory spans a hierarchy ranging from the registers within the CPU to offline memory such as magnetic tape. The general purpose registers are the fastest type of memory in the computer, but they are expensive so there are relatively few of them. The next fastest component of the hierarchy is the main memory. The main memory consists of RAM and is a separate functional element associated with the CPU. Many computers have a small, faster type of memory between the registers and the main memory, called a cache. A cache is usually high speed RAM within the CPU, which holds a copy of a small portion of main memory. After the main memory, the components of the memory hierarchy consist of the peripheral memories such as magnetic discs, optical discs and magnetic tape. These components have the disadvantage of being slower than registers and main memory. However, peripheral memory has the advantage of being less expensive and providing much larger amounts of storage space. Table 15–2 lists typical access times and storage capacities of the most common members of the memory hierarchy.

CONTROL AND DATA PATHS

Circuits associated with the main memory include control lines, data input and output lines and address lines. These circuits allow the memory to communicate with its external environment. The control lines are used to determine the type of operation, read or write, and hence the direction of data flow. The data input lines provide a path for the external environment to store (write) data into the memory. Conversely, the data output lines provide the path for the external environment to retrieve (read) data from the memory. The address lines specify the particular memory word to be accessed by providing the input to a decoder.

The size of the memory specifies the number of address lines required to access all the memory words. For example, a memory of 1024 (2^{10}) words requires 10 address lines. Two registers are associated with a memory unit. They are the memory address register (MAR) and memory buffer register (MBR). MAR stores the address of the memory word to be accessed. The MBR is used to store all information transferred to or from the memory unit. Figure 15–8 illustrates the relationship between the components of the memory unit.

INPUT/OUTPUT

Computers must have a method of communicating with the external environment. A computer must receive programs and data from the user and transmit the results of its computations back to the

Table 15–2. CHARACTERISTICS OF MEMBERS OF THE MEMORY HIERARCHY

Memory	Access Time	Size (Bytes)	Usual Contents
Registers	<750 ns	256	Intermediate processing results
Main memory	250 ns–2 μs	512 K–256 M	Currently executing program instructions and required data
Magnetic disc	10–100 ms	20 M–1 G	Program instructions and data not immediately required
Magnetic tape	Seconds	Up to 200 M	Archival storage of programs and data, back up of discs
Optical disc	83 ms	650 M, 1.2 G	Archival storage of large data sets (e.g., images)

ns = nanosecond, 1 billionth of a second; μs = microsecond, 1 millionth of a second; ms = millisecond, 1 thousandth of a second; K = kilo, multiply by 1024 (e.g., 1 K bytes = 1024 bytes); M = mega, multiply by 1,048,576; G = giga, multiply by 1,073,741,824.

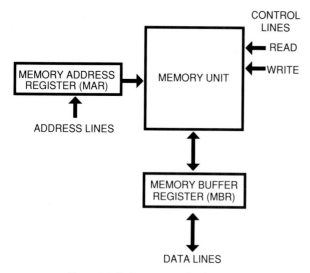

Figure 15–8. Components of main memory.

user. The input and output devices, called peripherals, provide the means for this communication. Common peripherals include card readers and punchers, terminals, printers and plotters. Other more specialized peripherals may be used in some applications, such as image display devices used in digital radiology.

INTERFACE

Peripherals are often electromechanical devices and usually operate at much slower rates than the CPU. This difference in speed requires synchronization between the operation of the CPU and memory and the operation of the peripherals. Also, the peripherals must perform translation of data formats. Synchronization and translation are achieved by connecting the peripherals to the computer through interfaces.

These interfaces may be connected to a data bus, which is also connected to the CPU, or they may be connected to a special I/O controller, which isolates the peripheral devices from the CPU. When an I/O controller is used, the CPU communicates with the I/O controller, which then sends and receives information from the peripheral device. In computer systems using a bus, the peripheral devices are usually memory mapped. In memory mapped I/O, accessing the control registers of the

devices employs the same instructions used to access memory; whereas systems using an I/O controller need special instructions for performing I/O operations.

TRANSFER OF DATA

The transfer of data between the CPU and the I/O devices may be accomplished in two different ways. The first is under program control. In this method, each data transfer is the result of an instruction executed by the processor and the processor must check a status register in the device's interface to determine when the next transfer can be made. Generally, the data is transferred between the device and one of the registers in the CPU. The second method, DMA, transfers data directly between the peripheral device and memory. The processor loads control registers in the device's interface with the length of the transfer and the starting memory location to/from which the data should be transferred. The device then transfers data to/from sequential memory locations until the specified amount of data has been transferred. While the data transfer is taking place, the CPU is free to perform other operations.

BASIC COMPUTER SYSTEM ARCHITECTURE

The basic hardware components of a computer system were discussed above. The relationship of those components is summarized in Figure 15–9. The following discussion of the operation of a simple computer system considers the principles that are applicable across the entire spectrum of computers, from personal computers to supercomputers. The computer discussed is a general purpose digital computer that executes programs stored in memory.

PROGRAM

To perform useful work, the computer must be told what to do and in what order it should be done. This is accomplished by a program, which is

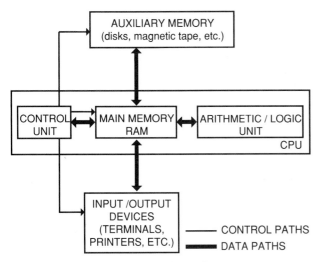

Figure 15–9. Relationship of fundamental system components.

an ordered list of instructions. Every digital computer has a set of executable instructions or operations. For example, the computer can add the contents of a memory location, M, with a register called the AC, by the following instruction: Add M,AC. Instructions are binary values interpreted by the control circuits of the computer. The instructions usually have several fields, or groups of bits, that specify the action to be performed and what data should be used. Figure 15–10 shows the format of two simple instruction words. In Figure 15–10, the opcode specifies the operation to be performed. The source and destination addresses specify the location of data to be operated on (the operands) and where the results will be placed, respectively.

To execute the program stored in memory, the computer performs a cycle of four phases: fetch, decode, indirect and execute. This cycle is repeated for each instruction in the program. The fetch phase is a sequence of operations during which the instruction is read from memory and brought into an instruction register within the CPU. During the decode phase, the opcode portion of the instruction register is decoded and the ALU is set up to perform the specified operation. In the indirect phase, the control logic determines if the operand is in the instruction or must be fetched from memory. If the instruction specifies an indirect address, the operand is read from memory. In the final phase, execute, the specified operation is performed. Depending on the type of operation, the results remain

in a register or are written to memory. This is achieved by the program counter.

A special register called the program counter maintains the address of the next instruction to be executed. The program counter loads the MAR when an instruction is fetched and moves in increments to contain the address of the next instruction. The sequence of the operation of the program counter may be modified through branch instructions.

Branch instructions are usually conditioned on the results of a previous operation. For example, a subtraction operation may be followed by a branch instruction to change the program counter if the result of the subtraction is 0. The result of the last operation performed by the processor is determined by using a special register called the processor status word (PSW). The PSW uses bits to indicate the result. One bit in the PSW is called the Z bit and it is set to 1 if the last operation resulted in the value of 0. When the branch instruction is executed the PSW is checked. If the Z bit is set (1), the result was 0 and the program counter needs to change. Thus, an offset is added to the program counter to move it to another section of the program. However, if the Z bit is not set, the result is a value other than 0 and the program counter is left unchanged. Consequently, the next instruction after the branch instruction is executed.

SINGLE REGISTER INSTRUCTION

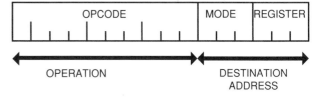

TWO REGISTER INSTRUCTION

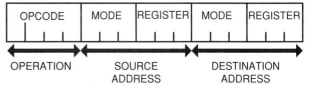

Figure 15–10. Examples of instruction word formats.

ACCUMULATOR REGISTER

In the computer program discussed above, the accumulator (AC) register is the workhorse. The arithmetical and logical operations are all performed on the data contained in the AC registers. Data are moved into the AC from memory, operated on and moved back to memory in a sequence of three instructions such as the following:

LDA A ;LOAD DATA FROM MEMORY LOCA-
TION A INTO AC
ADD B ;ADD DATA FROM MEMORY LOCA-
TION B TO AC
STA C ;STORE NEW CONTENTS OF AC AT
LOCATIONS C

The particular syntax of these instructions is specific to the target computer. Additional information on computer programs is discussed under Software. When the AC is always involved in operations, the use of the AC is implicit and it is not necessary to list it explicitly in the instruction syntax.

Generally, computers have many registers that are equivalent to the AC, as well as others that provide different capabilities. Commonly, a computer has eight or more general purpose registers, much like the AC, and the same number of floating point registers, which are used for floating point operations (decimals) rather than integer operations. Alternatively, a computer may have a set of data registers that can be used with either floating or integer operations and a set of address registers that are used only to hold memory addresses. The configuration of registers depends on the particular architecture of the computer.

THE REPRESENTATION OF DATA

Because computers are applicable to many tasks besides numerical computations, they must also work with alphanumerical data. This includes upper and lower case letters, digits and special characters such as exclamation marks and parentheses. These symbols are assigned a binary code that the computer can understand. Assigning these codes in order allows for an arithmetical comparison of one code value with another. This is useful in determining the alphabetical order of the corresponding characters. The most common coding is the American National Standard Code for Infor-

mation Interchange (ASCII). This code uses 7 bits and appears in Table 15–3. Similar codes have been developed, using 16 bits, to represent the characters of nearly every alphabet in the world, as well as the ideographic characters used in Chinese and Japanese.

To perform arithmetical operations, binary numbers must represent positive and negative integers. This requires that a bit be allocated to represent a positive and a negative sign. For positive numbers, the bit is 0, whereas the bit for negative numbers is 1. Several methods are available to represent the negative value of a binary fixed point (stationary decimal point) number. The most common method is signed 2s complement. The signed 2s complement of a number is formed by inverting all of the bits (change each 1 to 0 and vice versa) then adding 1. For example, 010011 (19) becomes 101100 + 1 for a signed 2s complement of 101101 (−19). Adding the two binary numbers in this example results in a value of zero.

$$
\begin{array}{r}
010011 \ (\ \ 19) \\
+ \ 101101 \ (-19) \\
\hline
000000
\end{array}
$$

Note that the sign bit is the leftmost bit. Also, two 1s added together results in 0 with a 1 carried to the next position to the left. The other two possible methods to represent a negative value, signed magnitude and signed 1s complement, have the disadvantage of allowing two representations for zero (+0 and −0).

Besides positive and negative integers, floating point numbers (floating decimals) must be represented. To do this, two parts are required, the mantissa and the exponent. The mantissa is usually considered to be a fixed point fraction and is often called the fraction part. The exponent designates the position of the decimal. Both parts have a sign bit to represent positive and negative fractions and exponents. Floating point represents a number in the form:

$$f \ (b^e)$$

The base, b, and the fixed point position, f, are assumed. The hardware that performs operations on floating point numbers must be designed using the assumed base and point position for correct

Table 15–3. SEVEN BIT ASCII CODE

Code	Character	Code	Character	Code	Character	Code	Character
00	NUL	20	SP	40	@	60	
01	SOH	21	!	41	A	61	a
02	STX	22	"	42	B	62	b
03	ETX	23	#	43	C	63	c
04	EOT	24	$	44	D	64	d
05	ENQ	25	%	45	E	65	e
06	ACK	26	&	46	F	66	f
07	BEL	27	'	47	G	67	g
08	BS	28	(	48	H	68	h
09	HT	29	)	49	I	69	i
0A	LF	2A	*	4A	J	6A	j
0B	VT	2B	+	4B	K	6B	k
0C	FF	2C	,	4C	L	6C	l
0D	CR	2D	–	4D	M	6D	m
0E	SO	2E	.	4E	N	6E	n
0F	SI	2F	/	4F	O	6F	o
10	DLE	30	0	50	P	70	p
11	DC1	31	1	51	Q	71	q
12	DC2	32	2	52	R	72	r
13	DC3	33	3	53	S	73	s
14	DC4	34	4	54	T	74	t
15	NAK	35	5	55	U	75	u
16	SYN	36	6	56	V	76	v
17	ETB	37	7	57	W	77	w
18	CAN	38	8	58	X	78	x
19	EM	39	9	59	Y	79	y
1A	SUB	3A	:	5A	A	7A	z
1B	ESC	3B	;	5B	[	7B	{
1C	FS	3C	<	5C	\	7C		
1D	GS	3D	=	5D	]	7D	}
1E	RS	3E	>	5E	^	7E	~
1F	US	3F	?	5F	__	7F	DEL

result. The hardware used to implement floating point operations is more complex than that required for integer operations and is beyond the scope of this text. Floating point operations require longer execution times than fixed point operations. Older generations of computers used software to emulate floating point operations using fixed point arithmetic. Current computers often use floating point coprocessors, which are designed to perform these operations quickly.

SOFTWARE

BASIC SOFTWARE CONCEPTS

Computer programs, or software, are detailed instructions that tell the computer what to do and when to do it. The computer takes these instruc-tions literally, performing each operation as instructed. For the computer, these instructions are simply groups of bits that form valid opcodes. When decoded, the opcodes result in the proper configuration of circuitry to perform the intended operation. The data operated on are simply, from the computers point of view, a group of bits to be manipulated. The logical design of the circuits, and the encoding of the data ensure that well-formed operations provide meaningful results.

However, it is not convenient for humans to work with information encoded in the form suitable for the computer. Likewise, it is not efficient for humans to write instructions directly in the form in which the computer sees them. The form the computer understands, called machine language, consists of the direct specification of opcodes and addresses as they should appear in memory. This type of programing was used for early computers, but it was quickly realized that to make computers more useful other methods were needed.

The first tool to simplify programing was the assembler. Assemblers are programs that read other programs, written in an assembly language, and produce a machine language version as output. Assembly language provides a syntax, e.g., load, store, and add, that is easier for humans to understand than binary codes. However, when one is writing assembly programs, every step of the program must be explicitly specified and the process is tedious for large complicated tasks.

The development that provided a dramatic increase in the applicability of computers was the introduction of high level languages. These languages also use a syntax, but one of a higher degree of abstraction, which more closely resembles the notations used by humans. A single statement in a high level language is much more powerful than an assembly language instruction. Therefore, a high level language program can represent a complex task much more concisely and in a manner more fitting for human interpretation.

High level languages are made possible by programs called compilers. A compiler reads the high level language program and translates it into assembly language instructions. The resulting assembly language program is then read by an assembler, which produces the machine language code for the computer to understand. Some of the earliest high level languages developed, FORTRAN and COBOL (*common business oriented language*), are still widely used. FORTRAN is oriented toward scientific and mathematical work and provides an algebralike syntax. COBOL is geared toward business programing and is more proselike than FORTRAN. There are many high level languages, and each has a syntax style that is suitable for the types of programing that the language is intended to support.

SYSTEM SOFTWARE

Recall that the earliest computers used hard wired programs for specific computing applications. To change the programing of the computer, the wiring needed to be altered. This process was time consuming and cumbersome. The introduction of stored programs simplified the programing process.

However, in both wired and stored programs, the computer performed a single computing task or was idle. This meant that the user could not perform another task until the computer completed the previous task. About the time that high level languages were developed, it was recognized that to increase the utilization (perform multiple tasks simultaneously) and manage the resources of the computer (e.g., the CPU and I/O devices), a comprehensive operating system was needed.

An operating system is a set of programs that provides an environment to execute the computer user's programs. The operating system controls the resources of the system and allows a user's programs to have access to the resources. Early systems were primarily batch systems in which a user's programs were submitted on punched cards. As operating systems progressed, the concept of time-sharing became possible.

In a time-shared system, many users' programs execute concurrently. Each user's program gets to use the processor for a short period of time, called a quantum. When the quantum has expired, the next user's program executes for its quantum. Because computers can process thousands of instructions each second, each user's program responds as if it is the only program executing on the computer. This is possible because programs perform I/O operations that are generally slow relative to the processing speed of the computer. This time difference allows the time-sharing processor to continually execute instructions. For example, when a program stops to wait for I/O operations, the processor "works" on another program.

Besides the operating system, other important components of the system software include the file system, network communications, assembler, compilers, linkers, editors and debuggers. The file system provides the means to organize information stored in the computer's disc and tape storage. A file may contain any type of information from alphanumerical text to binary data. The file system usually provides a hierarchical directory structure, allowing files to be grouped in meaningful ways. Network communications are provided by software that utilizes special communications hardware, allowing the computer to communicate with other computer systems. Compilers and assemblers, discussed above, support the programing task by converting high level programs to machine language programs. One of the linker's primary functions is to resolve references to variables and subroutine names. The linker also allocates memory space for data and allows the program to use software services provided by the operating system. Editors allow a user to enter and alter programs. Debuggers enable the user to step through programs one instruction at a time and to display the contents of program variables. This is useful in determining why a program is not operating correctly.

APPLICATION SOFTWARE

System software provides the general foundation for users of the computer. However, the computational tasks are supported by application software. As with computer hardware and system software, there is a wide range of application software. Application software deals with specific problems such as accounting, mathematical modeling and spread sheets. Application programs include programs written by the user and packages that can be purchased from software vendors. Some applications are general and available for many types of computers, whereas others are limited to specific computers.

The development of application software, especially commercial software, has undergone a great deal of growth in the recent past. Currently, the development of efficient, reliable software is costly and time consuming. Thus, there is a strong interest in methods to decrease the time required to develop applications while increasing their reliability. This interest has led to the development of manual design tools, structured design methodologies, computer aided software engineering (CASE) tools and application generators. Of these aids, CASE and application generators are the most common. CASE tools allow portions of the software design cycle that were performed manually to be developed by using graphic tools on a computer. They also allow libraries of information about the design specification to be compiled. CASE tools can use the information in these libraries with the graphic design data to check design consistency. By automating manual portions of software design and providing tools to rapidly check the quality of the software design, CASE greatly increases the productivity of software developers. However, CASE tools are still fairly new, are quite expensive and have a steep learning curve. Current tools are also somewhat geared toward software for business applications.

Application generators are another tool available for applications software development. To develop the application program, the generator takes graphic design information and program specification entered by the user and generates code. Tools of this kind offer businesses the hope of generating application software without the need for a programing staff. As with CASE, current application generators available are directed primarily at business. Figure 15–11 illustrates the relationship of the various types of software discussed in this chapter.

TECHNOLOGY TRENDS

Few technologies have grown as quickly as computer technology. Even fewer have had a rapid increase of power coupled with dramatic decreases in cost. The evolution of computer technology, both software and hardware, is continuing at a rapid pace. Massively parallel computing is promising for complex problems such as weather modeling. In the past, supercomputers were applied to these

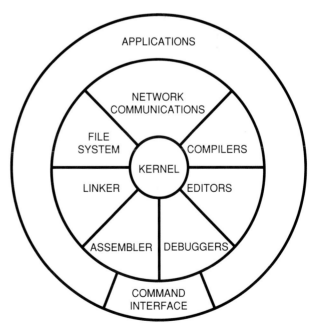

Figure 15–11. Relationship of software components.

large problems, but parallel computers are supplying greater computing power at lower cost.

An important set of tools for increasing software productivity and reliability are object-oriented programing and expert systems. Currently, the dramatic increase in desktop computing power at costs close to those of personal computers have occurred as a result of reduced instruction set computers (RISC). The power of personal computers has increased significantly, decreasing the gap in power between personal computers and workstations.

The availability of inexpensive computing power, coupled with networking technology, is changing the nature of computing. In the past, users time-shared the available computing power by employing terminals connected to a central computer. Currently, computer networks allow users an easy exchange of information. The computing power available per user is great enough to provide the use of computing intensive applications such as publishing software, graphic design tools and expert systems.

Because users have so much computing power and a wide range of software available, computer hardware and software vendors are increasingly pressured to standardize both hardware and software. Currently, standards exist for many aspects of computing, e.g., networking, operating systems and graphics. Standardization allows the equipment to interact and communicate with other equipment, enabling users to employ hardware and software from many vendors.

Two additional items expected to revolutionize computerized imaging are artificial intelligence (AI) and fuzzy logic. AI describes attempts to develop computer programs that exhibit attributes associated with human intelligence. These attributes include the capability to reason, understand relationships between objects, discover meanings and learn. Fuzzy logic is an emerging technique in which computers can make decisions in the face of uncertainty, effectively guessing. Both AI and fuzzy logic will be increasingly applied in imaging to allow computers to recognize and understand images. These techniques may eventually allow computers to scan radiographs to aid in the diagnostic process.

The trends discussed here, increased computing power at decreasing cost, standardization and interconnectivity, are greatly affecting the application of computers throughout society. These trends will dominate the near future of computing and are expected to continue to improve computer use in solving business and scientific problems.

Bibliography

Baer, JL. Computer systems architecture. Rockville, MD: Computer Science Press, 1980.

Barron, DW. Assemblers and loaders (3rd edition). New York: American-Elsevier, 1978.

Bushong, SC. Radiologic science for technologists (4th edition). St. Louis: Mosby, 1988.

Cullinan, AM. Producing quality radiographs. New York: Lippincott, 1987.

Hunter TB. The computer in radiology. Rockville, MD: Aspen, 1986.

Kuni, CC. Introduction to computers and digital processing in medical imaging. Chicago: Year Book Medical, 1988.

Mano, MM. Computer system architecture (2nd edition). Englewood Cliffs, NJ: Prentice-Hall, 1982.

Ralston, A and Reilly, ED, Jr. Encyclopedia of computer science and engineering (2nd edition). New York: Van Nostrand Reinhold, 1983.

Ritenour, ER and Hendee, WR. Computers in diagnostic radiology, lesson 1, section A. Slide/audiotape. Denver: Multimedia, 1983.

Siewiorek, D, Bell, CG and Newell, A. Computer structures: Principles and examples. New York: McGraw-Hill, 1982.

Wilkes, MV. Time sharing computer systems (3rd edition). New York: American-Elsevier, 1975.

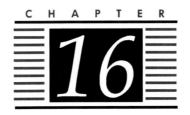

DIGITAL IMAGING OVERVIEW

WILLIAM J. DALLAS

INTRODUCTION

I arrived at my new job and immediately confronted mild disorientation. On the view box was an x-ray film being read and analyzed by a group of radiologists. Even with my lack of medical training, I could see that not everything was in order. The heart, or at least what should have been the heart, contained a large steel spring. The murmurs of satisfaction and astonishment emanating from the tight knot of people were not because the subject of this radiograph was an artificial heart—which had become commonplace at the University of Arizona Medical Center—but rather because this was a digital image and it was in the process of demonstrating one of its tricks. At first, the image was ugly and, worse, it was unreadable. Then, at the touch of a button, it was beautiful. At the conclusion of the demonstration of modern image processing magic, the technologist exhibited the state of the art in data communications by scurrying down the hall with the picture to the waiting team of surgeons. This is an example of one product of modern technology.

Hospitals are drowning in the flood of information they produce. As technology offers better tools for generating diagnostic information, the floodgates open wider. It is ironic that the revolution taking place in medical imaging is drawing us toward information gridlock. A moderate sized hospital presently generates about 1 gigabyte of picture information per day. Hospitals are legally bound to hold this information for 3 to 7 years. In some cases, e.g., silicosis or black lung disease, this period is extended to some 30 years. Warehouses are full of pictures and written reports. They are gold mines of information for analysis of patient histories, comparison between patients, analysis of the progress of disease—useless information because accessing it is simply too complicated.

As early as the mid-1960s, some visionaries saw in the computer a solution to this information overload problem. Let the computer transport, store, route and retrieve the data. However, while it was possible, in principle, to have computer-managed information systems, the necessary hardware, software and data management techniques were not yet available. As the 1980s drew to a close, the required technology began to appear. Research institutions are beginning to make their first attempts at implementing fully computerized imaging departments. This chapter discusses some of the related concepts of digital imaging. It concentrates primarily on picture archiving and communications systems (PACS).

INFORMATION HANDLING SYSTEMS

To understand digital information handling in the hospital of the future it is necessary to discuss the current state of affairs. There are several disjointed information systems, each of which concentrates on a more or less well-defined set of tasks. These systems are mainly manual: people, typewriters and index cards. More and more imaging departments are implementing computers to improve efficiency. Four common systems are the hospital information system (HIS), radiology information system (RIS), PACS and teleradiology system.

HOSPITAL INFORMATION SYSTEM

The highest-level information system is the one that takes care of admitting, tracking and billing patients in a hospital. It is known as the HIS (pronounced hiss). The HIS (see Chapter 17, Computerizing Administrative Tasks, for more information) was the first information system to be computerized. Many hospitals now have operational HISs composed of computers, terminals, printers and, importantly, software packages. Many commercial firms are offering HISs, and cobbled-together, quasi-research prototype systems are being replaced by commercial offerings.

RADIOLOGY INFORMATION SYSTEM

Moving down the hierarchical organization of information is the RIS (pronounced riss). The RIS (see Chapter 17 for more information) manipulates the information circulating in the radiology department. It does not handle the pictures themselves but rather information about pictures and patients. The RIS manages the scheduling of examination rooms, patients, technologists and radiologists as well as managing the film archive and issuing printed requests for films. Some functions of the RIS, such as billing, overlap or duplicate those of a HIS. This overlap is a symptom of a real problem: incompatibility. Getting a HIS and RIS to directly exchange information with one another is a major undertaking. Instead of the two systems being interfaced, one highly sophisticated digital information management system generates paper, the paper is read by human beings and the humans enter data into the second highly sophisticated digital information management system.

PICTURE ARCHIVING AND COMMUNICATIONS SYSTEMS

The third information system, the PACS, is a totally electronic picture handler. Unlike the HIS and RIS, the PACS handles pictures, not words. The PACS stores, retrieves, distributes and displays pictures. No longer must a librarian venture into the film archive and shuffle through endless shelves of 14×17 inch film envelopes. By simply typing a code and pressing a button, the collection of images that the diagnostician wishes to view appears.

To provide an idea as to the amount of information an imaging department produces, it is appropriate to perform a short calculation to determine how many words are the equivalent of a picture. An average word has 5 letters. One letter is represented by 8 bits. Therefore, a word has 40 bits ($5 \times 8 = 40$). A x-ray film of the chest contains 4316 lines. A line has 3556 points and each point has 12 bits. Thus, a picture contains $4316 \times 3556 \times 12 = 184{,}172{,}352$ bits. Because a word equals 40 bits, dividing by 40 determines the equivalent number of words in a picture, or $184{,}172{,}352/40 = 4{,}604{,}308.8$ words. A picture is worth more than a thousand words.

It can be readily seen by the preceding example that the quantities of information that a PACS must handle are enormous. PACS must also handle the information quickly and conveniently. This combination of large data volume, speed and user-friendliness is usually associated with something feared by hospital administrators: expense. Partially because of cost and partially because critical technology is only now becoming available, PACSs installed at the present time are too slow and small to handle the major portion of a department's image traffic.

TELERADIOLOGY SYSTEMS

The above discussion refers to a hospital as an isolated unit. This is overly simplistic. Many areas outside the hospital need the imaging information.

Thus, the pressures are mounting to communicate and integrate. The experts cannot be everywhere, physically, but pictures can. The method used to send the images to other locations is teleradiology. In teleradiology, the pictures in digital form are transmitted over channels between the acquisition and diagnostic sites. The picture transmission uses one of several channel technologies. In order of increasing sophistication, these technologies are standard telephone lines, high speed telephone lines, fiberoptic telephone lines, microwave links and, finally, satellite links.

PRESENT DAY PICTURE MANAGEMENT

The lack of appropriate input modalities is one of the impediments to introducing large scale PACSs. Conventional (film) x-ray units still produce about 80% of the image data in a hospital. A suitable digital replacement is a prerequisite to introducing complete PACSs. The closest modality to plain film replacement is computed radiography (CR). The replacement has not yet occurred because of poor image quality and difficult logistics. At present, film images have about twice the spatial resolution of CR. Although film's additional spatial resolution is not utilized in most examinations, CR's reduced image quality is a deterrent to its introduction. The most serious drawback, however, is cost. Because the image plate reader is expensive, the number of plate readers is limited to one or two. This limit means that the plates must generally be carried long distances from the examination rooms to the processor. Should CR's cost come down significantly, PACS development would be given a strong stimulus. Note, however, that CR is seen as only a temporary substitute for direct digital sensors. These sensors would be built into the examination tables and obviate the need for transporting cassettes to reading machines; only the digital data would be transported.

An additional difficulty is that even the digital modalities, nuclear medical imaging, computed tomography (CT), magnetic resonance imaging (MRI) and digital subtraction angiography (DSA), have traditionally had no digital outputs. The pictures are converted to video signals in the machine and the video images are photographed onto film. The present picture management systems are based on film. Film is also the display medium. The radiologist receives films while sitting, or standing, in a reading room. It is unclear whether reading rooms will remain after departments become totally digital. The environment has the advantage of easy exchange of information and opinions; it has the disadvantage of interruptions and distracting activities, e.g., other radiologists explaining findings to individuals and groups.

The radiographs are viewed by placing them on lighted panels. These panels are in one of two types of systems: light boxes (fixed view panels) or alternators (movable bank of view panels). Light boxes are simple mechanisms consisting of a frosted glass plate rigidly affixed to a box. Inside the box are several fluorescent tubes that provide the illumination. Films are mounted under pressure strips on the face of the light box by the radiologist. Typically, the films, in envelopes called film jackets or folders, are stacked on a table by the light box. The radiologist takes the film or group of films from the jacket, mounts the film, reads it, dictates the report into a tape recorder, takes the films down and proceeds to the next case. Comments about the case are written on the jacket or on attached sheets of paper. It happens, not infrequently, that a note is illegible or incomplete or that a piece of film is missing. The radiologist must then interrupt the reading to trace the missing information. Unlike the digital information of the future, film and paper are available to only one person at a time. If the referring physician or a specialist needs to see the film, it is checked out from the film library or other area. One of the less obvious causes of missing film is someone else's interest in it; if the case is interesting the film may be removed for incorporation into a presentation or publication.

Compared with light boxes, alternators are much more complex devices; they store films and present them, properly illuminated, on command. Inside the alternator, 200 radiographs are attached to frosted glass or plastic panels and stored. A tap on a foot pedal causes a whole new panel of four radiographs to be mechanically moved into view. Eight radiographs, two panels, are visible simultaneously. The alternators are loaded by individuals from the film library before the reading session. If an additional film is necessary for the diagnosis, one is removed from the alternator by the radiologist and is replaced by the new film.

The alternator is the standard by which PACS

display stations will be judged. The alternator displays several images simultaneously, changes a set of images within seconds, delivers the high resolution of the film display medium and even allows rudimentary image processing: magnification and density range windowing. To change the image's apparent magnification the radiologist moves nearer to the film, takes the film from the panel and moves it nearer or uses a magnifying glass. To see the details in a particularly dark area of the film, the radiologist takes the film from the view box and holds it in front of a bare bulb of an incandescent lamp. The bulb is called a hot light.

PICTURE ARCHIVING AND COMMUNICATIONS SYSTEMS

Digital picture handling is the task assigned to the PACS. The PACS consists of units that perform six elemental functions:

1. Acquisition
2. Distribution
3. Storage
4. Processing
5. Display
6. RIS-HIS interfacing.

ACQUISITION

Pictures are created by image acquisition modalities. Some examples of modalities, including commonly used abbreviations, are
Conventional x-ray film units
X-ray computed tomography (CT)
Computed radiography (CR)
Nuclear magnetic resonance imaging (MRI)
Nuclear medical isotope imaging (NM)
Digital subtraction angiography (DSA)
Cineangiography (CA)
Ultrasound (US) imaging
Acquisition modalities may be divided into two groups: those modalities that directly deliver pictures in digital form and those that are nondigital. The following briefly discusses the nondigital conventional x-ray film units; the digital units discussed are nuclear medical imaging, CT, CR, and DSA.

Conventional X-ray Film Units

Conventional units based on plain film are the oldest of the nondigital acquisition modalities. The film is used in a projection radiology unit in which a point x-ray source on one side of the patient irradiates a film screen on the other side. After development, the film carries an image of the patient. The image is most often produced using an intensifying screen. The intensifying screen converts the x-rays to visible light; the light then exposes the film. Because one x-ray produces many visible photons, the efficiency, i.e., the probability that the film will be exposed by an incident x-ray, increases dramatically. The double sided emulsion film is usually held in a flat cassette sandwiched between two intensifying screens to maximize efficiency. Plain film, which gets its name from being ordinary and not enhanced in any way, acts as both the detector and the picture display medium. This dual function makes the task of optimizing the final image difficult, although a hundred years of refinement has resulted in excellent compromises. A typical film has a resolution of 5 line pairs per millimeter and a size of 14 × 17 inches, giving an equivalent of 3300 × 4100 pixels (picture elements).

It is possible to convert the image on the film to a computerized image. This requires application of a film digitizer. A film digitizer, or scanning microdensitometer, is a machine that accepts the standard film formats (14 × 17, 10 × 12, 8 × 10 inches), scans the films and converts the optical density values into digital form. Scanners have been based on a variety of operating principles: video digitizers, linear photodiode array scanners, mechanical flatbed scanners, drum scanners and laser scanners.

As orientation for the following brief descriptions of these scanners: the standard resolution required for examinations using 14 × 17 inch film is 2.5–5 line pairs per millimeter, which translates to approximately 1500 × 2000 points to 3000 × 4000 points per image. The density range encountered varies greatly from department to department with the film preferences and recording techniques; the greatest range is approximately an optical density (OD) of 3 (3 OD is a factor of 1000 in intensity transmission).

Video digitizers consist of a light box, imaging optics, a video camera and electronics. Video digitization is fast, up to television frame rates of 1/30 second, but of relatively low spatial resolution, 512 × 512 or 1024 × 1024 points. The resulting pictures are also relatively noisy; they appear as though they were sprinkled with pepper.

Linear array scanners contain illumination optics, imaging optics and a camera head. In this head is a linear charge coupled device (CCD) or photodiode array of 1000 to 4000 elements, which is mechanically scanned over the image. Linear array scanners are slower than video scanners but still relatively fast, generally completing a scan in a few seconds. Their spatial resolution is medium to good at 2048 × 2048 or 4096 × 4096 points. The drawback is the limited density range that such scanners usually accommodate. Linear array scanners are usually limited to about 2 OD.

Mechanical flatbed and drum scanners generally illuminate a single point on the film using a microscope objective and collect the light from that single point with a second microscope objective. A photomultiplier tube measures the film density, giving an excellent density range. The illumination and light collection optics or the film, or both, are then moved into position for measuring the next point on the film. The highest resolution flatbed scanners can give 30,000 × 40,000 points on a 14 × 17 inch film but are slow, sometimes taking several hours to scan one film. Rotating drum scanners are faster but are still too slow for use in radiologic procedures. They can scan a plain film at 3000 × 4000 points in about 15 minutes.

The scanner of choice is becoming the laser scanner. This device moves a film across a slit that is being scanned at relatively high speed by a gas or solid state laser. The scanning is usually done by galvanometer mirrors, although acoustic cell deflection has been used. Laser scanners give resolutions of up to 4000 × 5000 points and penetrate an optical density of 3. It is common to have the digital output densities provided to a depth of 10 or 12 bits. At present, several companies are introducing new laser scanners for radiologic applications.

Nuclear Medical Imaging or Isotope Imaging

Nuclear medical imaging was one of the first clinically used imaging modalities to deliver an electronic image. For this reason, it was the first modality that relied on digital image handling. Nuclear medical imaging makes use of the fact that certain elements collect in specific types of tissue. If the element is also radioactive, the emitted radiation can be used to form an image of the tracer element's distribution. In an examination, an appropriate tracer, also termed a radiopharmaceutical, is first injected into (or ingested by) the patient. After the tracer has had time to collect in the targeted tissues, a gamma camera is used to image the tracer.

The gamma camera is generally of the Anger variety. An Anger camera consists of four elements: the collimator, the detection crystal, the photomultiplier tube (PMT) array and the electronics. The collimator serves the same purpose as the aperture in a pinhole camera. It forms a map between the patient and the detector crystal; each point on the crystal responds to a narrow, pencil shaped volume of activity. The detector crystal is generally thallium doped sodium iodide. Its function is to convert impinging gamma rays into optical photons. Each gamma ray acts as an optical point source. The light resulting from each point falls on several photomultipliers. The photomultiplier array consists of 20–40 PMTs covering the face of the detection crystal. The PMT entrance windows may be round, hexagonal or square. The PMTs are run in integration mode rather than in photon counting mode; the signals from the PMTs do not distinguish between gamma events. This fact is important in understanding the image assembly technique realized in the electronics.

The electronics form the image by additive interpolation of the PMT signals. Traditionally, this interpolation has been done by a resistor grid. The grid typically consists of 64 × 64 nodes, where adjacent nodes are connected by resistors. Input of the PMT signals occurs at the nodes corresponding to the PMT locations. The image signals are then taken from all nodes and digitized to form a 4096 point image from the 30 nodes driven by PMT signal amplitudes. Recently, the resistor grid has been replaced by direct signal digitization and microcomputer processing. The images from a nuclear medical system are relatively small, 64 × 64 pixels, and shallow, 6 bits deep. The small format suited nuclear medical images well for the early computers.

Computed Tomography

In the early 1970s, CT became the second modality to rely on the digital computer. In the early days, CT was sometimes known as computerized axial tomography (CAT). The word axial was included because the image formed was a slice perpendicular to the patient's central axis. The word tomography is compounded from the Greek words for slice and picture. A CT image has, typically, 512 × 512 pixels of 12 bit depth.

CT is revolutionary for two reasons:

1. The image is free from the superimposed structures of a projection image.
2. The discrimination between x-ray absorption coefficient values is much better than with conventional radiography.

The CT machine consists of four parts: the gantry, the x-ray source, the linear detector array and the electronics. The gantry supports the rigidly connected x-ray tube and detector array and allows that assembly to rotate about the patient's axis. To perform a CT scan, the assembly is cocked (rotated) to its start position. Then a scan is performed by rotating the assembly 180 degrees. The machine is cocked again, the patient table moves a few millimeters and another scan is performed. The cocking action is necessary to avoid destroying the data transmission and high voltage cables connected between the gantry and the source-detector assembly. There are several variations in CT scanning geometry. One is used in the newly available continuous rotation machines, which have nonrotating, full circle detector arrays. Another variation is used in fast, special purpose machines that have no mechanical motion but rather produce the x-rays by scanning an electron beam over an anode that surrounds the patient.

Computed Radiography

General radiology, using projection x-radiography and plain film, produces the highest volume of picture data in the hospital. In the early 1980s, a potential replacement for plain film was brought onto the market. The system, CR, replaces the traditional film-screen combination found in x-ray cassettes with an imaging plate. The composition of this plate is similar to that of an intensification screen. When the plate is exposed to x-rays, the crystal imperfections in the plate are excited to a higher energy level. The free decay of these sites is quite slow. However, they can be caused to decay immediately by laser beam illumination. On decaying, the molecules emit the energy that they have stored as optical photons of a wavelength different from that of the laser. This stimulated emission is collected, converted to an electrical signal by a photomultiplier and digitized in synchronization with the scanning. The images are typically 1760 × 2140 pixels by 10 bits. Higher spatial and exposure resolutions are being pursued. The original motivation for this invention was to have a direct replacement for plain film. Examination procedures and equipment would remain the same; the only change would be that, instead of a film processor, an image plate scanner would make the latent image visible. An additional advantage has since become apparent. The exposure latitude of the CR imaging plate is far greater than that of film. This increased latitude translates into almost no retakes. Not having retakes is especially important for portable examinations, in which the exposure conditions are usually difficult, and for pediatric patients, for whom the amount of radiation dose is critical.

Digital Subtraction Angiography

In the late 1970s, digital hardware was increasing in speed to the point at which digitization of television frames could be combined with simple real time processing. One of the applications of this technology was in imaging blood vessels (DSA). A DSA machine consists of four parts: the x-ray source, an x-ray image intensifier, a television camera and a frame grabber. The x-ray intensifier is a large vacuum tube for converting x-rays to optical images. The entrance window is between 6 and 22 inches in diameter. The inside of the entrance window is coated with a scintillation layer, which converts the incident x-rays to light, and a photocathode layer, which converts that light to electrons. The electrons are accelerated through the tube and focused on the exit window. The exit window is coated with a phosphor, which converts the electron image to a small, bright, optical image. High efficiency optics image the phosphor onto the television camera's target. The frame grabber digitizes the video signal and stores the frame. Since the resulting picture is a "still-life," the process is sometimes called frame freezing. The subtraction feature is then used (see Chapter 20, Film, Film Processing and Photographic Techniques, for specific information on subtraction). The first frame is of the patient's blood and all surrounding detail. Contrast medium, a radiopaque substance, is then injected into the blood near the area of interest. The second frame contains everything the first frame did but, in addition, contains the contrast medium filled vessels. On subtraction, all surrounding detail is suppressed and the vessels appear in sharp detail. Digital subtraction angiography gives pictures of 512×512 or 1024×1024 pixels and 8 bit depth.

DISTRIBUTION

At present, almost all picture information is present as films in folders or film jackets. These films may be located in several different areas. The flow of film requires that the envelope be picked up from where it is and carried to where it should be. Within a building, "running with the film" is sometimes referred to as the Keds network. The Keds network is a local area network (LAN) of a sort. For medium range and long haul distribution (transporting images to another building or geographical area), the alternatives, taxi and airplane networks, are used. The average capacity of these networks is high, but the delays are long.

It is possible to connect computers to send film images from one area to another. This configuration is called a distribution network. The present-day distribution network architecture and hardware are straightforward. There are electronic analogs to all three of these network categories, i.e., the local area, medium haul and long haul networks. With PACS, the LAN is the network of choice.

Networks

Networks consist of two parts: channels and nodes. Information travels through the channels and is manipulated at the nodes. The channel hardware is cable. The node hardware is the electronic black box. For PACSs, the nodes are display stations, acquisition devices, data archives, etc.

There are three types of networks in the PACS: the LAN, the wide area network (WAN) and the global area network (GAN) or teleradiology system.

There are many proposals for dividing the communications load among these networks, especially between the LAN and the WAN. The following is a brief description of the function of these networks.

The core network of the PACS is the LAN, which carries pictures between acquisition nodes, data base archives and display stations. Such a LAN supplies connectivity within one department or clinical section. The communications links between sections are supplied by the WAN. The picture transmission between hospitals and to remote sites is over the teleradiology system. The technology used for realizing the LAN and WAN is fiberoptics.

Teleradiology differs somewhat from the LAN and WAN. Teleradiology is diagnosis at a distance: the pictures, in digital form, are transmitted over channels between the acquisition and diagnosis sites. These sites may be in adjacent buildings or halfway around the world. The picture transmission uses one of several channel technologies. In order of increasing sophistication, these are standard telephone lines, high speed telephone lines, fiberoptic telephone lines, microwave links and, finally, satellite links. There are standardization projects proceeding within the electrical engineering community for defining actual GANs that will, at some point in the future, be suitable for teleradiology.

Channel Technologies

Networks are connected by cables. There are many cable types that can be used in constructing a network. Four commonly used in medical applications are twisted pairs, baseband, broadband and fiberoptic.

The term twisted pairs refers to pairs of garden variety wires that are twisted about one another in pairs. Several of these pairs are bound together in a cable. Twisted pairs is the type of cable used for computer terminal connections.

Baseband and broadband are ways of using coaxial cable. In baseband systems, the signal is sent directly into the cable. Broadband systems first use the signal to modulate a high frequency carrier signal and then inject the total signal into the cable. The baseband approach is considerably faster than the twisted pair approach. The broadband approach allows higher data transmission speed than even the baseband coaxial cable. Of course, the cost goes up as the speed increases.

Fiberoptic cable allows for the highest speed of data transmission. The fibers' small size and immunity to electromagnetic interference are additional advantages. The decreasing cost and increasing speed indicate that fiberoptic cables are the best hardware for PACS. A network topology is the layout of the connections between nodes or black boxes. Common topologies are mesh, tree, ring, dual ring, bus, star and star cluster.

Packet Routing

The information being transmitted is broken into packets. The path determination is called packet routing. Three common types of packet routing are broadcasting, circuit switching and packet switching. A broadcasting network sends all information to all nodes. The circuit switched network decides where the information should travel and then establishes a circuit, a pathway, over which a group of packets travel. At the end of the transmission, the circuit is dissolved. The telephone system is a good example of a circuit switched network. The packet switching is the newest form of packet routing. Each packet of information has a few bits attached as a header. This header contains a destination node address and sometimes a return address. When the packet arrives at a node, that node determines whether it is the addressee or where to forward the packet. Examples of packet switched networks are the computer networks such as GTE's Tel Net or Tymshare's Tymnet.

Logical and Physical Properties

Physical properties are tangible items, e.g., cables and black boxes. Logical properties are intangible (exist in the mind's eye), e.g., channels and nodes. A broadband cable may be carrying several signals, each impressed onto a different carrier frequency. So, although physically there is just one cable connecting two black boxes, logically there may be many channels involved.

Designing systems to contain physical and logical properties is not an academic exercise—it is essential in designing efficient systems. The physical location requirements and constraints on data routing can be quite different.

Network Interfaces

To get the pictures into and out of the network, equipment interfaces are necessary. If a unit com-municating with a viewing console contains a computer, there is a reasonable expectation that the data will be available when needed elsewhere, e.g., in a HIS, RIS, and especially PACS. Sometimes, there is difficulty in the communications if the equipment components sending and receiving the information are devices from different manufacturers. It is common for different equipment to be incompatible. This is done to protect company secrets and to help prevent competitors from taking advantage of new developments. Designing equipment that is unique to a specific company hinders the development of a universal standard interface.

However, attempts are made at standardizing interfaces between pieces of radiological equipment. One of these attempts is the interface standard developed by the American College of Radiology (ACR) in conjunction with the National Electrical Manufacturers Association (NEMA) (American National Standard Institute, 1985).

The ACR/NEMA standard is a specification for a point to point connection between pieces of medical imaging equipment. The specification is organized into layers. The lowest is the hardware (physical medium) layer; the higher layers are software that progresses toward the application connected to the interface. The hierarchy of layers (beginning at the top) are application, presentation, session, transport/network data link, physical and physical medium.

The specification goes into a reasonable amount of detail about the physical to session layers. At the lowest level (physical medium), the specification describes a 50 pin connector, the wiring of that connector to a cable and the signals that are to be sent to and received from that cable. The physical medium is in parentheses in the preceding list because it is different in nature from the other layers and in the standard it is not listed as a layer. Above the session layer, there is much creativity but little compatibility in developing network connections. However, the standard is relatively new, and the ACR/NEMA committees are considering what should be done about the upper layers and other bits of vagueness that have been discovered as various groups have begun implementation of the software described by the standard.

To understand how the system works, imagine a quantity of data being produced by the imaging equipment at the top. The data are organized into a packet and given an appropriate header by the application layer hardware-software to pass to the presentation layer. The packet is passed downward through the layers, growing a little bit at each layer through the addition of header information, until it is in the proper, standard form. The packet is then sent, travels across the cable, is received and begins a trek, upward, through the ACR/NEMA layers of the receiving equipment. At each layer, the packet is stripped of information, like an onion being peeled, until it arrives in a format that the receiving device can understand.

STORAGE

Hospitals generate a large volume of picture information. A typical hospital generates about 3 gigabytes of picture data per day for each 1000 beds. There are many ways to visualize this quantity of data. One way is to translate the number of bytes into the height of a stack of floppy discs that would be needed to store the data. A personal computer–type floppy disc has a 360 kilobyte storage capacity. A stack of 11 floppy discs is 1 inch high. A stack of floppy discs with a storage capacity of 1 gigabyte is 22 feet high. The daily picture data production of an average medium to large (1000 bed) hospital is equivalent to a stack of floppy discs 66 feet high, roughly the height of a seven story building. Storing the total, 5-year, archived picture data of a medium to large hospital would require a stack of floppy discs 120,450 feet high, i.e., the height of a 12,000 story building. For comparison, the Empire State Building is 102 stories high.

In a PACS environment, storage subsystems, or database archive systems (DBAS), must provide for this information. Access to the stored data must be convenient and rapid. To meet speed requirements and minimize cost, PACS DBASs are generally discussed as being multilevel, hierarchical storage units containing mixed storage technologies. The motivation for this construction is drawn from the operation of the present day film based departments. Film stores information quite densely, but even so, warehouses are still required to house the film archive. The film archive consists of three portions: immediate, short term and long term. The immediate portion consists of those films mounted on film alternators and contained in stacks of envelopes next to light boxes. The short term portion consists of those films stored in the film library.

The film library, where film jackets are stored on shelves, is usually located adjacent to the reading room. The long term portion resides in basements and distant warehouses. This partitioning is natural because the degree of demand for a given film is correlated with its age.

The film is read soon after it is made; the demand for that film is high. It is put on the alternator for reading. The access time is short: a few seconds when the film is read in its normal order on the alternator. After this initial reading, access to the film may be needed a few times during the patient's hospital stay, say for a week. During this time, the film is stored in the film library, the access time is reasonably short, a few minutes or hours, depending on the urgency. After the patient leaves the hospital, the film is needed only occasionally. After a year or so, the film is needed almost never. At this point, the film is transferred to the warehouse. In the unlikely event that a film in the warehouse archive is needed, it can be retrieved, although this process is quite time consuming (on the order of days).

By using this multilevel storage strategy, the average access time is kept low, while the total amount of stored data remains high. The cost is also minimized because the storage space is arranged in order of decreasing cost—alternator, film library, warehouse. Storage space is also arranged in order of increasing required capacity.

The analogous arrangement of storage technologies in a DBAS for a PACS (decreasing cost and increasing required capacity) is semiconductor memory, magnetic discs and optical discs. Semiconductor memory presently costs about $100 per megabyte. A typical winchester magnetic disc costs approximately $10 per megabyte. Optical disc jukeboxes store data for well under $1 per megabyte. Typical per image access times are a few milliseconds, a few seconds, and minutes, respectively. This design strategy is a clear analog to the present day film archive system. That is, store the immediately needed images in semiconductor memory, the not so immediately needed on magnetic disc and the warehoused images on optical disc. As an example of the floor space required: a present day film library, occupying a large room, can be stored in a cube shaped optical disc jukebox about 1 m across.

The efficiency of DBAS and LAN can be increased by exploiting an additional freedom: data fragmentation, whether the DBAS is centralized or distributed. At present, the images from different imaging modalities are read near those modalities. An imaging department may be divided into several section e.g., CT, digital (image intensifier) and MRI. The images generated by these sections most often spend their useful lives in that one section. To minimize the traffic in a PACS network, one strategy is to create miniarchives located geographically in each department section. This arrangement would exploit the low intersectional demand, minimizing intersectional traffic load and required design capacity. Also, although data generated in a specific section could be accessible by WAN to the entire system, the traffic at each miniarchive is much smaller than it would be for the centralized alternative.

IMAGE PROCESSING

Image processing has great promise but conceals a great danger. The dark side of image processing is the artifact: a detail that is not present in the original image but is introduced by the processing. Medical images must be handled with special care. Primarily, caution is limiting the speed with which image processing is being introduced to the medical community.

Some image processing is necessary in the PACS to prepare images for visual display. The cathode ray tube (CRT) is not film. It cannot display as much information simultaneously as film. Image processing functions are necessary to selectively enhance details of the images to adapt them for display on the CRT. There is a learning phase for radiologists in reading these processed images; the acceptability of this learning phase has a strong impact on the speed at which PACS is introduced. One image processing technique under intensive investigation is adaptive histogram equalization (AHE), which was developed at the University of North Carolina, Chapel Hill. This method and its derivatives hold promise for automatically compressing images' dynamic ranges for display on CRTs. The following is a discussion of two types of image processing for PACS: compression and contrast enhancement.

Compression

Image compression is a form of image processing that may have a significant impact on the develop-

ment of PACS; it affects PACS's cost directly. Compressing the images so that smaller amounts of information need be handled by the PACS allows reducing the system storage capacity and the transmission bit rate, without reducing the diagnostic performance of the system. There are two classes of compression algorithms: reversible and irreversible. A reversible coding allows exact recovery of the original image from the compressed version; irreversible coding does not. In general, the highest reversible compression ratio that can be obtained for a medical image is three; the compressed image occupies one-third of the space of the original. Irreversible coding can attain much higher compression ratios but does discard information. The diagnostic and legal acceptability of irreversible compression will be determined by extensive research and application. No final decision will be made until PACSs are in widespread use. The present tendency of emerging PACS realizations is to offer both uncompressed or reversibly compressed images and irreversibly compressed images, with the choice left to the user.

Enhancement

The second type of image processing necessary in a PACS is contrast enhancement or, more generally, image preparation for display. The necessity for this preparation comes from a weakness of CRT displays: they can render only a relatively limited number of distinguishable gray shades. The image information content must be adjusted to the display. One example of image processing for enhancement is high spatial frequency boost filtering. In this type of processing, fine structures and details are emphasized and global properties suppressed. Applying this type of processing to a chest image makes some finely structured details behind the mediastinum and heart visible; it also gives the normal fine lung structure the exaggerated appearance of diseased tissue as caused by lung infiltrates.

In spite of the difficulties caused by the artifacts, some simple processing is acceptable for certain modalities. One of the best examples is gray level stretching (the digital counterpart of brightness and contrast adjustment of CRT monitors). This method is also called windowing or level and window manipulation. The processing consists of selecting a narrow range of gray values and linearly stretching this narrow range to the full range of the display device. The center gray value of the narrow range is the level, and the width of the input range is the window. This technique is regularly applied to CT images. The artifacts introduced by windowing are now well understood by the radiologist and can be easily disregarded.

DISPLAY

The display station is a critical component because it is the radiologist's window into the PACS. To successfully compete with the alternator, the digital viewing station must offer high quality display, rapid image changing, simultaneous viewing of many images and simple image processing. Display stations of widely varying complexity exist in the PACS. This leads to a variety of names. There are viewing stations, display or viewing consoles, image workstations, review, diagnosis and analysis consoles, among others. The terminology is, unfortunately, not precise. The main components of a display station are one or more video monitors, video memory and an interface to the image network. Other components, such as large semiconductor memories, winchester disc storage, special image processing and analysis hardware, may be included. For instance, a review console may be a display station used by a referring physician to help visualize the radiologist's report. This console could be rather simple, with only moderate resolution and no image processing facilities. The analysis consoles, on the other hand, may be used for primary diagnosis and disease quantification. This console would have to be much more sophisticated, including all of the functions listed above.

The degree of image quality presented by the various viewing consoles is still a matter of discussion. There are many contributing factors to image quality, such as spatial resolution, image size, image brightness, contrast resolution, noise, flicker and phosphor persistence. Studies have begun showing that the required resolution depends on factors such as the examination type, the technique and the particular radiologist doing the reading. It appears that between 1000 and 2000 pixels across the screen are needed to support most diagnoses, though there is some evidence that even higher resolutions may be required in special cases, e.g., to see hairline bone fractures and pneumothoraces. The contrast resolution, or number and distribution of gray levels

at each pixel, varies by examination. However, the general requirement seems to be between 10 and 16 bits, which is equivalent to 1024 and 65,536 gray levels. The spacing of these levels is also important.

Image size also seems to be important; relatively large monitor screens, at least 19 inches diagonal, appear to be the most desirable. Monitors are becoming available that provide resolutions of 1536 × 2048 and 2048 × 2560 pixels with 60 to 72 Hz (refreshes per second). Whether the brightness, uniformity, contrast resolution and modulation depth of this new generation of monitors are sufficient for primary diagnosis is the subject of current research. Measuring the physical attributes of the images is necessary but not sufficient. Diagnostic accuracy is the targeted property. In conjunction with physical measurement, psychophysical measurements (such as questionnaire based studies) are being used to answer these questions.

The ideal display station is a complex machine whose characteristics are not fully understood at the present time. It appears now that film and CRT viewing stations will coexist for some time. The balance of readings will shift only slowly from film to CRTs.

CONCLUSION

At present, the environment of the hospital is in a state of rapid flux. Computerized images are having an impact in several ways. The separation of the acquisition and display stages of the imaging process makes for a much better, easier and more reliable diagnosis. The emergence of digital image handling systems promises to increase the efficiency of hospital operation.

In the next few years, it is anticipated that there will be many changes in medical imaging. Many of these changes are expected to be influenced and even made possible by the availability of computerized images.

Bibliography

Ahmed, N, Natarajat, T and Rao, KR. Discrete cosine transform. IEEE Transactions on Computers, C-23(1):90–93, January 1974.

American National Standards Institute. Fiber distributed data interface (FDDI). ANSI X3T9.5, Z3.139–1987.

American National Standards Institute. Digital imaging and communications. ACR/NEMA Standards Publications No. 300, 16–27; 16–28, 1985. Washington, D.C. National Electrical Manufacturers Association, 1985.

Arenson, RL, et al. Clinical evaluation of a medical image management system for chest images. American Journal of Roentgenology, 150:55–59, 1988.

Capp, MP, et al. The digital radiology department of the future. Radiologic Clinics of North America, 23:349–355, 1985.

Chandler, D. Hard drive busts gigabyte barrier. PC Week, 31:10, October 1988.

Chen, PPS. Database design based on entity and relationship. In Yao, SB, ed. Principles of database design. Vol. 1. Englewood Cliffs, NJ: Prentice-Hall, 1985, pp 174–210.

Chen, TM and Messerschmitt, DG. Integrated voice/data switching. Institute of Electrical and Electronics Engineers, Inc., Communications Magazine, 26 (6):16–26, 1988.

Chen, WH and Smith, CH. Adaptive coding of monochrome and color images. Institute of Electrical and Electronics Engineers, Inc., Transaction on Communications, COM–25 (11):1285–1292, 1977.

Cho, PC, et al. Clinical evaluation of a radiologic picture archiving and communication system for a coronary care unit. American Journal of Roentgenology, 151:823–827, 1988.

Davisson, LD. Rate distortion theory and application. Proceedings Institute of Electrical and Electronics Engineers, Inc., pp. 156–164, July 1972.

Deans, SR. The radon transform and some of its applications. New York: Wiley, 1983.

DeSimone, D, et al. The impact of a digital imaging network on physician behaviour in an intensive care unit. Radiology, 169:41–44, 1988.

Dwyer, SJ, III, et al. Local area networks for radiology. Journal of Digital Imaging, 1:28–38, 1988.

Elnahas, SE, et al. Progressive coding and transmission of digital diagnostic images. Institute of Electrical and Electronics Engineers, Inc., Transaction on Medical Imaging, MI–5:73–83, 1986.

Fajardo, LL, et al. Excretory urography using computed radiography. Radiology, 162:345–351, 1987.

FDDI token ring access control (MAC). SNSIX3.139 Standard, 1987.

Freeze, R. Optical disks become erasable. Institute of Electrical and Electronics Engineers, Inc., Spectrum, 25(1):41–45, February 1988.

Garcia, N, Munos, C and Sanz, A. Image compression based on hierarchical encoding. Proceedings International Society for Optical Engineering (SPIE), 594:150–1156, 1985.

Gitlin, JN. Teleradiology. Radiologic Clinics of North America, 24:55–68, 1986.

Goldberg, M and Sun, HF. Image sequence coding using vector quantization. Institute of Electrical and Electronics Engineers, Inc., Transaction on Communications, COM–34:703–710, July 1986.

Goodman, LR, Wilson, CR and Foley, WD. Digital radiography of the chest: Promises and problems. American Journal of Roentgenology, 150:1241–1252, 1988.

Gray, JE, et al. Digital radiography: Is it feasible? or desirable? American Journal of Roentgenology, 143:1345–1349, 1984.

Hillen, W, Schiebel, U and Zaengel, T. Imaging performance of a digital storage phosphor system. Medical Physics, 14 (5):744–751, 1987.

Hindel, R. Review of optical storage technology for archiving digital medical images. Radiology, 161:257–262, 1986.

Huang, HK, et al. Radiological image compression using error-free irreversible two-dimensional direct-cosine transform coding techniques. Journal of the Optical Society of America, 4 (5):984–992, 1987.

Huffman, DA. A method for the construction of minimum-redundancy codes. Proceedings Institute of Radio Engineers, 40:1098–1101, 1952.

Jain, AK. Image data compression: A review. Proceedings Institute of Electrical and Electronics Engineers, Inc., 69 (3):349–389, 1981.

Kangarloo, H, et al. Two-year clinical experience with a computed radiography system. American Journal of Roentgenology, 151:605–608, 1988.

Lo, SC and Huang, HK. Radiological image compression: Full-frame bit-allocation technique. Radiology, 155:811–817, 1985.

Lo, SCB, Krasner, B and Mun, SK. Impact of noise on radiological image compression. Proceedings International Society for Optical Engineering 1092:244–250, 1989.

Lux, P. A novel set of closed orthogonal functions for picture coding. Archiv fur Elektronik und Übertragungstechnik 31:267–274, 1977.

Lux, P. Redundancy reduction in radiographic pictures. Optica Acta 24:349–365, 1977.

MacMahon, H, et al. Digital chest radiography: Effect on diagnostic accuracy of hard copy, conventional video, and reversed gray scale video display formats. Radiology, 168:669–673, 1988.

Malek, M. Integrated voice and data communications overview. Institute of Electrical and Electronics Engineers, Inc., Communications Magazine, 26 (6):5–15, 1988.

Mankovich, NJ, et al. Operational radiologic image archive on digital optical disks. Radiology, 167:139–142, 1987.

Morris, PG. Nuclear magnetic resonance imaging in medicine and biology. Oxford: Clarendon Press, 1986.

Nasser, M, et al. Image coding using vector quantization: A review. Institute of Electrical and Electronics Engineers, Inc., Transaction on Communications, COM–36 (8):957–971, August 1988.

Natterer, F. The mathematics of computerized tomography. Philadelphia: Wiley, 1986.

Netravali, AN and Limb, JO. Picture coding: A review. Proceedings Institute of Electrical and Electronics Engineers, Inc., 68 (3):366–406, 1980.

Philips, BW. 'Floptical' disk drive stores 20.8 Mbytes of data. Electronic Design, 11:65–68, August 1988.

Roos, P, et al. Reversible interframe compression of medical images. Institute of Electrical and Electronics Engineers, Inc., Transaction on Medical Imaging, 7:328–336, 1988.

Ross, FE. FDDI—a tutorial. Institute of Electrical and Electronics Engineers, Inc., Communications Magazine, 24(5):10–17, 1986.

Seshadri, SB, et al. Satellite transmission of medical imaging. Proceedings of the SPIE—The International Society for Optical Engineering, Medical Imaging II. 914, February 1988.

Sonada, S, et al. Computed radiography utilizing scanning laser stimulated luminescence. Radiology, 148:833–838, 1983.

Taira, RK, et al. Design and implementation of a picture archiving system for pediatric radiology. American Journal of Roentgenology, 150 (5):1117–1121, 1988.

Tasto, M and Wintz, PA. Image coding by adaptive block quantization. Institute of Electrical and Electronics Engineers, Inc., Transaction Communications Technology, COM–19:957–971, 1971.

Tateno, Y, Iinuma, T and Takano, M (editors). Computed radiography. Tokyo: Springer-Verlag, 1987.

Tzou, KH. Progressive image transmission: A review and comparison of techniques. Optical Engineering, 26:581–589, 1987.

Wang, L and Goldberg, M. Progressive image transmission by transform coefficient residual error quantization. Institute of Electrical and Electronics Engineers, Inc., Transaction Communications, *36*:75–87, 1988.

Welch, TA. A technique for high-performance data compression. Computer, pp. 8–19, June 1984.

Wintz, PA. Transform picture coding. Proceedings Institute of Electrical and Electronics Engineers, Inc., *60* (7):809–820, 1972.

Wu, WK and Burge, RE. Adaptive bit allocation for image compression. Computer Graphics and Image Processing, *19*:392–400, 1982.

Ziv, J and Lempel, A. A universal algorithm for sequential data compression. Institute of Electrical and Electronics Engineers, Inc., Transaction Information Theory, *IT–23*:337–343, 1977.

Ziv, J and Lempel, A. Compression of individual sequences via variable-rate coding. Institute of Electrical and Electronics Engineers, Inc., Transaction Information Theory, *IT–24*:530–536, 1978.

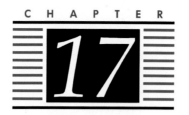

17

COMPUTERIZING ADMINISTRATIVE TASKS

ALAN L. RYAN

INTRODUCTION

The 1970s was noted for the rapid increase in computer use. Computers appeared in all areas of life, from microwave ovens to electronic banking machines. They were popular because they performed tasks normally done by humans or replaced older less efficient equipment. An efficient computer is able to perform tasks faster and with a higher degree of accuracy than a human. Because computers could do a better job faster and were cost effective, application of computers to industry flourished. Medical imaging departments also realized that computers were useful in performing tasks. Today, computer use in imaging departments is found in technical areas, e.g., computed tomography, magnetic resonance imaging and ultrasound (refer to Chapter 16, Digital Imaging Overview, for more information on this subject), and in administrative tasks. This chapter concentrates on the general design of a computerized administrative imaging department and uses of software modules.

ADMINISTRATIVE SOFTWARE AND THE IMAGING DEPARTMENT

A computerized radiology administrative system is referred to as a radiology information system (RIS). A RIS tends to save the department money and increase referral revenue. After an initial learning curve (3–6 months), a RIS helps direct the department's activities, smooths patient flow and allows the staff to become more productive. Implementation of a RIS allows managers to find time to accomplish tasks that they were unable to perform with a manual administrative system.

The basic functions of a RIS are to accumulate information, store data, manipulate data and produce informative reports. These functions are useful in facilitating more knowledgeable departmental decisions. There are many companies marketing a RIS. The more popular companies are National Medical Computer Services' (NMCS) ARM, DEC RAD, Dupont's Mars II, Dimension Systems' Maxifile and Hewlett Packard's (HP) Images. It should be stressed that a RIS is only as good as the application software program provided by the vendor and the staff operating the system.

Some traits of a good application software package are versatility, applicability and simplicity. A versatile program is able to perform a variety of tasks. For the software to be applicable, the software tasks must meet the department's needs. A program is simple in the sense that it is easy for a person to use. It should be noted that software that is simple to use is often complex from the standpoint of technical programming.

To maximize computer efficiency, individuals responsible for operating the software should familiarize themselves with all the capabilities of the package. Because software packages perform a variety of tasks, it is not unusual for a user to spend 3–6 months' training to master all the functions of the system. This training period is often frustrating. Sometimes this frustration becomes discouraging and can lead to departments' returning to less frustrating methods, namely reverting to the manual process. However, departments that are able to work through the frustrations find that the rewards of computerization greatly outweigh the benefits obtained from a manual system.

The primary benefits of a RIS include saving time, adding revenue and increasing referrals. To achieve these benefits, the computer software system should include modules for patient scheduling, patient tracking, film tracking, transcribing and word processing, maintaining teaching files, tracking inventory, automatic purging and reporting productivity.

MANUAL ADMINISTRATIVE TASKS

Before discussing administrative computer use, it is necessary to understand the flow of paper in a manually run department (Figure 17–1). In a manually run hospital radiology administrative system, the flow of paperwork usually begins with the hospital information system (HIS) in admissions. After completing the appropriate forms at the admissions office, the patient is given an x-ray requisition to take to the imaging department (this task may not be performed in private imaging centers or practices). When the patient arrives at the front desk (reception area) of the imaging department, a staff member receives the requisition and searches the card file for the patient's history card. History cards are notorious for becoming lost, misfiled or incorrect, causing a good deal of wasted time as staff members look for the card. Time and motion studies reveal that it is not unusual for patients to wait at the front desk for 5 minutes while the clerk searches for a history card. After the card is located (or not located, if the patient was never at the facility before), and depending on the comprehensiveness of the HIS, the clerk returns to the reception desk and types a pull slip, flash card and label.

The pull slip is used to pull the master jacket or subjacket, which contains the previous films of the patient. These films may be transported to the reading room or to the quality control area or may accompany the patient.

The flash card, label and requisition travel with the patient and technologist to the examination room where the procedure is performed. On completion of the examination, the flash card is used to imprint the patient's information on the films. The completed examination films are then placed in the patient's film folder (jacket). The label may be placed in one of several areas, e.g., on the film jacket or the daily log sheets (the actual location of the label is determined by the individual imaging department). The completed films and requisition are taken to the reading room where the physician dictates the report.

The dictation tapes and requisitions for all patients are transported from the reading room to the transcription area. Transcriptionists type the reports. After the report is typed, it is returned to the physician for approval and signature. Reports needing editing are returned to the transcriptionist, corrected and sent back to the physician. Unedited reports are sorted relative to the patient's floor (if the patient is admitted to the hospital) and the referring physician. The paper flow (reports) ends at several locations. The sorted reports are sent to the patient's floor (if applicable) and the physician. Other areas receiving a copy of the report are the medical records department and the patient's film jacket.

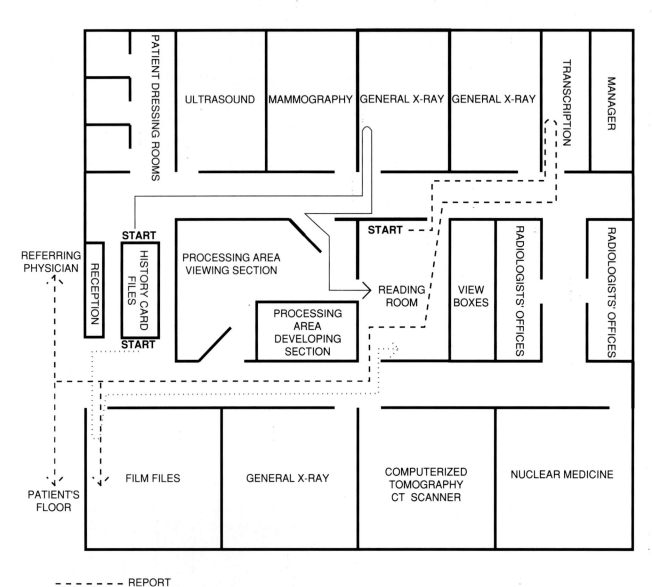

Figure 17–1. Manual paper flow in an imaging department. (From National Medical Computer Services.)

HOSPITAL INFORMATION SYSTEM

Many hospitals use a computer based HIS, which allows the admitting staff to enter (key in) patient demographic and billing information for use within the hospital. Imaging departments operating in a manual mode must hand type the same data that was typed by a computerized HIS.

HISs usually operate on either a mainframe or a minicomputer. HIS may be designed as a centralized system. That is, all hospital departments have terminals that operate off the hospital's main computer (Figure 17–2). This type of system eliminates the need for departments to have their own computer network. Advantages of a centralized HIS are

- No interface is required.
- The hospital deals with a single vendor.
- Financial support is the responsibility of the hospital administration.
- Hardware is standardized.
- Data processing personnel are responsible for computers.

The disadvantages of a centralized HIS include

- Software is usually for hospital administrative work instead of imaging needs.

- Multiple users can result in slow system response time.
- The entire hospital is dependent on one central processing unit.
- Choices of HIS vendors are limited relative to ancillary departments.
- Priorities for updates, changes and enhancements are usually made at the hospital administrative level rather than imaging department level.
- The system is expensive.

HIS may also be designed as a decentralized system. In this type of system, each department is autonomous, often functioning by using an individual system, e.g., RIS. Some systems operate on minicomputers and some on microcomputers. There are many advantages of installing RIS software. These include

- There is better support for the imaging department.
- Software is more relevant to the department's needs.
- Enhancements, updates and changes of software relate to departmental needs.
- The department may choose the vendor.
- There is flexibility in that the computer may stand alone or be interfaced with other hospital computers.

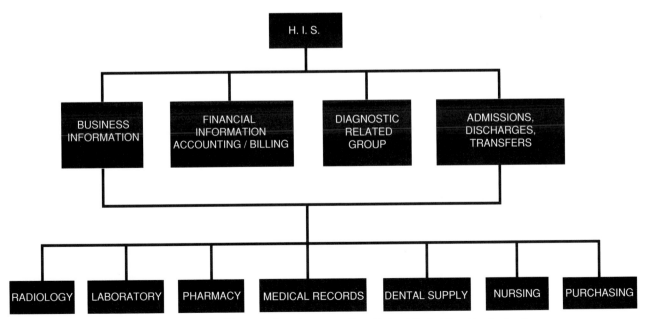

Figure 17–2. Centralized hospital information system. (From National Medical Computer Services.)

RISs are not without their drawbacks. Some disadvantages of a RIS are

- The cost of an interface with a HIS may be high.
- The hospital usually has multiple computer vendors, increasing costs.
- Financial support comes from the departmental budget.

Communication of a RIS with the HIS is obtained through an interface. The interface allows patient information keyed into the HIS to become available to the RIS. For example, for a patient requiring a radiologic procedure, the medical records number of the patient is entered in the imaging department computer. This allows the RIS to have access to the information previously keyed in admissions. This method saves time by eliminating redundant data entry. Another method of interfacing is called a one way interface. In the one way interface, the data being transmitted to the department's printer can be split and diverted to the RIS, eliminating the need for a complicated two way interface.

RADIOLOGY INFORMATION SYSTEM

As mentioned previously, a RIS performs many tasks. The following is a brief summary of the software modules associated with the various tasks.

PATIENT SCHEDULING

Hospitals, imaging centers, and private practices schedule some or all of their procedures. In a manual administrative system, each modality's schedule is usually kept separately, requiring a number of scheduling books to be maintained. Some facilities have one central location that does all the scheduling, whereas others allow each modality to schedule their own appointments, e.g., ultrasound and CT. Scheduling can be a major effort within the imaging department (not to mention other hospital departments trying to schedule a patient at the same time the imaging department wants that patient). Scheduling on a manual basis can be time consuming and error prone. Most scheduling RIS modules provide a number of functions designed to save time and improve efficiency.

These include inquiring, checking for conflicts, logging in the patients, logging the procedures (daily log), scheduling the patients and producing management reports.

The first step in scheduling patients with a RIS is for the staff member to enter the patient's name into the computer. When the patient's name appears on the screen, the staff member verifies that the information is correct by checking the birth date, social security number or other reliable data with the patient. This takes place in seconds rather than the minutes it usually takes to look through the card file manually. For first time patients (patients who have not been to that department before), the patients' data can be entered either by the imaging staff or through a HIS interface as mentioned above.

Normally, procedures to be scheduled are entered along with a starting time. A good scheduling system checks to see what resources are available for that particular procedure(s), e.g., room(s) and physician(s). Because schedules for all modalities are viewed simultaneously, the problems normally associated with manual scheduling of multiple procedures, e.g., procedural conflicts, are greatly reduced. Depending on policy, each modality can be autonomous and patients can be scheduled independently, if desired.

Most manual scheduling errors are in the form of procedural conflicts. One type of conflict occurs when two procedures are scheduled for the same time. Another involves the order in which procedures are scheduled. A scheduling safety feature built into the RIS software is to check for scheduling conflicts. For example, if one procedure cannot be performed immediately after another or must precede (prerequisite) another, the system alerts the user of the conflict. This reduces errors and assists in a smooth patient visit, increasing referrals to the department and hence revenue.

A time saving feature of a RIS is the automatic printing of flash cards, labels, pull slips and transportation slips. As previously mentioned, in a manual system, it is common for history cards to be lost or misfiled. A primary advantage of a properly used RIS is the elimination of lost or misfiled patient history records. This improved efficiency is due to the software's ability to prohibit the assignment of identical x-ray numbers to two different patients.

Another advantage of the patient scheduling

module is that a daily log is created as a by-product of keying in the patients with their corresponding procedures. Also, patient management reports are generated. These reports are vital to the proper functioning of a modern, well-run department.

In addition to scheduling the patient, producing a daily log sheet and generating patient management reports, this module captures charges. When the procedure is keyed in, the RIS stores the examination charge by procedure code. This links the correct charge to the procedure. This information may be used with the HIS or for private physician fees. Because many facilities interface the RIS to the HIS, accurate fee information is transmitted to the HIS for patient billing. Also, a system interfacing the HIS with the RIS makes the charges available to key hospital staff members. This eliminates the need to rekey billing data, saving time and eliminating errors. Most RISs have the ability to separate the technical fees from professional charges. The system can use this information to produce electronic media (floppy disc, tape), enabling the physicians to perform their portion of the billing.

PATIENT TRACKING

Many hospital patients undergo multiple examinations involving several departments. It is common for departments or physicians to seek information regarding the examination status of a patient undergoing imaging tests. A patient status report helps other departments or physicians plan or readjust their schedules. The patient tracking module of a RIS tracks the patient and informs the user of the present status of the patient, e.g., waiting room for 12 minutes, examination completed 5 minutes ago and appointment pending in 10 minutes. This type of information allows the staff to rapidly determine the status of the patient, saving the staff time in trying to locate the patient. Consequently, staff members can respond to a referring office more quickly than when using the manual method, increasing the service level of the department.

Each patient's status is electronically time stamped and is available for productivity reporting. This information may be used as a quality control mechanism to determine the time the patient spent in the examination room, the average time spent by the patient in the waiting room, the orderly transportation time and the average time to perform certain procedures.

FILM TRACKING

Another feature of a RIS is film tracking. In a manual film tracking system, a person hand writes the name of the individual checking out the film, the date, the expected return date, possibly the address and perhaps a phone number. Also recorded is the patient number and which studies are checked out. After films are checked out, there is a manual follow-up process to determine if the films have been returned. A letter is sent to those individuals who have not returned films. This process is time consuming and involves some form of a card filing system or logging method.

Computerizing film tracking saves a great deal of time and eliminates the need for a card file. To use the film tracking module, the file room clerk searches the patient's file by name, birth date or x-ray number (medical record numbers can also be used). When the name appears on the screen, the clerk is aware of the film's location by reading the patient's record. To check out an individual study or an entire patient master jacket, the clerk passes a bar code wand over the bar code label located on the master, subjacket or film. After the examinations are recorded, the wand is passed over the location label, which identifies where the films are going. Location labels are kept in a file for quick access. The areas where films can be checked out to are unlimited. The location can range from a specific room within the imaging department to a medical center thousands of miles away. Most RISs allow the department to define the film check-out locations.

A good film tracking module records how long the film has been checked out and generates follow-up letters requesting that the films be returned. This saves a tremendous amount of staff time and reduces the amount of lost and missing films. Many systems can limit the number of films to be checked out to certain people or locations. Also, some systems enable the user to track films within their facility that have been borrowed from other facilities. Unreturned films can result in legal problems, especially if the films are needed as evidence in a court case. Because more films tend to be returned when using a RIS than with a manual system, there is an increase in the number of stored films. Thus, more films are available for disposal when they become legally obsolete. Disposing of more film increases the amount of silver recovered, increasing revenue. Improving the film return rate increases the probability that the films are available for review in the event that the patient has additional studies performed at that facility.

TRANSCRIPTION

Hospitals use some form of transcription whether the reports are transcribed within a hospital typing pool or in the imaging department itself. The report process includes typing the report, a physician's signing the report and distributing the report to the hospital floors (where applicable), master film jackets and referring physicians. However, unless each report is manually compared with the procedures that were logged and billed, lost charges can and do occur. This is a laborious task but is necessary to eliminate lost charges. To help avoid lost charges, some form of integration must take place between the logging of a patient and the transcribing of a report.

An integrated transcription module within a RIS is important for this reason and from an inquiry standpoint. In a RIS, the transcribed reports are correlated with the procedures logged to determine if any procedures were added, changed or deleted. Corrections are made if there is a discrepancy between the procedures logged and the typed reports. Integrating the first step of dealing with the patient, logging the procedures to be performed, with the last step, transcribing the report, eliminates nearly 100% of all lost charges, thereby increasing department revenue.

An integrated transcription module can also provide the referring physician with immediate access to patient reports. To receive reports immediately, the referring physicians must have a terminal, printer or facsimile machine in their office. With facsimile capabilities, a RIS dials the referring physician's telephone number and sends the document without any human intervention. The result is better service to the referrer and fewer status calls to the department, saving both the imaging staff and the referring physician time and money. Physicians who do not own a terminal, printer or facsimile machine can obtain a verbal report by calling the imaging department. Because the RIS can provide access to patient records by x-ray number, patient name, radiologist or referring physician, the user can refer to a report using any one of these items. The information is displayed in a matter of seconds. Most RISs also have a method to alert the staff if the report has not yet been transcribed and this information can be relayed to the referrers.

The report itself is representative of the imaging department to the referring office and is the imaging department's product. Besides being diagnostically accurate, the report should be professional in appearance, e.g., no misspelled words. Word processors may be linked to a RIS to improve the appearance of a report. A word processor allows the user to enter (input) data and view the information on a screen before printing on paper. The many functions of word processing systems provide the user a great deal of flexibility. These options facilitate corrections (e.g., add, delete) and provide a rapid method for data movement and most offer a "spell check" capability to reduce spelling errors. The quality of printing is a function of the type of printer used. Two printers that produce professional looking reports are the letter quality printer and the laser printer. Care needs to be taken to ensure that the word processor and the printer are compatible. Some systems allow the users to format their own reports. The reports may be designed to offer letterhead reports to clinics or chart formats for the imaging department records.

PURGING

Purging is a method of deleting old patient history cards and films from the respective file. The length of time a patient's records are kept on file is usually determined by state laws. Removing old cards provides the imaging department with more space. Eliminating old films increases space and increases department revenue through silver recovery sales.

To manually purge a card file, each card must be reviewed. Manual purging of the film file requires someone to look at every master jacket, removing the legally obsolete folders. Even with color coding or other manual methods, this takes a good deal of time.

The RIS's purging feature prints a chronological listing of all jackets to be pulled. There is an option for the user to determine whether or not to purge a file. Those patient files purged can be recorded on some form of electronic media, e.g., tape and floppy disc. The use of a RIS purging module eliminates the need for a card file used in manual purging.

TEACHING FILE

Radiologists frequently review interesting cases. Sometimes this is required for instructing others, such as in a teaching environment, and other times reviewing cases is necessary to prepare for a speech. Whatever the reason, on a manual method it is extremely time consuming for the staff to find a particular case study when the procedure was possibly performed many months or years ago. It could take days to bring together the information required by the physicians in these situations.

A RIS has an option for the user to maintain a teaching file or interesting case file. By entering the American College of Radiology pathology codes or other data, e.g., key words, a person can easily gather the required data requested by the physician.

INVENTORY

Inventory is a necessary process of all imaging departments. The manual inventory process requires the time consuming task of having someone count and record the number of supplies. The RIS inventory module integrates the number and type of procedures performed with the number of supplies remaining. This is beneficial because supplies used for a procedure automatically reduce the quantity on hand. Thus, by knowing the number of procedures performed and the number of supplies, it is possible to have the RIS advise the user when to reorder. The inventory system does not eliminate the need for manual inventory. Manual inventory is required because it is possible that items may be used and not recorded on the computer, e.g., multiple injections for a procedure. However, the frequency of inventories is greatly reduced when using a computerized inventory system.

PRODUCTIVITY REPORTS

Numerous helpful reports are readily available from a RIS. The reports are especially useful in providing data for a quality assurance program. The

Table 17–1. EXAMPLE OF PRODUCTIVITY REPORT

Shift Activity Report for NMCS Radiology Management

11:30:58   07/13/91

DEPT	SHIFT	DESCRIPTION				Start	Time End	Days SMTWTFS									
1	1	First shift				07:00	16:00										
Pt Type	Period	Visits	Procs	Tec Units	Rad Units	Reports	Words	Type	Tran Time	Late Arvl	Wait Time	Late Exam	Exam Time	Long Exam	Post Exam
In-pt	Day	14	22	182	51				46	40	−40	0	31	7	11
Out-pt	Day	0	0	0	0				0	0	0	0	0	0	0
Emergency	Day	0	0	0	0				0	0	0	0	0	0	0
Out-surgery	Day	0	0	0	0				0	0	0	0	0	0	0
All types	Day	14	22	182	51	0		0	46	40	−40	0	31	7	11
In-pt	PTD	17	36	266	96				40	30	−31	0	53	7	12
Out-pt	PTD	1	4	49	12				0	0	0	0	75	10	15
Emergency	PTD	0	0	0	0				0	0	0	0	0	0	0
Out-surgery	PTD	0	0	0	0				0	0	0	0	0	0	0
All types	PTD	18	40	315	108	0		0	38	29	−29	0	54	7	12
In-pt	YTD	17	36	266	96				40	30	−31	0	53	7	12
Out-pt	YTD	1	4	49	12				0	0	0	0	75	10	15
Emergency	YTD	0	0	0	0				0	0	0	0	0	0	0
Out-surgery	YTD	0	0	0	0				0	0	0	0	0	0	0
All types	PTD	18	40	315	108	0		0	38	29	−29	0	54	7	12

From National Medical Computer Services.
Pt Type = patient type; Procs = procedures; Tec Units = technologist units; Tran Time = transportation time; Late Arvl = late arrival; In-pt = in-patient; Out-pt = out-patient; PTD = period to date (the department specifies the period); YTD = year to date.

following is a list of some more popular reports produced by a RIS:

Canceled appointment schedule reports
Inpatient transportation schedule
Radiology appointment schedule
Radiology room schedule
X-ray record request
Daily activity summary
Daily activity detail report
Film utilization by shift
Room activity report
Patient detailed report
Film quality report by procedure
Film quality report by room
Film quality report by technologist
Film reject report by procedure
Film reject report by shift
Film reject report by technologist
Procedure summary report
Film utilization by technologist
Physician activity report
Film quality report by shift
Shift activity report
Film reject report by room
Procedure activity report
Staff activity report
Film utilization by procedure
Film utilization by room

With the use of a report generator, many database systems allow the users the flexibility to extract any data that are in the system and print that data in many different formats (Table 17–1). User definable formats for both transcribed reports and daily reports are available with some systems. Also, most systems allow the user to "download" file data for use with certain standard microcomputer based programs.

CONCLUSION

There are four primary advantages of a RIS. One advantage is the saving of personpower hours. Time spent on maintaining inventory, film filing, etc., is reduced substantially. A second advantage of a RIS is the decrease of errors. Fewer scheduling conflicts, errors in charges, etc., are recorded with a RIS. As a result of decreased errors, the third advantage of a RIS is better patient care. The last advantage of a RIS is the increased revenue. There are many ways that a RIS increases revenue. The most common methods include the cutting of current costs and the increased physician referral as a by-product of improved departmental patient care and management.

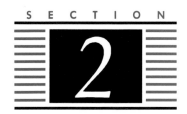
FILM PROCESSING AND PHOTOGRAPHIC TECHNIQUES

It is possible for a radiographer to use the x-ray equipment properly but to have to repeat a film because of processing problems. Because radiographs from several areas of the department are developed in a centralized processing area, when processing problems arise they affect all the areas using the processor. Consequently, it is essential to ensure that the processing area is functioning properly to minimize the number of repeat films needed and to limit the unnecessary radiation absorption by the patient or technologist.

Discussion of film processing is also important because the recovery and sale of silver is a source of income.

This section contains detailed information about the design of a processing area, automatic processor function, film processing and silver recovery. Unlike other texts this includes information on quality control (QC), and specific chapters that discuss QC or chapters in which learning is reinforced by practical laboratory experience contain cross-references to laboratory experiments in the laboratory manual, *Concepts in Medical Radiographic Imaging*.

Highlights of this section include information of first and third order subtraction, stereoradiography and film duplication.

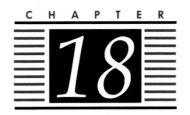

PROCESSING AREA DESIGN AND QUALITY CONTROL

INTRODUCTION

The advent of computer technology has changed the manner in which imaging departments function. Computers play an important role in both the administrative and technological aspects of imaging. In the past, administrative tasks, such as typing of requisitions, calculating budgets and determining the availability of examination reports, were performed by the employees. Today, many of these time consuming person-hours are performed by computers (refer to Chapter 17, Computerizing Administrative Tasks, for discussion of administrative uses of computers). The technical aspect of imaging has also experienced dramatic changes created by computer technology. Computers are commonly used to produce images in computed tomography (CT), magnetic resonance imaging (MRI), nuclear medical imaging and ultrasound. Computer technology is being used, to a lesser degree, in conventional radiography. Most of the computer imaging equipment in use today makes limited use of film processing areas (the film processing area is commonly referred to as the darkroom).

The processing area consists of a section in which film is developed (developing section) and a section to view the film (viewing section). Modern day imaging departments make extensive use of conventional radiography and subsequently extensive use of processing areas. Some professionals predict that, within the next 10–20 years, computers will become the primary source of imaging. If this is true, computers would essentially eliminate current conventional radiography methods and decrease processing area use and film storage needs by an estimated 80–90%.

This chapter addresses processing area and quality control. Because most imaging departments use automatic processors, this chapter concentrates on processing areas utilizing automatic processors and contains information on film development using a daylight processing system. Specific information about the related areas of processors, film processing, sensitometry, silver recovery and reject film analysis are found in other chapters.

PROCESSING AREA DESIGN

LOCATION

Ideally, the location of the processing area is determined during the planning stages (architectural design) of the imaging department. However, to meet growth needs, departments already constructed expand by renovating the existing facility. As a result, it is common for the processing area location to be limited to areas where plumbing or electricity is or can be made available. Placing a processing area near plumbing and electricity is essential. However, to locate a processing area solely by the availability of water and electricity tends to compromise other factors needing consideration when selecting an appropriate location. Besides water and electricity, two other primary considerations in determining processing area location are the size of the department and the type of imaging modalities being used. Some questions that need to be answered relative to department size and type of imaging modalities are

1. How many rooms are in the department?
2. What type of rooms exist, e.g., for angiography and nuclear medical procedures?
3. Do any rooms require rapid film development or are they apt to utilize the processor for an extended period, e.g., angiography?
4. Where are the rooms physically located?

Increasing the size of the department increases the need for multiple processing areas. A common factor used to determine the specific number of processing areas is the number of imaging rooms it is designed to service. A centralized processing area may service four to six conventional radiography rooms (Figure 18–1). Smaller, more localized processing areas (decentralized) tend to service two x-ray rooms (Figure 18–2). Thus, the number of processing rooms depends on the philosophy of the departmental leaders regarding the preference for a centralized or decentralized system. It is not unusual for part of the department to be decentralized and part centralized. Each system has its advantages and disadvantages.

The advantages of a centralized processing area include

Lower start-up costs
Better quality control
Fewer operating expenses
Easier determination of patient examination status.

A centralized processing area decreases equipment and purchasing costs because fewer processors are required. Also, electrical and plumbing requirements are fewer, resulting in decreased costs. Quality control is increased because fewer processors are used. This results in increasing uni-

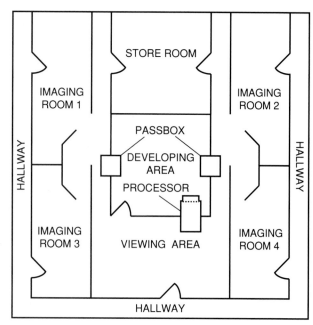

Figure 18–1. Centralized processing area.

formity of film development. Operating costs are decreased as a result of fewer processing area personnel and fewer processors to maintain. Lastly, because the number of processing areas is limited, individuals seeking x-ray reports or a status check on their patient need only to contact one area to determine examination status.

Decentralized processing areas have the advantages of

Increasing the life span of the processor
Reducing the amount of people traffic in the department
Saving the technologist steps
Decreasing the number of or need for quality control technologists.

There are fewer films developed per automatic processor in imaging departments with a decentralized processing system. The decreased processor workload increases the life span of the processor (note: the processor must be used sufficiently to avoid deterioration of chemical residue build-up on rollers). Also, whereas centralized processing areas require the majority of technologists to process their films in one area, decentralized processing areas increase the number of areas available for film processing. Consequently, decentralized processing areas decrease the amount of people traffic. This

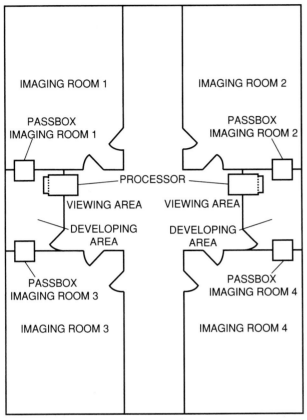

Figure 18–2. Decentralized processing area.

2. Fluoroscopic (F)
3. Radiographic and fluoroscopic (R and F)
4. Ultrasound
5. Nuclear medicine
6. Angiographic (including cardiology)
7. Tomographic
8. Computed tomographic
9. Magnetic resonance imaging

When determining the location of the processor(s) by room type assessment, it is important to also consider the workload or need for immediate products (films) created by the room (question 3). In general, rooms used for procedures that may "tie up" the processor for an extended period (e.g., angiographic serial filming) or have a need to see the films immediately should have a processing area of their own or share the processor with one other room. Rooms producing a low volume of films, e.g., ultrasound, usually operate best when sharing a processor with high volume rooms.

Lastly, the physical location of the imaging rooms needs to be considered (question 4). Many imaging departments are designed to locate modalities using similar imaging methods (e.g., ultrasound and nuclear medicine) in their own respective area. These specialty areas function almost as a minidepartment within the main department. Most of these specialty areas make considerably less use of film processing areas relative to conventional radiography. When determining the processing area location(s) in departments with minidepartments, consideration is given to the amount of processor usage and the distance a technologist must walk to develop films. For low volume specialty areas, care should be taken to avoid having the technologist walk significant distances to develop films for the purpose of sharing a high volume processor.

ENTRANCE DESIGN

Regardless of the location or number of processing areas, a common problem encountered in film processing is the accidental exposure of films to white light (light striking). Exposure to white light blackens or fogs the film in the area where the film was subjected to white light. The light striking of films of an examination or part of an examination mandates that the fogged films be retaken. Repeated filming for procedures utilizing ionizing ra-

saves technologists unnecessary steps, which would otherwise be used walking back and forth to a centralized area. Because fewer patient radiographs are developed per processor with decentralized imaging departments, technologists are more apt to see their finished film products. This eliminates the need to have a quality control technologist handle all radiographs and advise the technologist of the status of their radiographs.

Besides determining the number of rooms in the department and whether to have a decentralized or a centralized processing area, the second question needing to be answered when determining the location of the processor is the type of rooms within the department. Many types of rooms are possible in imaging departments. The type of room depends on the type of equipment installed in the room. There are numerous equipment combinations that can occur. The following is a list of some types of rooms found in imaging departments.

1. Radiographic (R)

diation (as opposed to other forms of imaging, e.g., ultrasound) causes unnecessary radiation absorption by the patient. If the film bin (storage place for unexposed films) is light struck, all fogged films must be replaced. Because film bins are designed to store a minimum of 600 films, the replacement of fogged films can potentially cost the department thousands of dollars. The two most frequent ways films are accidentally exposed to white light is by opening a door leading into the developing section and by turning on a white light in the developing section during film development. The latter cause is easily prevented by placing a microswitch on the film bin so that white lights are automatically turned off when the film bin is opened. Proper design of the entrance door of the developing section helps eliminate the former cause of film fogging.

There are four common types of developing section entrances. They are
1. Single door
2. Double door
3. Revolving door
4. Maze (labyrinth).

The type of entrance built depends on the amount of money available for construction and the amount of space available. Regardless of the type of entrance used, all entrances should be designed to prevent unwanted opening of the door during film development.

The simplest entrance is the single door (Figure 18–3). To prevent unwanted opening of the door, there is a lock on the developing side of the door (there should be some system to allow for the unlocking of the door from the outside in case of an emergency, e.g., fire and illness of person in developing section). Individuals entering the developing section lock the door before beginning film development. If there is no full time processing area staff member, each individual technologist develops his/her own films. This limits the use of the processor to technologists who may enter the developing section at the same time. Others wishing to process films cannot develop their films until the individuals in the developing section have finished their film processing. Some systems are designed with a passbox to pass exposed, but undeveloped, films to individuals in the developing section (see under Basic Processing Area Construction for more information about passboxes).

The use of a passbox when individual technolo-

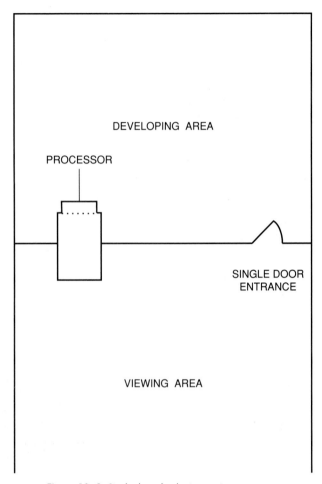

Figure 18–3. Single door developing section entrance.

gists develop their own films requires cooperation on the part of all individuals. Care needs to be taken to avoid filling the passbox with films so that the individuals in the developing side do not spend an extended period of time processing other technologist's films, hindering their own work efficiency. Also, if individuals on the developing side do not process films left in the passbox, this information should be transmitted to the technologist who placed the films in the passbox. Failure to advise technologists that their films need developing may result in an extended time delay before the films become processed.

A more efficient developing section entrance than the single door method is the double door system (Figure 18–4). The doors are built with an electrical interlocking system. The interlocking system is designed so that only one door can be opened at a time. The technologist is able to open the outer door while the inner door is locked (Figure 18–4A). The technologist can open the inner door only when the outer door closes. The outer door locks on the opening of the inner door, preventing light from leaking into the developing section. This system allows people to enter and leave the developing section as needed, eliminating the need to wait for someone to finish developing films, as is the case with the single door entrance.

The revolving door also allows people to enter and exit the developing section at will. The revolving door is cylindrical (the opening represents about 25% of the cylinder). The door is mounted on an outer support system (Figure 18–5), which has

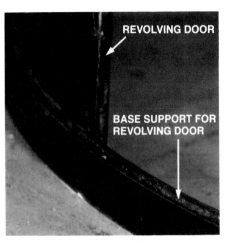

Figure 18–5. Revolving door entrance door mount.

grooves to allow the door to revolve. The support system also has full length curved sides. Half of the curved side support is on the developing side and half is on the viewing side. To enter the developing section, the individual (1) moves the door opening to the viewing side (Figure 18–6A); (2) steps inside the opening (Figure 18–6B); (3) while standing still, turns the door so that the opening is on the developing side (Figure 18–6C) and (4) steps into the developing area (Figure 18–6D). This process is reversed when the technologist wishes to leave the developing section. As can be seen in Figure 18–6, regardless of the door position, white light is unable to enter the developing section.

The maze or labyrinth requires a lot of physical space (Figure 18–7). It is built so it makes a U-turn because white light travels in straight lines and is unable to turn corners. The efficiency of the labyrinth entrance is improved if (1) black paint is used for the walls and ceilings, (2) the height is no greater than 7 feet, (3) the length of the passages is no less than 10 feet and (4) the width of each hallway is not more than 3 feet. The maze eliminates the need for doors. Doorless entrances makes it easier for the technologist to enter the developing section, especially if he/she has his/her hands full carrying items. Some mazes have a white line painted at eye level to help the individual with direction. It is important that individuals entering or leaving the maze keep to the right, reducing the possibility of hitting each other while entering or exiting the developing section.

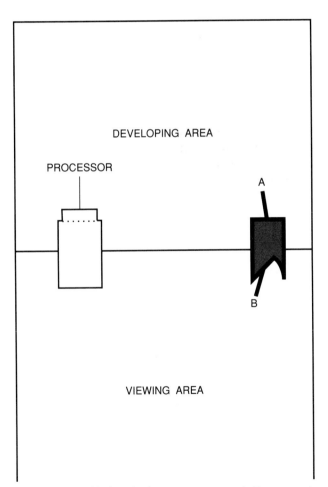

Figure 18–4. Double door developing section entrance locking system. A, Inner door locked; B, outer door unlocked.

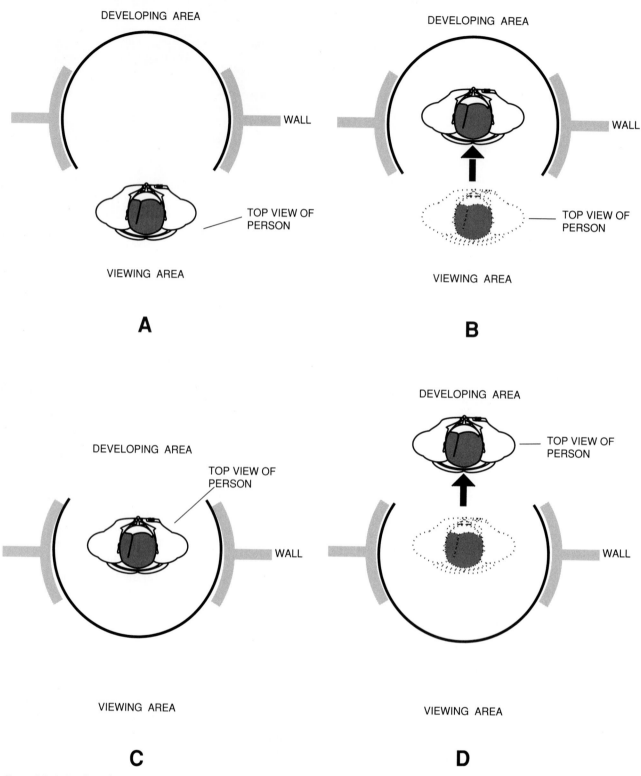

Figure 18–6. Revolving door use. *A,* Move opening to viewing side. *B,* Step into opening. *C,* Move door to developing side. *D,* Step into developing area.

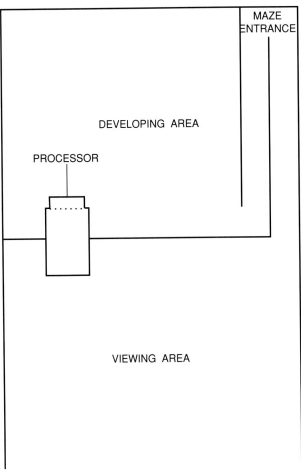

Figure 18–7. *Maze entrance.*

BASIC PROCESSING AREA CONSTRUCTION

Floor, Counter Top and Wall Material

The processing area differs significantly from other rooms in the imaging department. For example, the developing section is enclosed and has equipment utilizing caustic chemicals. Thus, it is important to construct a processing area to maximize environmental safety. The processing area contains a processor with caustic chemicals (developer and fixer), and sometimes the chemicals spill on the floor, counter tops or walls. Thus, it is recommended that the floor, counter top and wall be made of material that is unaffected by the chemical properties of the developer or fixer. A safe floor is made of a nonporous material that is resistant to staining by chemicals and does not become slippery when wet. Examples are substances containing a high proportion of asphalt, porcelain and natural clay tiles. This material can also be used to protect walls. When wall tiling is unavailable, it is advisable that walls be coated with a high quality waterproof paint. Enamels or epoxy paints with a matte finish are safe to use. The color of the wall should be able to reflect light emitted from the safelight. Reflected light helps increase illumination without adversely affecting the film.

Ceiling

The ceiling carries the risk of particles falling off and into a cassette or chemical solution. When one is selecting ceiling paint, it is important to avoid paints that are apt to flake or peel. Plasters should be avoided, as they tend to peel away with time. A drop, or false, ceiling is recommended for rooms in which water pipes or other items enter the room at the ceiling level. These items should be above the false ceiling.

Ventilation

The developing section is an enclosed room. Thus, unless the room is properly ventilated, air in the room tends to get stale. The best type of ventilation is a centralized heating and cooling system. All ventilation systems need to ensure that sufficient air intake and exhaust exists. Such systems often employ vents. If vents are used, they need to be light tight to protect film from becoming fogged. Some type of filtering system is recommended to prevent outside air particles from being drawn into the room by an intake air system (e.g., fan). An adequate ventilation system keeps the developing section at a temperature range between 68 and 70° F and a humidity range of 40–60%.

Passbox

Technologists not working with daylight processing systems need a means for transferring exposed films to the developing personnel without having to enter the developing section. This is most commonly performed through the use of a passbox. Passboxes are built into the wall (about 4 feet from the floor) and connect the developing section to a hallway or room located on the opposite side of the wall. A passbox contains two compartments. One compartment is for exposed film holders; the other is for unexposed film holders. Each compartment is labeled relative to its respective content. The height of the passbox is about 20 inches to easily accommodate large film holders, e.g., 14 × 17 inches (35 × 43 cm). The width of each compartment is about 8 inches, enabling the technologist to place several film holders in the passbox at one time. This is important because most x-ray procedures require multiple film exposures. Passboxes are lightproof and are often lined with lead to protect against radiation. An interlocking device is used to ensure that both sides of the passbox are not opened at the same time (Figure 18–8).

A common device to prevent simultaneous opening of the passbox doors is a movable rod. The rod passes through the compartment divider and is able to protrude on either side of the wall. To open the passbox, the technologist pushes the rod inward (Figure 18–8B). This extends the rod to the opposite side, preventing someone from opening that side. After the rod is pushed inward, the handle is turned to a vertical position (Figure 18–8C). Turning the handle accomplishes two things: frees the doors so that they may be opened and prevents anyone from opening the doors on the other side of the passbox. If a technologist attempts to push the rod inward and meets resistance, the doors are probably

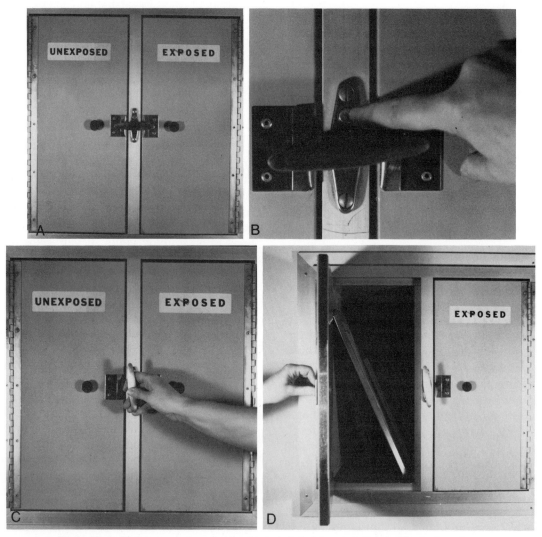

Figure 18–8. Passbox use. *A,* Door closed and locked. *B,* Push in rod. *C,* Turn handle. *D,* Open door.

opened on the other side. Thus, the technologist must wait for the doors on the opposite side to be closed before retrying to open the doors. The movement of the rod and doors tends to make noise; therefore, being aware of sounds informs the technologist whether the doors are opened on the opposite side.

Radiation Protection

To protect both the film and personnel from radiation, the processing area should be protected from radiation. For example, x-ray rooms adjacent to the processing area should never have the x-ray beam's primary ray directed at the processing area wall. Radionuclides are best stored a safe distance from the processing area. Some other common methods used to protect the processing area from radiation include lining the walls, floors or ceiling with at least 2 mm of lead and using a solid brick wall a minimum of 8 inches thick or at least 6 inches of concrete. It is also important to periodically monitor the processing area for radiation. Monitoring is best performed by a physicist or other qualified personnel.

CONTENTS OF THE DEVELOPING SECTION

The developing section is where unexposed and exposed film is handled. Contents vary from institution to institution. The contents are determined by the size and type of imaging department that the processing area is servicing. However, some of the items located in the developing section are universal to all processing areas regardless of the size or type of imaging department. These items include a workbench, lighting, film storage bin and film storage area.

Workbench

The workbench or counter is where most processing tasks are performed. The counter is used to load and unload the film holder, open a box of films, clean cassettes, etc. The top of the counter should be made of material that is resistant to being chipped by cassettes, does not produce static and is easily cleaned. A hard wood, e.g., teak, or thick linoleum meets these conditions. A safety feature for the prevention of static on film is to ground the

counter top. To optimize working conditions, the counter top should be long enough to accommodate several large film holders lying side by side. It is useful to have shelves or another type of storage built underneath the counter. The shelves can be used to store a minimum of a week's worth of unexposed film, tools for preventive maintenance or repair of equipment and cleaning material. If the storage area is multipurpose, care needs to be taken to store unexposed film where it will not be damaged by other items, e.g., liquids from cleaning materials.

Lighting

The lighting in the developing section consists of general white lights and safelights. White light is used to perform preventive maintenance or repair work on equipment, clean the room, store unexposed film or accomplish other tasks requiring good visibility. The most efficient lighting is overhead mounted fixtures. During film handling, the white lights are off and room illumination is achieved by safelights.

Illumination by safelights may be direct or indirect (Figure 18–9). Indirect lighting is more intense than direct lighting and is used for general illumination. Indirect safelights face the ceiling so that the light is reflected from the ceiling. Thus, the ceiling must be painted a color that reflects light and be at least 10 feet high. Direct safelights face downward toward the work area. They are usually mounted on the wall or by the processor film feed tray at a distance of at least 4 feet from the working area. Lights mounted near the feed tray are connected electronically to go off when a film is fed into the processor. The light intensity of bulbs should meet the standards recommended by the company making the safelight. This is usually between 15 and 25 W. All safelights must emit a color allowing an individual to work with the film for about 1–1 1/2 minutes without fogging the film. The color of the safelight depends on the type of film used. Information on the type of light to use is available from film companies. Common colors used are orange-red and green (see under Quality Control for safelight test information).

Film Storage

The developing section has two areas for film storage. One area stores films for immediate use

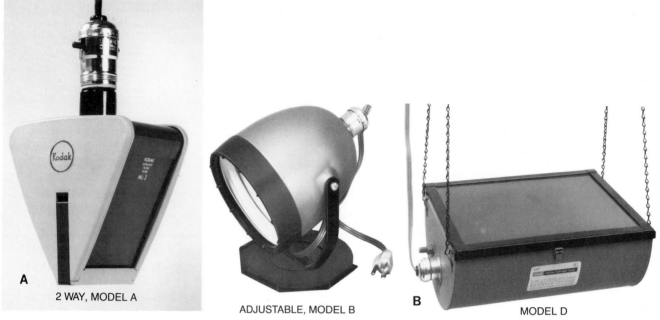

Figure 18–9. Type of safelights. *A,* Direct; *B,* indirect.(© Eastman Kodak Company. Reprinted courtesy of Eastman Kodak Company.)

and is called a film bin. The other area is used to store films needed to replenish the bin. The film bin is mounted under the counter. A film bin is a large lighttight drawer hinged at its lower end (Figure 18–10). The bin holds a variety of film sizes. Each film size is located in its own slot and can hold one box of film (about 100 films). Films are positioned in decreasing size from the front of the bin to the rear. A warning not to open the film bin in white light should appear on the outside of the bin. To prevent accidental opening of the bin in white light, a microswitch designed to turn off white lights should be attached to the film drawer. Thus, when the drawer is opened, the microswitch turns off all white lights.

CONTENTS OF VIEWING SECTION

The viewing area is designed as a temporary place to store films before the radiologist dictates a report regarding the radiographic findings. Thus, the viewing area is designed for sorting, dispensing and maintaining quality control of radiographs. Dictating of reports and long term filing of completed examinations is performed in an area other than the viewing section.

The size of the viewing area depends on the volume of work, the number of people working in the area and the number of processors servicing the viewing section. In general, an increase in square footage is indicated if the workload is large, if a significant number of people enter and leave the viewing area or when more than one processor services the viewing section.

High volume departments have a significant amount of activity dedicated to film dispensing and film sorting. This increases the number of people using the viewing area when compared with that for low volume departments. As a result, people traffic is heavier in the high volume department. To avoid people bumping into one another, the viewing room has to be large enough to allow individuals to freely pass each other while they perform their tasks.

The processor is placed where there is sufficient room to permit individuals to repair or perform routine preventive maintenance without interfering with the viewing of radiographs.

Contents of the viewing section vary from institution to institution. However, some items are recommended for all processing areas. The viewing area should contain a minimum of white lights, a place to store films and film folders, film illuminators, a counter or table and a telephone or intercom.

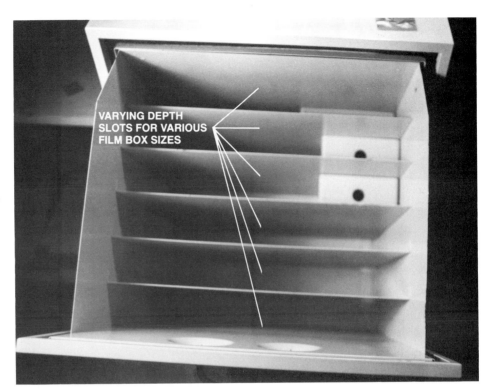

VARYING DEPTH SLOTS FOR VARIOUS FILM BOX SIZES

Figure 18–10. Empty opened film bin (top view).

Lighting

Because processor repair or maintenance is a necessity, white lights should be bright enough to allow processor personnel good visibility while working on the equipment. It is recommended that the lighting be overhead. Fluorescent lights are often used as the overhead illumination. They tend to be inexpensive to operate and provide excellent illumination. One disadvantage of fluorescent lighting is that individuals working for extended periods of time, e.g., quality control technologist and work supervisor, may develop headaches or become tired. These individuals should use incandescent lighting.

Film Storage

The primary tasks performed in the viewing area include storing the previous examinations of the patient, checking the current films as they are processed for quality control, filing the films in the appropriate patient folder and placing the folder in the designated area for the radiologist to dictate a report. These tasks require sufficient space and correct equipment for the individual(s) performing the tasks to work effectively.

A shelf is often used in the viewing area for the temporary storage of films. The shelf's height and depth are enough to store the patients' film folders in an upright position. There are vertical dividers (slats) in the shelf, allowing a patient's folder to be placed in any one of the variety of slots created by the dividers (Figure 18–11). The slots may be labeled with letters for filing patient folders alphabetically or with numbers for separating folders on the basis of the x-ray identification numerical code. The shelf should be located where it is easily accessible and does not interfere with the other activities of the viewing area, e.g., sorting films.

Illuminators

Another necessity of the viewing room is film illuminators, often referred to as view boxes. It is recommended that the view boxes be mounted on the wall at eye level in an area close to the processor. The distance from the processor to the view boxes is such that the number of steps needed to transport the film from the processor to a view box is minimal.

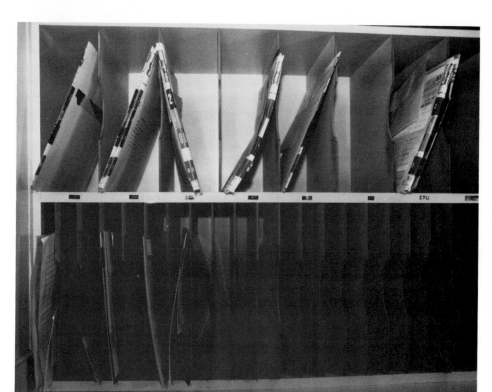

Figure 18–11. Film storage shelf with slots for patient folders.

Also, the location of the view boxes should not hinder the flow of people traffic.

Workbench

Technologists need some sort of workbench, e.g., a counter or table, in the viewing room to perform their tasks. Ideally, the workbench is located so that it is accessible from all sides. This helps facilitate the movement of traffic. However, oftentimes there is insufficient space to permit the placing of the workbench to allow easy access from all sides. Rather, the workbench generally takes the form of a counter and is mounted on the wall (Figure 18–12). The top of the counter can be horizontal or vertical. It is advisable for counters with vertically positioned tops to have a ledge at the bottom to prevent items, e.g., films and pencils, from rolling off. Horizontal tops are advantageous because the user is able to place items in a variety of locations, eliminating the possibility of their rolling off. Supervisors or quality control technologists spend much time bending over horizontal counters to do paperwork. Thus, horizontal tops may create back

problems. The angle of the vertical top permits individuals to write while in an upright position, reducing stress on the spine.

It is not unusual for the view boxes to be mounted on the wall above the counter. If the view boxes are attached to the wall above the counter, they should not extend the full length of the counter. Mounting view boxes in this manner restricts viewing traffic to a specific section of the counter area. Instead, the supervisor and the quality control technologist should be able to perform their tasks at a section of the counter not containing the view boxes without being disrupted by others.

Communication

Most departments have one technologist stationed at the viewing area during the time of the heaviest workload of the department. To properly perform tasks, the technologist needs access to paperwork and some form of communication system. Thus, part of the counter should provide a space for items needed to complete paperwork (pencils, papers, film sticker labels, etc.) and a telephone or intercom system. The use of an intercom allows the technologist to have his/her hands free while communicating with others. However, such a system has the disadvantage of not being able to provide a private, two way conversation. Using a telephone as a means of communication requires the technologist to hold the receiver of the telephone with one hand while talking, therefore restricting the use of his/her hands. If a telephone is the communication system of choice, the cord attached to the receiver should be at least 12 feet long. The long cord allows the technologist to move around the viewing area, gathering information that may be needed to answer the caller's questions. Unlike the intercom, the telephone does provide for private, two way conversation.

ADDITIONAL ITEMS

Four additional items are essential to any processing area. They are chemical storage tanks, a silver recovery unit, a sink and a film identifier.

These items can be located in places other than the processing area.

Chemical storage tanks (replenishment tanks) are where the developer and fixer reserve supply is kept. The supply is used to replenish the chemicals used during film processing. There are several areas where chemical storage can be located. They include the developing section, the viewing section and an isolated area away from the processing area. Chapter 19, Automatic Processor and Preventive Maintenance, contains detailed information regarding chemical storage tanks.

Located near the replenishment tank is a silver recovery unit. There are several types of silver recovery systems available. The objective of a silver recovery unit is to reclaim, for resale, as much silver leaving the fixer as possible. Chapter 22, Silver Recovery, contains detailed information regarding the various types of silver recovery systems and their function.

A sink is a valuable asset to the processing area. It should be located as close as possible to the processing area without getting in the way of the

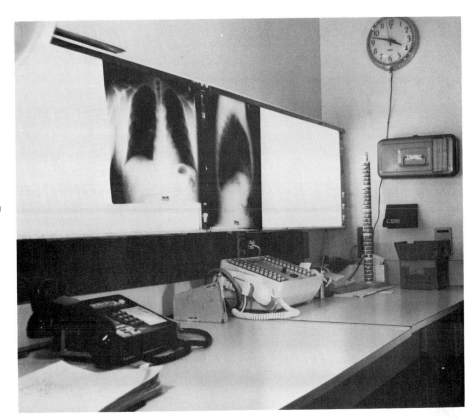

Figure 18–12. Counter area of viewing section.

normal workflow. The faucet of the sink should be able to accommodate the attachment of a hose. The hose can be used to clean the parts of the processor that are unable to be removed. The primary use of a sink is for washing items, e.g., processor racks. Because the sink is used to clean processor racks, its depth, width and length must be great enough for the largest processor rack to fit comfortably. It is advisable to have a drain board attached to the side (or sides) of the sink. The board is used to hold items and allow the excess water to drain off items.

The film identifier is a mechanical device used to imprint the patient's name on the film (Figure 18–13). Some identifiers are constructed to include a clock. During the patient information card exposure, the clock imprints the current time adjacent to the patient information. To operate a film identifier, the patient information is typed or printed on a card. The card is inserted in the slot of the identifier (Figure 18–14). When a cassette is inserted in the film identifier, the window of the cassette is opened (Figure 18–15), uncovering the film. A light is transmitted through the information card, exiting at varying intensities, and strikes the film. The varying intensities (the darker areas of the card, e.g., typed information, absorb more light than the lighter regions) result in the imaging of the appropriate information on the film. After exposure the cassette window is closed and the cassette is removed.

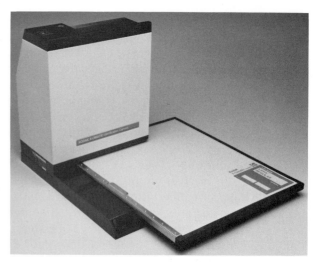

Figure 18–13. Film identifier. (© Eastman Kodak Company. Reprinted courtesy of Eastman Kodak Company.)

DAYLIGHT FILM PROCESSING SYSTEM

Conventional means of film processing require a lot of space and a processing area to handle films in a special light controlled environment. Under this system, during a typical 8 hour day, technologists alternate between working in normal room light and in a darkened room scores of times. They are continually adjusting and readjusting, e.g., eye sensitivity to light, to daylight and darkness numerous times in a day.

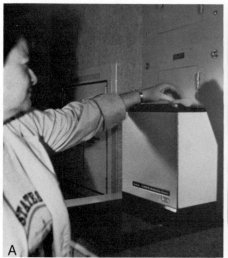 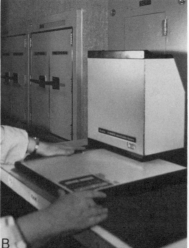 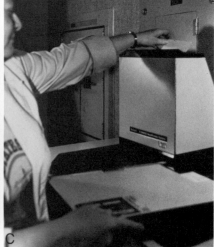

Figure 18–14. Film identifier use. A, Insert card. B, Insert cassette. C, Remove cassette and card.

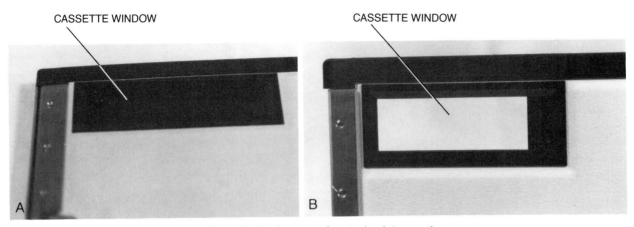

CASSETTE WINDOW

CASSETTE WINDOW

Figure 18–15. Cassette window. A, closed; B, opened.

Daylight film processing provides a means of loading and unloading film under normal room lighting conditions. The advantages of daylight systems include allowing technologists working alone to maintain contact with the patient during film development, saving time, improving the environmental conditions for the technologist and eliminating the need for a developing section. A disadvantage of daylight systems that automatically transport the film to the processor is the stopping of all film exposures (work) when the processor is undergoing repair or preventive maintenance. Another drawback of daylight processing is that nondaylight films (e.g., mammograms, dental x-ray films and odd sized films) must be developed in a conventional processing area. Consequently, provisions need to be made for nondaylight film, e.g., a conventional processing area to process nondaylight film.

There are two types of daylight systems. One uses special equipment to load and unload cassettes. The other operates on the concept of cassetteless handling of films. Cassetteless systems transport film in the absence of any type of film holder. During this process, film movement from storage to development is a function of the equipment. The technologist is responsible for patient positioning, setting the radiographic technique and making the exposure. Chest radiography commonly uses cassetteless daylight processing (Figure 18–16). In this system, films are sheet fed from the storage area to the exposure area. After entering the exposure area, the films are compressed by intensifying screens. The technologist makes an exposure during film compression. After the exposure is completed, the intensifying screens open, releasing the exposed film. The exposed film is then transported to the processor for development or to a film magazine. Use of a film magazine requires

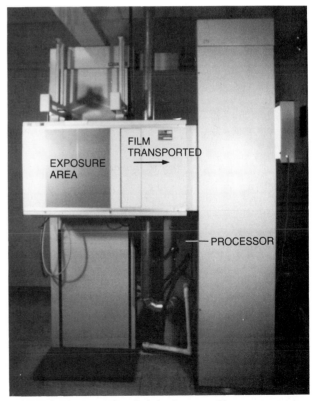

FILM TRANSPORTED

EXPOSURE AREA

PROCESSOR

Figure 18–16. Cassetteless daylight chest unit. Film is transported to exposure area. The exposed film is transferred to a processor located behind the chest unit.

the technologists to develop the film in a conventional processing area.

Cassette daylight systems employ special equipment and cassettes designed to enable the technologist to load and unload film in normal room lighting (Figure 18–17). Cassettes used for daylight systems are of the same basic design as cassettes used for conventional radiography. The difference between the daylight and conventional cassette rests in the daylight cassette's having a slit on one edge that can open or close automatically for film loading or unloading. To fill or empty daylight cassettes, a film loader and unloader are needed. The film loader and unloader may be self-contained in one unit or a separate unit for each respective function may exist.

Film loading machines are designed to load either one particular size of film or several different film sizes. Film loaders have two different types of film storage. One allows the loading of film in regular room lighting. The other uses a film magazine that is loaded and unloaded in the developing section

of the processing area. The cassette loader is constructed so that it is light tight and protected from radiation. The ideal cassette loader/unloader is easy to operate and is able to load and unload cassettes quickly. The optimum location of a daylight loading and unloading machine is where the equipment can service two or three x-ray rooms. To load a cassette with film, the cassette is placed inside the film loader. The film loader automatically opens the cassette, inserts the correct size of film and closes the cassette.

To unload an exposed cassette, the cassette is placed in the unloader machine. The unloader automatically opens the cassette and removes the film. Depending on the design of the unloader, the film is either transported to the processor at the time of unloading or is deposited in a film magazine. Units using a film magazine require the magazine to be manually removed to the developing section where the films are processed.

Regardless of whether a cassette or sheet feeding system is used, there exists a need to imprint the

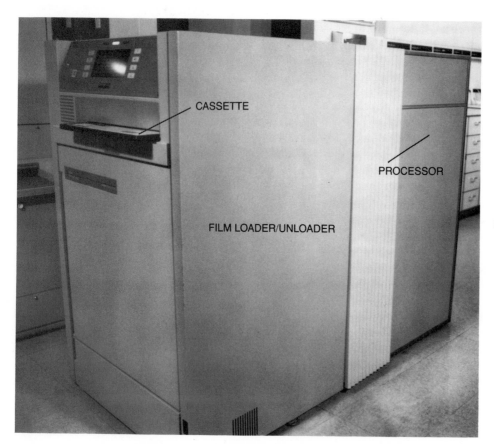

CASSETTE

PROCESSOR

FILM LOADER/UNLOADER

Figure 18–17. Daylight system.

patient information, e.g., name and age, on the radiograph. This information may be put on the film in two ways. One method is similar to the conventional method of film identification. In this method, the information to be recorded is typed or printed on a card. The card is placed in the photographic marker. The photographic marker illuminates, causing light to pass through the patient information card and exit at various intensity levels. Light exits at a lower intensity in the areas where the patient card has printed information and at higher intensities in nonprinted areas. The exiting light strikes and exposes the film. The more light intensity exposing the film, the blacker that area is. The other method of film identification is the identification printer. The printer is a hand held device that illuminates when the user presses a button. To use the printer, patient information is written or typed on a thin sheet of paper. The paper is placed on a light plate and inserted in the cassette and an exposure is made by depressing the light button. The illumination prints the patient information on the radiograph.

QUALITY CONTROL

Processing areas play a major role in the quality of the image produced. One processing area is responsible for the processing of hundreds of films daily. The actual number of films developed depends on the number of imaging rooms the processing area services and the workload of the department. Malfunctioning automatic processors or other problems, e.g., light leak, cause fog or artifacts to appear on the film. These unwanted images create unreadable films. The only way to make unreadable films diagnostic is to repeat the film. Repeated films using modalities producing ionizing radiation result in unnecessary radiation absorption by the patient, wasted time and increased departmental costs. Repetition of films using nonionizing modalities, e.g., ultrasound, increases departmental costs and wastes time. Consequently, it is important to implement a quality control program designed to prevent problems from happening. However, it is not always possible to detect trouble before it occurs. Sometimes, processing area problems are identified only after developed films display fog or artifacts. The specific processing area quality control

program utilized by an imaging department depends on the complexity and contents of the area. At a minimum, the following processing area quality control tests or rules should be implemented:

1. Inspections for foreign substances and contamination
2. White light check
3. Temperature control check
4. Radiation test
5. Safelight test
6. View box inspection
7. Film storage check

This chapter concentrates on the quality control of the developing and viewing sections of the processing area. Quality control relating to the automatic processor is discussed in Chapters 19, 21 and 22.

FOREIGN SUBSTANCES AND CONTAMINATION

An easy problem to resolve is the prevention of foreign substances. Foreign substances are items that do not belong in the processing area. Most foreign substances are caused when individuals eat, smoke or drink in the processing area. Therefore, an important rule to follow is no eating, drinking or smoking allowed in the processing area. Engaging in these behaviors may cause food particles, ashes or liquids to fall into cassettes or the processor chemicals. Objects that fall into cassettes create artifacts on the film. These artifacts require the films to be repeated. If foreign objects find their way into the processor chemicals, they contaminate the solutions. Solutions may also be contaminated when chemicals spill into tanks other than their proper container, e.g., the developer spilling into the fixer. Contaminated solutions are undesirable because they inhibit proper film development. Improperly developed films must be repeated. The only way to clean contaminated chemicals is to drain the solutions and replace them with fresh chemicals. Replacement of processor chemicals is costly and time consuming.

FOG

A common cause of film artifacts is fog. Fog is unwanted exposure of the film. The exposure may be the result of light, radiation or heat. To prevent fog, the processing area needs to be light tight, radiation protected and temperature controlled.

The following is a test to determine if unwanted white light is penetrating the developing section. Turn on all the white lights in the rooms and hallways surrounding the developing section. Enter the developing section. Shut off all white lights and safelights. Wait 5–10 minutes to allow the eyes to adapt to the darkness. After the eyes have adapted, look around the room to see if any light is entering. Make sure to visually inspect the area around doors, the processor(s) and pipes. These are the most common places for light to enter. Areas where light is entering should be repaired. Avoid temporary repair jobs, e.g., tape, as these are transient solutions.

Another cause of film fog is radiation exposure. Thus, periodic radiation tests should be performed by a qualified person. The degree of sophistication of the test varies with the expertise of the individual performing the test. Tests may range from the placing of a film badge in the developing section for a period of time to the use of sensitive radiation monitoring equipment. Generally, the use of sensitive monitoring equipment should be performed when the processing area is first installed, especially if it is located near radiation rooms. Additional use of monitoring equipment is indicated when adjacent radiation rooms are renovated or new equipment is installed. After the processing area has been identified as radiation safe, periodic monitoring via use of a film badge–type system is sufficient.

Temperature is another factor that may cause film fog. The optimum temperature for film storage is 50 to 70° F. As a rule, most facilities in the United States are able to maintain this range during the winter months. However, not all institutions have centralized air conditioning, so temperature may become a problem during summer months. Facilities not having centralized air conditioning need to provide some form of cooling for the film storage area. Because many processing areas have no windows, a window air conditioning unit becomes impractical. Two options for these departments include storing the film in a cool basement or the construction of an air conditioning system for the film storage area. To check the room temperature, a thermometer should be attached to the wall. This is not usually a problem, as most facilities have a thermostat with a thermometer attached to the wall. No cooling system is indicated in locations that do not exceed 70° F.

Safelights are another potential source of film fogging. The safelight is designed to allow individuals to see what they are doing while performing the tasks associated with film development. The color of the safelight or the filter over the safelight is a hue to which the x-ray film is insensitive. The intensity of safelights are safe to the extent that the individual does not spend an extended period of time handling the film. Extended exposure of the film to a safelight will eventually fog the film. There is no standard regarding the length of time a film could be exposed to a safelight without being fogged. However, practical experience seems to dictate that 2 minutes is sufficient time for an individual to perform the tasks necessary for film development. Thus, safelight tests should reveal that the light is safe (does not fog the film) for no less than 2 minutes. Imaging departments may select different time standards to suit their individual needs.

There are a variety of safelight tests; the following represents one type.

1. Enter the developing section and turn off all the safe lights.
2. Load a cassette with the fastest speed film used in the department.
3. Exit the developing section and enter an x-ray room. Place the cassette on the x-ray table. Cover half of the cassette *lengthwise* with a strip of lead (Figure 18–18).
4. Expose the cassette to obtain a density between 0.5 and 0.8.
5. Reenter the developing section, taking the exposed cassette and three pieces of heavy paper or other opaque material.
6. While the safelights remain off, unload the cassette. Place the film on the counter top underneath the safelight to be tested. Position one piece of opaque material *lengthwise* on the film so it covers one-fourth of the outer edge of the film. Place a second piece of opaque material *lengthwise* on the film to cover the opposite one-fourth of outer edge of the film (Figure 18–19A).
7. Place the last piece of opaque material *crosswise* on the film about 1 inch from the top of the film (Figure 18–19B) and turn on the safelight.
8. Every 30 seconds move the paper that is *crosswise*

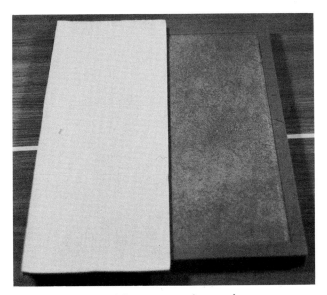

Figure 18–18. Safelight test position of cassette for x-ray exposure.

down the film approximately 1 inch until the film has been completely exposed to the safelight.

9. Turn off the safelight and process the film.

Using an 8 × 10 inch (20 × 25 cm) film for the safelight test results in 4 rows having varying exposures and 10 sections of safelight exposure time (Figure 18–20). Row A represents an area of no exposure (this area was covered by the lead during x-ray exposure and paper during the safelight exposure). The second row, B, was exposed only to the safelight (it was protected by lead during the x-ray exposure). Row C was exposed to both x-ray and the safelight. The last row, D, was exposed

only to x-rays (it was covered during the safelight exposure). The row with no exposure, A, is used to measure the film base fog. The density in row D is used to ensure that the x-ray exposure range was between 0.5 and 0.8. Rows B and C are used to determine the longest length of time the film is able to be handled under the safelight before the film is fogged by the safelight. The top section (1) is exposed for the longest time. For a film exposed with 10 sections each for 30 seconds, the top section is exposed for 300 seconds. It is possible to determine the safe time that a film can remain under the safelight before being fogged by measuring the density difference between rows B and C. The section where the density difference exceeds 0.05 above the base film fog represents the first unsafe time. For example, given that base film fog is 0.25 and the first section where the density in rows B and C is 0.05 above base film fog (or 0.25 + 0.05 = 0.30) is section 6, section 7 represents the maximum safe time. The exposure time of section 7 is 120 seconds. Thus, this test demonstrates that the film can be exposed to the safelight for 2 minutes (120 seconds) before becoming fogged. Sometimes, the test results are less than the base fog plus 0.05 density difference. If this occurs, the safe time is the maximum time the film was exposed.

ILLUMINATORS

After film development, films are viewed by hanging them on a film illuminator (view box). There are many different view box designs. Three

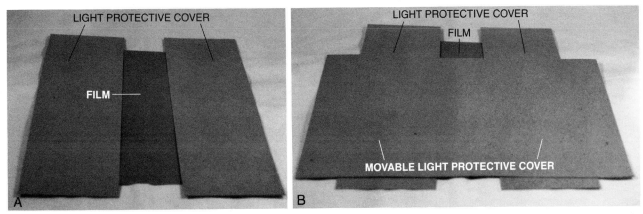

Figure 18–19. Safelight test. *A,* Film covered on outer edges; *B,* placement of movable paper.

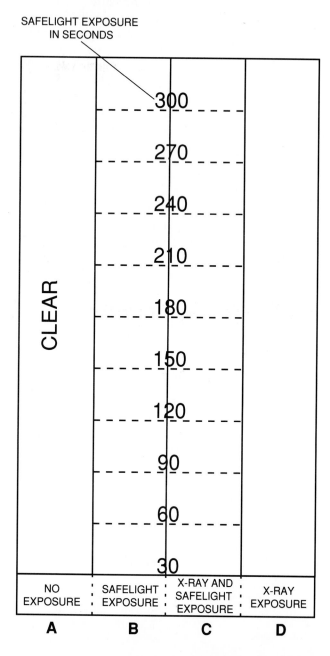

8 INCH BY 10 INCH FILM

Figure 18–20. Various exposure sections of film for safelight test.

common designs are single, stationary bank and movable bank (Figure 18–21). Located inside view boxes are fluorescent bulbs and reflective material. A Plexiglas front is used to cover the bulbs. The light emitted should be uniform and have an intensity of a minimum of 500 foot-candles. The intensity may be measured using a photographic light meter.

Dust may accumulate on the Plexiglas, inhibiting light transmission. Thus, the Plexiglas should be cleaned regularly. Care should be taken to avoid using cleaning agents that interact with the composition of the Plexiglas, e.g., acetone. To maintain uniform light emission in bank view boxes, when one light bulb burns out, all bulbs within the bank

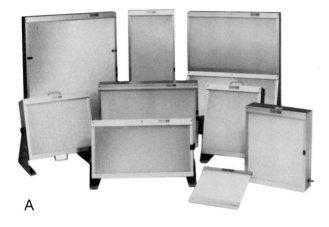

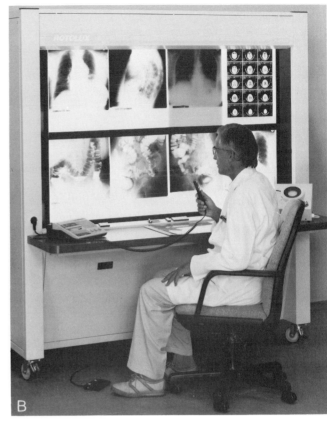

Figure 18–21. View boxes. A, Single and multiple fixed bank; B, movable bank. (From American Medical Sales, Inc.)

are replaced. Replacement bulbs are of the same brand and tone of lamp.

FILM STORAGE

To prevent the possibility of film fogging, films are stored in a room with a temperature between 50 and 70° F and a humidity range between 40 and 60%. Because hot air rises, temperatures are best measured by placing a thermometer at the level of the highest place where film is stored. In arid regions where the humidity is well below 40%, a humidifier may be used to increase the moisture in the air. Those areas where humidity exceeds 60% may employ a dehumidifier to lower air moisture.

Films tend to deteriorate with age. All films are supplied with a date of expiration stamped on the outside of the box. Films should be stored on end and so that the oldest films are used first. Flat storage causes pressure marks (artifacts) on the film. It is possible to extend the life of film by refriger-

ating it. Thus, if the imaging department has a low volume, it is possible to extend the usefulness of the film by putting it in the refrigerator. Film that is refrigerated needs to be placed at room temperature for 8 to 12 hours before opening the box. This prevents condensation from forming on the film.

LABORATORY EXPERIENCE

Individuals wishing to expand their knowledge in this area can perform Laboratories 27, Processing Area Design, and 28, Processing Area Quality Control, in *Concepts in Medical Radiographic Imaging: Laboratory Manual*. The Processing Area Design laboratory enables learners to familiarize themselves with the design and physical set-up of the processing area. Participation in the laboratory requires individuals to investigate the layout of their processing area. They also are responsible to locate and record the various contents and equipment in the area.

In the Processing Area Quality Control laboratory, the investigator actively participates in inspecting or testing processing area items. The objective of the laboratory is to identify potential problems that may exist.

Bibliography

Bushong, SC. Radiologic science for technologists (4th edition). St. Louis: Mosby, 1988.

Chesney, DN and Chesney, MO. Radiographic imaging (4th edition). Boston: Blackwell Scientific Publications, 1981.

Cullinan, AM. Producing quality radiographs. New York: Lippincott, 1987.

Fuji Photo Film Co., Ltd. Control of the photographic properties of medical x-ray films processed in automatic processors. (Medical x-ray products technical handbook reference number XM3–34E. -74.4-OB.3-1). New York: Pyne X-ray Corporation.

Fuji Photo Film Co., Ltd. The fundamentals of automatic processors for medical x-ray films. (Medical x-ray products technical handbook reference number XM3–35E. -74.5-OB. 3-1). New York: Pyne X-ray Corporation.

Fuji Photo Film Co., Ltd. Processing and handling of medical x-ray films. (Medical x-ray products technical handbook reference number XM3–3E. -73.11-OT.3-3). New York: Pyne X-ray Corporation.

Gray, JE, et al. Quality control in diagnostic imaging. Baltimore: University Park Press, 1983.

McKinney, WEJ. Radiographic processing and quality control. Philadelphia: Lippincott, 1988.

McLemore, JM. Quality assurance in diagnostic radiology. Chicago: Year Book Medical, 1981.

Selman, J. The fundamentals of x-ray and radium physics (7th edition). Springfield, IL: Thomas, 1985.

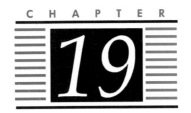

AUTOMATIC PROCESSOR AND PREVENTIVE MAINTENANCE

INTRODUCTION

After x-ray exposure of a part, the film is processed to visualize the image. Original film processing techniques (manual processing) were time consuming. Thus, patients and physicians waited several minutes for the film to be processed before a diagnosis could be made. This was not only an inconvenience, but in some cases, e.g., patient under general anesthesia, undesirable. Consequently, a need arose to design a system of rapid film processing.

This chapter discusses the development of rapid film processing, components of an automatic processor and preventive maintenance for automatic processors. Refer to Chapter 21, Sensitometry and Processor Quality Control, for information on processor monitoring. Chapter 20, Film, Film Processing and Photographic Techniques, provides information on the chemical process of image formation. Chapter 22, Silver Recovery, discusses processor silver recovery.

EVOLUTION OF AUTOMATIC PROCESSORS

Up until the 1950s, the majority of film development was performed manually. The processing time from a dry film to a dry radiograph was about 1 hour. Besides being time consuming, manual processing was also limited by the following:
1. A large space was needed for the equipment.
2. The film needed to be attached to a hanger.
3. The number of films processed (workload) during the workday was low.
4. Someone was needed to perform the various processing steps.

Film processing methods changed dramatically in 1944 when Pako designed the first generation automatic processor. The Pako automatic processor was a hanger-type design. It required films to be attached to hangers for transportation through the solutions. The hanger processor eliminated a lot of the manual labor. However, the total processing time did not decrease significantly. Also, there was still a need for film hangers, someone to put the film on the hangers and a lot of space for the processor. In 1955, Eastman Kodak Company introduced the roller automatic processor, which greatly improved on past systems.

A major advantage of the roller system was to simplify film processing by eliminating the need for film hangers. Other advantages of the roller automatic processor included film processing time was substantially decreased (to about 8 minutes), a large quantity of films could be developed within the normal workday and film quality increased. Decreasing the processing time allowed for a faster diagnosis. The increase in the number of films developed provided a means of increasing the workload of the department. The quality of the film increased because the normal human variations associated with manual film processing no longer existed. Also, the automatic processor was consistent in its processing method from one film to the next.

From 1955 to 1964, a variety of improvements were made to the original roller processor. The two most significant changes were the decreased space needed for the processor and the reduction in processing time. By 1964, film processing time was down to 3.5 minutes.

Another milestone in automatic processors occurred in 1967 with the introduction of the rapid film processor. The rapid processor produces a dry radiograph in 90 seconds. Since 1967, many improvements relative to the efficiency of the processor have occurred. However, to date, no major changes or new advancements have occurred.

SUMMARY OF MANUAL PROCESSING

The sequence of manual processing is similar to that of automatic processing. Thus, before discussion of the rapid automatic processor, a brief summary of manual processing is in order (a more in-depth discussion of manual processing is located in Chapter 20).

Manual film processing begins at the developer. The function of the developer is to change the film's latent (invisible) image to a manifest (visible) image. There are four components of the developer solution. They are the developing agents, preservative, accelerator and restrainer. The most common developing agents are metol and hydroquinone. The developing agents reduce the exposed silver halide crystals of the film to metallic silver. A preservative (sodium sulfite) is added to the developer solution to prevent oxidation. The accelerator (sodium hydroxide or sodium carbonate) is an alkali used to help the developing agents penetrate the film emulsion. This is usually achieved by swelling the emulsion. The restrainer (potassium bromide) prevents the developing agents from acting on the unexposed crystals.

After the film has been developed, it is submerged in the wash water to remove as much of the developer solution as possible. This helps prevent crossover contamination of the developer and the fixer when the film is placed in the fixer solution. Sometimes a weak acid is added to the wash water (stop bath) to help neutralize the developer and stop the action of the developing agents.

From the wash, the film is placed in the fixer to remove unexposed silver halide crystals and harden the film. The fixer contains four components. They are the fixing agent, preservative, acidifier and hardener. The fixing agents (hypo) are usually sodium thiosulfate or ammonium thiosulfate. The fixing agent dissolves and removes unexposed and undeveloped silver halide from the film. The fixer preservative serves the same purpose as the developer preservative. This is the one element common to both the fixer and developer solutions. The acidifier (acetic acid) has several functions. One function is to maintain an acidic level of the fixer, which neutralizes the action of the developer. The acidifier also prevents potassium alum (hardener) from precipitating. Lastly, the acidifier helps in the hardening process by suppressing the swelling of the emulsion. The function of the hardener (potassium alum or chrome alum) is to prevent physical damage to the emulsion and harden the emulsion.

After fixing is complete, the film is put in the wash water to remove the fixer solution before drying the film. When the film has completed the wash cycle, it is placed in the dryer where hot air is circulated over the film to dry it.

CONVERSIONS FROM MANUAL TO AUTOMATIC PROCESSING

The basic theory behind rapid film processing is to increase the solution temperature (which decreases the time needed for film processing) and provide a means of film transportation (rollers). Although this appears to be simple, raising the temperature of the solutions and using a roller film conveying system creates new problems. These problems are

1. Finding a substance that prevents chemical fogging of the film caused by the high temperatures of the solutions
2. Stopping the film from sticking or jamming in the processor during transportation
3. Preventing the emulsion from peeling off the film
4. Maintaining proper chemical concentration of the developer.

To solve these problems, the composition of the developer and the construction of the film used during manual processing were changed.

DEVELOPER COMPOSITION

The automatic processor developer contains three additional items absent from the manual developer solution. One, a hardener (e.g., glutaraldehyde), prevents the film from sticking to the rollers and stops physical damage to the film caused by the swelling of the emulsion during development. Antifogging agents, such as aldehydes, are also added to prevent chemical fog created by the high temperature. Lastly, sulfate compounds are added to minimize the swelling of the emulsion.

In addition to an altered chemical composition of the developer, the chemical concentration of the developer in a rapid processor differs from that in manual processing. This occurs because of a build-up of bromide ions from the reduction of silver halide. Bromide ions act as a restrainer, hindering normal film development. To counteract this effect, the contents of the manual processing replenisher are altered by increasing the quantity of accelerator, decreasing the amount of restrainer or increasing the alkali level.

FILM CONSTRUCTION

The composition of the emulsion and base of films used for manual processing presented many problems when used in automatic processors. Thus, the construction of the film used for manual proc-

essing underwent three changes to resolve the problems arising from roller transportation and rapid processing at high temperatures. The first alteration was to make the film emulsion thinner to prevent the film from jamming during transportation. The emulsion was also made harder to withstand the pressure from the rollers and sustain high temperatures. The last alteration was to change the base material to be strong, be stable and have low water absorption properties (a current material used is polyester).

BASIC AUTOMATIC PROCESSOR DESIGN

The components of an automatic processor vary from company to company. Also, design changes exist among different models within the same company. Regardless of the potential differences, there are common components necessary for all automatic processors. These include

1. A system of rollers for film transportation
2. A mechanism to circulate the solutions
3. A means to regulate proper temperature control for the various sections
4. A method of developer and fixer replenishment
5. A dryer system.

FILM TRANSPORTATION

The function of the film transportation system of an automatic processor is to move the film at the correct speed through the various processor solutions and dryer section. The film must move through the processor without slipping or jamming in the transportation system. As the film is conveyed from solution to solution, the transportation system also serves to remove (squeeze) excess chemicals from the film before the film enters a new solution, e.g., remove developer solution before the film enters the fixer. The film transportation system consists of the following:

1. Motor
2. Feed tray
3. Crossover racks
   a. Entrance
   b. Developer-fixer (D-F)
   c. Fixer-wash (F-W)
   d. Squeegee

4. Deep racks
   a. Developer
   b. Fixer
   c. Wash
5. Receiving bin

The heart of the transportation system is the motor (usually a fractional horsepower motor). The motor is used to turn a main drive shaft, which rotates the rollers. The speed of the motor is faster than the rate needed to turn the rollers. A system of gear reductions is employed to reduce the speed to an acceptable rate (10–20 revolutions per minute). Many motors are designed with an adjustable speed control. More efficient processors have a motor that automatically goes on standby or shuts off during idle times (when no films are being processed) of 3 minutes or longer. This helps conserve energy and increase the life span of the processor.

When the motor is energized, the rollers rotate to transport the film through the processor. Film travel begins at the feed tray and continues to the entrance rack where the film exits into the developer rack. From the developer rack, the film enters the D-F crossover rack and is conveyed to the fixer rack. The film leaves the fixer rack, is transported to the F-W crossover rack and moves to the wash rack. From the wash rack, the film enters the squeegee rack, passes through the dryer rollers and finally comes to rest in the receiving bin (Figure 19–1).

Recall that film travel begins at the feed tray. The feed tray is a polished stainless steel flat tray (Figure 19–2). The sides have guide rails to ensure that the film is aligned properly (straight) relative to the entrance roller. The feed tray is usually adjustable. Its movements include up, down, left and right. The tray is adjusted so the edge of the film enters the processor straight and hits the lower roller of the entrance rack, lifting the film off the feed tray.

The entrance rack (Figure 19–3) is considered a crossover rack in that the film crosses from the feed tray into the developer. Besides transporting the film, the entrance rack often contains the detector system and regulates the replenishment system. The detector system makes an audible sound (usually a bell) advising the user that the film has entered the developer and another film may be safely fed into the processor. Another audible sound (usually a buzzer) is activated if two or more films are entered simultaneously and overlap each other. The entrance rack may also regulate the

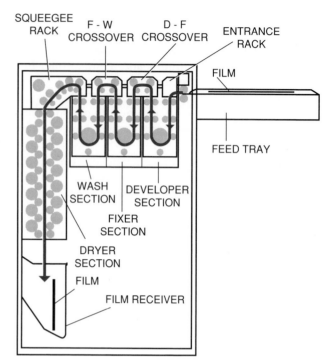

Figure 19–1. Film travel in an automatic processor.

replenishment pump. The replenishment pump is turned on as a film moves through the entrance rack and replenishment stops (pumps are turned off) when the film is completely in the developer. Processors with safelights above the feed tray have the safelight circuitry regulated by the entrance rack. No current flows to the safelight (turned off) when a film enters the entrance rack. Current is resupplied to the safelight (turned on) when the film exits the entrance rack. All of the entrance rack functions are regulated when the top roller of the entrance rack moves up, activating one or more microswitches.

Other crossover racks are the D-F, F-W and squeegee (Figure 19–4). The D-F and F-W cross-overs have the same construction. Both direct the film's movement from one tank to another, e.g., developer tank to fixer tank. This is achieved by employing a series of rollers and guide shoes (deflector plates). Besides moving the film, the rollers of the D-F and F-W also remove (squeeze) excess solution from the film. The solution (obtained in the tank from which the film exits) is removed to avoid contaminating the tank in which the film is about to enter. The squeegee rack contains several

FILM GUIDE ASSEMBLY

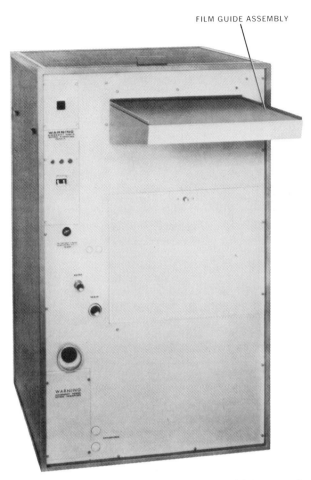

Figure 19–2. Feed guide assembly. (© Eastman Kodak Company. Reprinted courtesy of Eastman Kodak Company.)

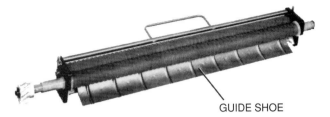

GUIDE SHOE

Figure 19–3. Entrance rack. (© Eastman Kodak Company. Reprinted courtesy of Eastman Kodak Company.)

more rollers than the D-F and F-W crossovers. Because the squeegee rack moves the film from the wash tank into the dryer, more rollers are needed to remove the maximum amount of water from the film to facilitate film drying.

Crossover racks are usually separate from the deep racks. Unlike the deep racks, the crossovers are not submerged in a solution. Because the crossovers are out of solution, they tend to dry out. To help prevent them from drying out, a plastic fume hood (Figure 19–5) is placed over the D-F and F-W crossovers. Also, when the processor is shut off for 2 hours or longer, the chemicals may condense on the crossover rollers. Thus, the crossover rollers should be cleaned before restarting the processor.

There are three deep racks located in the processor. They are the developer, fixer and wash racks

(Figure 19–6). Each rack is located in its respective solution tank, e.g., the developer rack is in the developer tank. The racks are easily removed from the tank for cleaning, maintenance or repair. Deep racks are constructed similarly but tend to vary in length.

Deep racks contain rollers, guide shoes and a turnaround. Most roller diameters range from 3/4 inch to 3 inches, with the most frequent diameter range being 3/4 inch to 1 inch. As with the crossover racks, the deflector plates function to guide film travel. The turnaround alters (or turns around) the direction of film travel by 180 degrees.

The material from which rollers are constructed varies. The material may be hard (e.g., stainless steel) or soft (e.g., rubber). Hard rollers are easy to clean but create more pressure on the film, increasing the possibility of artifacts. Soft rollers are more apt to wear with excessive cleaning or use of abrasive cleaning materials. However, they do not create as much pressure on the film as hard rollers. It is common to find a variety of roller materials, both hard and soft, within the same processor. The roller material used depends on the function of the roller, e.g., remove excess water.

Roller configuration is either staggered (zigzag) or opposing (face to face). A staggered configuration is designed so the rollers are off-centered to one another (Figure 19–7A). The rollers of a face to face configuration are directly opposite one another (Figure 19–7B). Each configuration has advantages and disadvantages. The staggered design is advantageous because it decreases the pressure on the film, reducing the incidence of possible artifacts. However, the staggered configuration is more prone to transportation (film jamming) problems. Conversely, the opposing configuration is more stable in its film transportation. However, the opposing configuration creates more pressure on the films

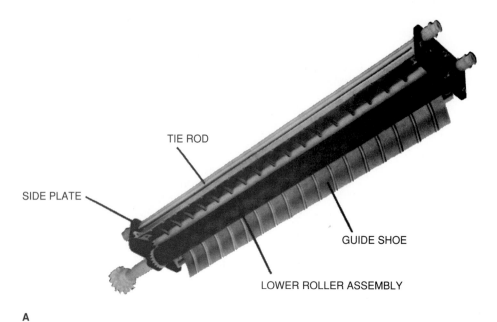

Figure 19–4. Crossover racks. *A,* Developer-fixer rack. (© Eastman Kodak Company. Reprinted courtesy of Eastman Kodak Company.) *B,* Squeegee.

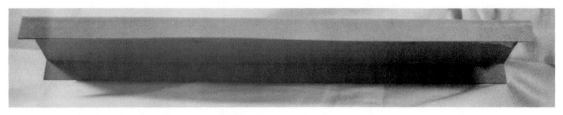

Figure 19–5. Fume hood.

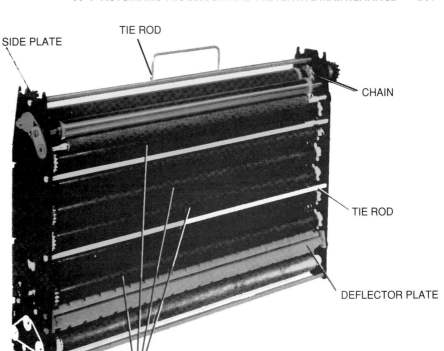

SIDE PLATE

TIE ROD

CHAIN

TIE ROD

DEFLECTOR PLATE

ROLLER ASSEMBLY

A

Figure 19–6. Deep racks. *A,* developer; *B,* fixer.
Illustration continued on following page

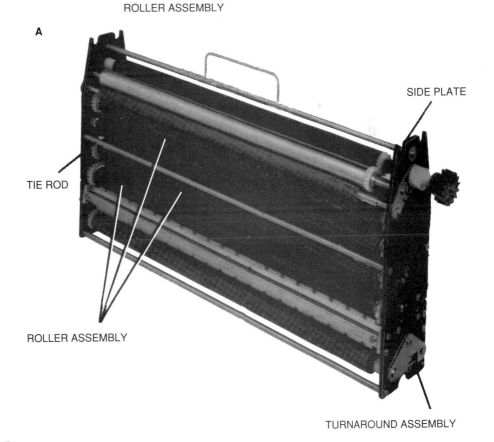

SIDE PLATE

TIE ROD

ROLLER ASSEMBLY

TURNAROUND ASSEMBLY

B

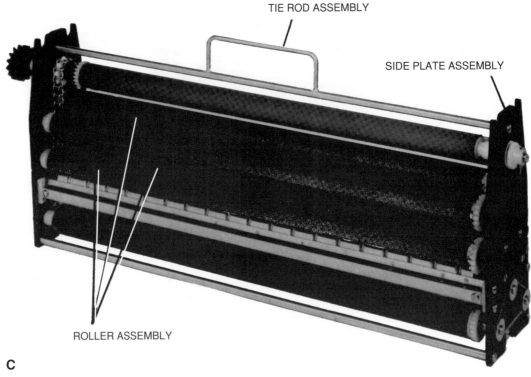

TIE ROD ASSEMBLY

SIDE PLATE ASSEMBLY

ROLLER ASSEMBLY

C

Figure 19–6 *Continued C, wash.* (© Eastman Kodak Company. Reprinted courtesy of Eastman Kodak Company.)

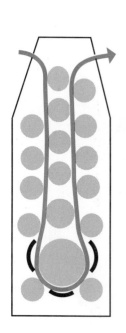

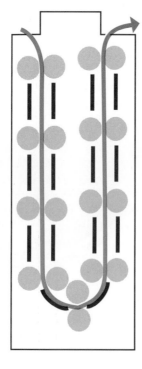

Figure 19–7. Roller configuration. *A,* staggered; *B,* opposing.

A   B

than the staggered configuration, increasing the probability of artifacts.

Turnarounds are located at the bottom of the deep rack and change the film direction from a downward movement to upward travel (Figure 19–8). This is achieved by a series of rollers and deflector plates. Often, a large roller (2–3 inches in diameter), called a master, is used in conjunction with several smaller 1 inch rollers (cluster).

All racks use deflector plates to help guide the film from one area to another. These plates are made of aluminum and are placed between the rollers (Figure 19–6). The space between the deflector plate and the film is wide at the point of film entry and narrow at the exit point. The wide opening makes it easier to catch a misaligned film, whereas the narrow opening directs the film to the proper path.

CIRCULATION SYSTEM

The circulation system works in conjunction with the temperature control system. The solution flow for circulation begins when the solution exits the respective processor tank from an outlet and enters the circulation pump. The solution is pumped through a heater (the fixer may not use a heater) and to a filter (the fixer rarely has a filter) and returns to the respective processor tank through an inlet (Figure 19–9). The four functions of the circulation system are

1. To provide a means of temperature control
2. To maintain correct chemical activity of the solutions
3. To achieve filtration
4. To agitate the solution.

The temperature of the solutions tends to decrease as cooler replenisher chemicals enter the tank. Consequently, a need exists to circulate the solution past a heater to warm it to the correct temperature (see under Temperature Control).

Replenishment solutions also contain a higher pH value than the chemicals in the processor. Because the solution is circulated, the activity of the chemicals is more uniformly distributed.

A filter is used primarily for the developer. Some filters are disposable and others are reusable. The objective of the filter is to prevent gelatin, which may have been removed from the film, from damaging or clogging the pump. The size of the particle trapped depends on the construction of the filter. Regardless of whether a disposable or a reusable filter is used, it is important to select a filter that removes the correct size of particles. A filter with large pore openings permits debris to pass through the filter. If the pore openings are too small, the filter may clog, reducing solution agitation and possibly causing damage to the circulation pump.

Solutions are agitated to provide even distribution of the chemicals on the film surface for uniform development. Agitation is more critical in 3 minute processors than in 90 second processors. The former move the film through the developer more slowly, necessitating solution movement for better film surface to chemical contact. However, the film transportation in a 90 second processor is so fast that the speed at which the film travels though the solution accounts for a pseudoagitation and uniform development.

TEMPERATURE CONTROL

Temperature control in a processor is critical. Temperatures above or below normal produce im-

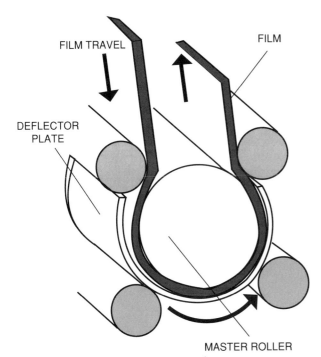

FILM TRAVEL

FILM

DEFLECTOR PLATE

MASTER ROLLER

Figure 19–8. Turnaround.

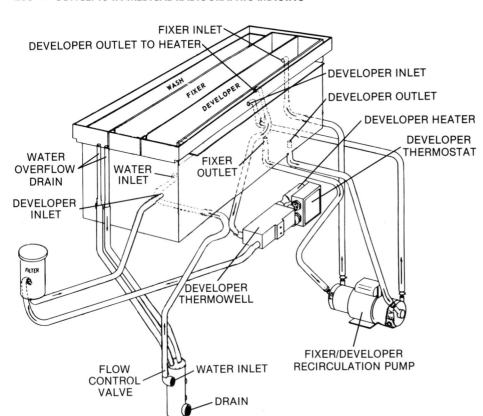

Figure 19–9. Flow of solutions in the circulation system of an automatic processor. (© Eastman Kodak Company. Reprinted courtesy of Eastman Kodak Company.)

properly developed films. Proper film development occurs with correct developer, fixer, wash and dryer temperatures. Several methods are used to regulate the temperature of these areas. A common method to sustain the appropriate temperature of the developer is through a heat exchanger. The fixer usually maintains its temperature from the heat convection of the adjacent tanks (developer and wash). The wash water temperature control is regulated by a water mixing valve (cold water processors rarely have mixing valves installed). Heat regulation for the dryer is via the dryer thermostat and heater.

Figure 19–9 demonstrates the circulation of the solutions. Recall that the developer flows through the outlet of the developer tank, passing through the circulation pump to the heat exchanger. The heat exchanger is a device used to warm or cool the developer solution. There are two heat exchanger designs. In one design, the developer flows through a cluster of small tubes, which are located in a larger compartment containing water (Figure 19–10A). The other design is the dual compartment (Figure 19–10B). One compartment of the dual compartment heat exchanger houses a heating element and developer solution. Adjacent to this compartment is a water compartment.

In the tube cluster heat exchanger design, the developer solution passes through the tube clusters. The larger compartment contains preheated water (heated by the water mixing valve) flowing around the tubes containing the developer. If the temperature of the water is less than that of the developer, the water cools the developer. Conversely, a water temperature higher than that of the developer solution heats the developer. This type of heat exchanger usually prevents heat build-up in the environment, e.g., room temperature. It is common in the tube cluster heat exchanger for the developer to travel through another, more accurate, heating system.

The dual compartment heat exchanger is controlled by a thermostat. The thermostat has a temperature sensing device (usually located at the bottom of the developer tank) and a place to adjust the temperature (located external to the developer

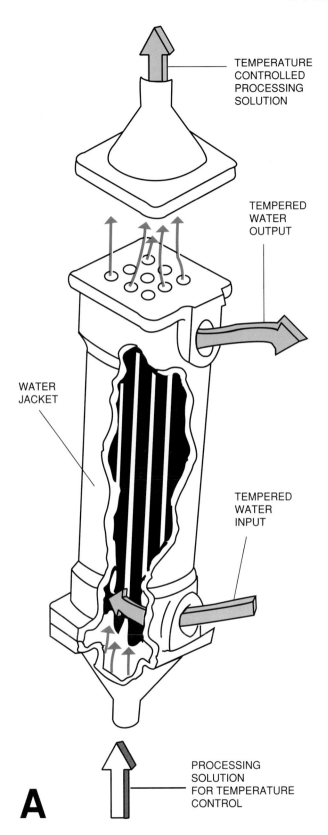

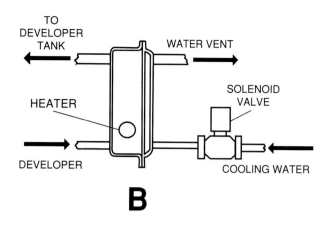

Figure 19–10. Heat exchanger. A, Tube (© Eastman Kodak Company. Reprinted courtesy of Eastman Kodak Company.) B, Dual compartment. (From Fuji Medical Systems, USA, Inc.)

tank). If the developer solution entering the compartment is too cold, the heating element is energized, warming the solution. Also, the solenoid for the water flow stops the flow of water to the adjacent compartment. When the developer solution entering the compartment is too warm, the heating element is deactivated and the solenoid opens the water valve, allowing cool water to flow through the adjacent compartment, thus decreasing the temperature of the developer. The heating element and solenoid operate so that when one is on, the other is off, and vice versa.

After the developer is heated to its correct temperature, it passes through a filter. Any particles, e.g., gelatin, in the developer are removed by the filter. After passing through the filter, the developer returns to the developer processing tank.

As mentioned above, the temperature of the fixer is usually maintained by convection of the adjacent developer and wash tanks. However, some processors circulate the fixer through its own heat exchanger unit. Also, some processors circulate preheated water through a compartment located below the fixer tank (Figure 19–11). It should be noted that some processors may heat the developer by circulating the water below its tank.

The wash water is regulated by a mixing valve (the exception being cold water processors) located

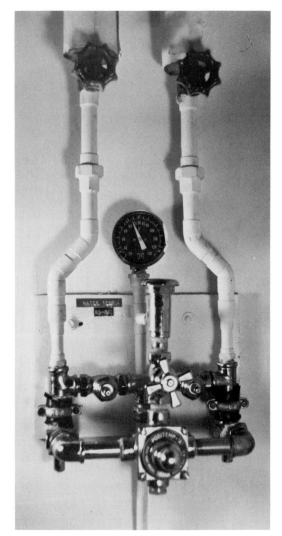

Figure 19–12. Mixing valve.

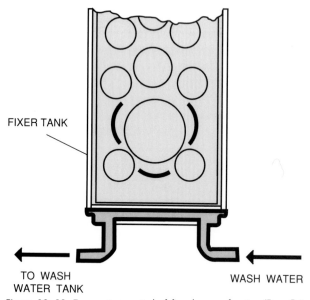

FIXER TANK

TO WASH WATER TANK

WASH WATER

Figure 19–11. Temperature control of fixer by use of water. (From Fuji Medical Systems, USA, Inc.)

on the plumbing of the incoming tap water. The mixing valve is commonly located on the developing side of the processing area. The mixing valve is designed to blend or mix hot and cold water to obtain the desired temperature. This is achieved by having the cold water enter through one pipe and the hot water enter from a second pipe. The hot and cold water converge at the mixing valve and are blended to achieve the desired temperature. The mixed water leaves through one mutual pipe (Figure 19–12). For the mixing valve to operate properly, a certain amount of water pressure is necessary and the water is filtered. Areas with low water pressure may require an addition of a pump to obtain the correct pressure. The filter is useful in preventing dirt from entering the processor. However, the filter has no effect on the salt or other minerals that may be in the water. Thus, the composition of the water should be tested to determine if a need exists to soften the water.

The mixing valve is positioned after the water filter or softeners. The temperature is regulated by a temperature sensitive valve. When the valve senses that the water is too hot, it stops the flow of hot water. As the temperature falls below the desired level, the valve opens, allowing more hot water and less cold water to flow. The mixed water exits through a mutual outlet pipe. A thermometer bulb is often placed in the outlet pipe to record the temperature of the water. If the water exiting is not the desired temperature, there is a handle or knob located on the valve to adjust the hot and cold water mixture, changing the temperature of the outgoing water.

REPLENISHMENT

The replenishment system keeps the activity of the chemicals correct and maintains the proper quantity (full tank) of solutions. The critical solutions needing proper replenishment are the developer and fixer (Figure 19–13). As part of the circulation system, the wash tank has a continuous flow of water.

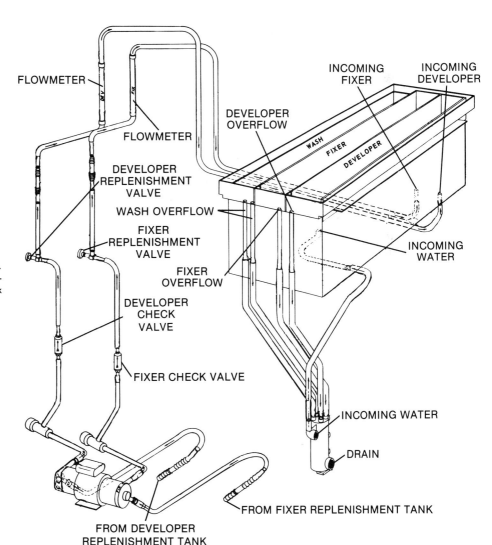

Figure 19–13. Replenishment cycle. (© Eastman Kodak Company. Reprinted courtesy of Eastman Kodak Company.)

The replenishment cycle begins at the reservoir (replenishment) tank. The replenishment tank may be located at the bottom of the processor or outside the processor. Reservoirs located inside the processor tend to have a small volume (2–3 gallons) and are useful in low volume departments. Replenishment tanks stored outside the processor are capable of holding much larger quantities of solution (10–50 gallons). These tanks tend to have a floating lid inside the tank to help prevent oxidation.

Replenishment solutions are pumped in the respective processor tanks. The pump is activated in one of two ways. One method is by mechanical detectors attached to the entrance rack. When a film enters the rack, the top roller rises, activating the detectors. The detectors start the replenishment pump. The detectors continue to function (pump solution) as long as they sense the film (until the film has completely entered the developer rack). The other method of energizing the replenishment pumps is by a timer and is called the flood method. In this method, every time a film is fed into the processor, a timer is activated (runs) until the film enters the developer (timer shuts off). With every new film entered, the timer runs, accumulating time until it reaches a preset duration (e.g., 15 minutes). When this occurs, the timer starts the replenishment pumps for several minutes (floods the solutions) and resets itself.

The film detector system operates the pump per film entered. The timer method does not energize the replenishment pump until several films are fed into the processor. Thus, the detector system is film area (film length times film width) dependent. The greater the film area is, the longer the replenishment is. However, the timer method replenishes a large quantity of solution on the basis of an average number of films.

Because the detector system is film area dependent, the method of film feeding is critical. For example, two common film sizes are 8 × 10 inches and 10 × 12 inches. The area of the 8 × 10 inch film is 80 square inches (8 × 10 = 80). The 10 × 12 inch film has an area of 120 square inches. Thus, the 10 × 12 film requires more replenishment owing to its larger area. However, if the 10 × 12 inch film enters the processor crosswise (so the 10 inch side is parallel to the feed tray guide) and the 8 × 10 inch film is fed into the processor lengthwise (so the 10 inch side is parallel to the feed tray guide),

the detectors sense that the films have the same area, replenishing the same amount of solution for each film. Thus, most processor manufacturers provide instructions as to the proper manner to enter films.

Besides the film area, the type of film emulsion and the amount of exposure on the film affect the rate of replenishment. Because these variables may change, there are controls on the processor to regulate the replenishment rate. The range of replenishment for the developer is 45 to 100 ml per 14 × 17 inch film size. The usual fixer replenishment range is 85 to 110 ml per 14 × 17 inch film. Exact developer rates can be determined by measuring the amount of bromide exiting the developer. A quantity of 8 g per L or greater signifies underreplenishment, whereas 4 g per L or less indicates overreplenishment. An underreplenished developer results in a loss of the shoulder portion of the Hurter and Driffield curve (refer to Chapter 21, Sensitometry and Processor Quality Control) with corresponding loss of contrast and density. Overreplenishment of the developer causes the Hurter and Driffield curve to move to the right and creates chemical fog. Measuring the bromide level has the disadvantage of necessitating a laboratory analysis of the solution.

It is easier to estimate the fixer replenishment rate. This is achieved by using silver estimating paper. If the estimating paper indicates that 4 g per L or less of silver is leaving the fixer, it is being overreplenished. A reading of 8 g per L or more of silver signifies underreplenishment of fixer. Overreplenishment wastes fixer solution. Underreplenishment results in poor fixing and hardening of the film.

DRYER SYSTEM

The dryer system is the last component of film processing (Figure 19–14) and is where the film is dried. The dryer system consists of a motor, blower, air plenum, heater, thermostat and air tubes.

A fractional horsepower motor drives the blower. The blower heats the air, circulates air and moves the moistened air out the exhaust. If the blower or motor stops functioning, there is a substantial increase in temperature. A special high heat thermostat is usually placed in the dryer system as a safety

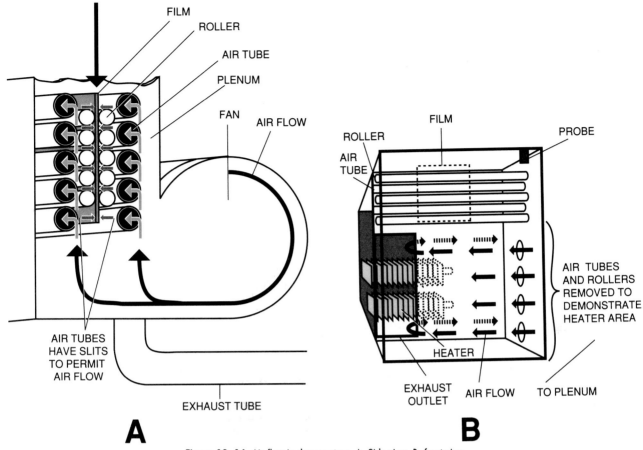

Figure 19–14. Air flow in dryer system. A, Side view; B, front view.

to prevent any overheating of the processor due to a malfunctioning dryer system.

The dryer system takes in room air through the blower. The composition of the room air is important. Ideally, the room air should be dry and free from dust. Dirt entering the blower can decrease air flow. It can also get on the blower blades, heater or thermostat, creating additional problems. Moisture in the room air is removed by the dryer system.

Often, the air entering the blower passes through a filter to remove dust particles. Air exiting the blower travels over a heater, where it is warmed to the desired temperature (120–150° F). The heater (Figure 19–15) is regulated by a thermostat, which turns on the heater when the entering air is cold and shuts the heater off when the air becomes too hot. From the heater, the air travels through the plenum to the air tubes.

An air tube is a long plastic vent with a narrow slit along its length (Figure 19–16). Air tubes are commonly located on either side of the film and blow hot air on the film as it moves through the rollers. The rollers are usually made of porous material, which collects the moisture from the film as the film is transported. The hot air from the air tubes assists in drying the film and moving the moist air through the exhaust.

STANDBY FEATURE

Many late model processors have a standby feature built into the processor. This feature is designed to conserve energy and increase the life span of the processor. Energy consumption is reduced by decreasing the water and deactivating the drive motor, blower motor and dryer heater(s) during idle times (when no films are processed) of 3 min-

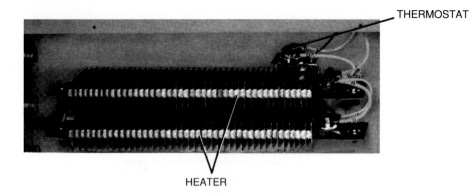

Figure 19–15. Dryer heater. (© Eastman Kodak Company. Reprinted courtesy of Eastman Kodak Company.)

utes or longer. This also increases the life span of the processor by decreasing the wear on moving parts.

To prevent the processor from getting too cool during the time when no film is processed, the motors and dryer heater(s) remain off for a preset time (usually 15 minutes) and then are reactivated until the desired dryer temperature is obtained. After the dryer reaches its temperature and if no film is fed in the processor for 3 minutes, the standby mode is reactivated. To process film while the processor is on standby, a switch (usually located near the feed tray) is pressed, restoring the processor to its normal operation.

Processors containing a standby feature have additional parts added to the unit. These are a control box and a water bypass. The control box regulates the standby intervals and contains the switch to restore normal operation of the processor. The water bypass regulates the flow of water to the processor.

MAINTENANCE

Automatic processors are electromechanical devices. As such, parts wear down, break, become misaligned, etc., causing the processor to malfunction. Consequently, it is important to implement a maintenance program to prevent potential problems.

Most processor manufacturers supply a list of tasks that should be performed routinely. The time intervals for each task list must be correlated with the amount of time the processor is used. For example, a department with a significant workload may need to perform a manufacturer's suggested monthly tasks more frequently, e.g., every 3 weeks. The time intervals suitable for a department are best determined by observation of the processor, sensitometry test results and a consultation with a processor service or technical representative.

Many institutions find it economically wise to contract out the tasks involved with processor care. It is not unusual for these contracts to be awarded to a local processor service company. If processor care is contracted out, the frequency of care and specific tasks to be performed should be identified in the contract.

Departments using service contracts often perform their own daily sensitometry tests. Thus, there is a need for the department and the service company to share information. For example, if the sensitometry tests indicate a problem, this information should be transmitted to the service people. Also, if service personnel work on the processor, e.g., use a system cleaner, this information should be provided to the department, especially because

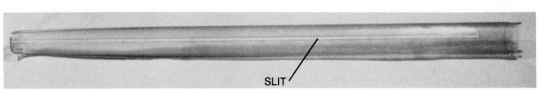

Figure 19–16. Air tube.

some types of maintenance affect sensitometry results. Sharing of information often occurs in a variety of ways. For example, an effective method of transmitting processor maintenance information is by posting a cleaning schedule (log) near the processor. Other information may be communicated by telephone, in notes, etc.

Regardless of whether a service contract exists, the department usually has daily tasks to perform on the processor. These are associated with the start-up and shut-down of the processor. These may vary from one processor model to another. The common tasks for the start-up and shut-down procedures are summarized below.

PROCESSOR START-UP

There are several tasks involved in the proper processor start-up procedure. The first task is to wash the D-F and F-W crossover racks with a nonabrasive cloth. The rollers are rotated to ensure that the entire surface area of each roller is cleaned. Next, the entrance and squeegee racks are wiped clean with a damp cloth. As with the D-F and F-W racks, the rollers are rotated during cleaning. The deep racks have several rollers that are located at the top and are out of solution (exposed to the air). These rollers are washed to remove any possible dirt or chemical condensation deposits. The racks are cleaned in the order of film travel (e.g., developer, fixer, wash). This helps decrease the possibility of cross-contamination. The other items needing cleaning are the fume hoods, splash guards and feed tray. To prevent artifacts, the feed tray is cleaned with an antistatic solution and dried with a cloth. Before the racks are returned to the processor, the solution levels of the tanks are checked to ensure that the tanks are full.

The developer and fixer drain valves remain closed until a need arises to change solutions. Thus, these tanks are full of solution, making it easy to check the level. The water in the wash tank is usually drained to prevent the accumulation of algae. It is recommended that the water tank drain valve be left slightly ajar, rather than continually opening and closing the water valve to drain and refill the wash tank. The valve is opened enough to drain the water at a *slower* rate than the rate at which the water enters the processor. Thus, when

the incoming water valve is turned on, the water tank fills. When the incoming water valve is turned off, the tank empties through the drain valve.

The next step in starting the processor is to turn on and adjust the temperature of the incoming water. This is performed with the top of the processor, crossover racks and fume hood off. Having these items off provides a means of checking to ensure that the water level and overflow are operating properly.

After all solution level checks are performed, the rollers and fume hoods are returned to their proper place in the processor. Care should be taken to make sure that the entrance rack is dry before placing it in the processor. With the racks in place and with the top lid of the processor off, the main power to energize the drive shaft is turned on (units with one main power switch also energize the recirculation pumps, replenishment pumps and dryer motor concurrently). After the drive shaft is on, a check is performed to ensure that all the rollers are rotating. If the rollers are rotating, the top lid of the processor is replaced and the recirculation pumps, replenishment pumps and dryer motor (the pumps and motor are already functioning in processors with one main power switch) are turned on.

The processor is allowed to reach its proper temperature level (warm up) before the next step of processing green film. With the processor at its correct temperature, several green 14 × 17 inch films are processed. Green film is recommended because it is unprocessed and undergoes the normal processing procedure. Also, it is more profitable to retrieve the film's silver content using the silver recovery rather than through the sale as scrap film (see Chapter 22).

While the film begins its travel (at the entrance rack), the following items are checked:

1. The safelight goes on and off when expected (if applicable).
2. The bell sounds when the film exits the entrance rack.
3. The replenishment pumps are functioning at the correct level and rate (this method is not useful in checking flood replenishment units). This may be performed by observing the flowmeters.
4. Film exits the processor (enters the receiving bin) straight and is free of debris.

PROCESSOR SHUT-DOWN

The processor shut-down procedure is not as time consuming as the start-up procedure but is equally important. The first step in the shut-down is to turn off all the electrical switches. Next, the incoming water valve is turned off. At this point, if the wash tank drain valve is not kept ajar, the respective drain is opened to empty the wash tank.

Next, the top lid of the processor is removed, exposing the racks and fume hoods. The fume hoods, D-F and F-W crossovers, entrance rack and squeegee rack are cleaned in the same manner as during the start-up procedure. After being cleaned, they are stored in a safe place, e.g., on a shelf free from possible damage or dust. Avoid returning the racks to the processor owing to possible condensation and chemical deposit build-up resulting from the processor cooling.

When all racks are removed, the splash guards and drive shaft are checked for debris and cleaned if necessary. Lastly, the lid is returned to its proper place and left ajar to prevent chemical deposits.

WEEKLY TASKS

Included in the weekly tasks are the daily procedures. Weekly processor maintenance tasks vary from one company to another. Owing to the rapid increase of service contracts, few departments actually perform these tasks themselves. Thus, only a summary of common tasks is presented here.

Weekly tasks generally involve removal, cleaning and inspection of the deep racks. There is some controversy relative to using system cleaners on the racks. Advocates of system cleaners believe that they are beneficial and, when used properly, can be completely removed from the rollers. Those opposing the use of system cleaners argue that the cleaning solution enters the racks, causing permanent damage, and can never be entirely removed from the rollers. If a department elects to use system cleaners, the manufacturer's instructions should be followed carefully. It is possible to inspect the racks while cleaning them. An inspection of the racks includes a check of the gears for wear or missing teeth and a check of the chains for wear and tension as well as a check to ensure that the rollers move freely.

While all the deep racks are out of the tank, the solutions are inspected for foreign bodies and the circulation pumps are turned on to check the solution circulation (make sure the pumps are turned off after checking the circulation).

Other weekly checks include inspecting the filters for dirt, cleaning the air tubes and checking the replenishment lines. The replenishment lines are inspected to ensure that there are no kinks, bends or debris in the tubing.

MONTHLY TASKS

As for weekly tasks, a brief summary of the common monthly procedures is presented here. Besides the normal daily and weekly tasks, monthly inspection includes

1. Check for feed tray alignment
2. Drain and clean all tanks
3. Lubricate gears as recommended by the manufacturer
4. Check to ensure that the detector switch is engaging and disengaging properly, adjust as needed
5. Check the tubing, especially where it attaches to motors, for leaks
6. Check the amount of replenishment and adjust as needed.

TROUBLESHOOTING

The complexity of an automatic processor means that there are hundreds of areas where possible malfunctions may occur. To help diagnose the specific cause of a problem and implement a solution, manufacturers often provide troubleshooting charts. These charts are inclusive, which results in a long document. It is important for technologists to have a working knowledge of how to use a troubleshooting chart.

A typical chart (Appendix C) lists problems by the various processor systems, e.g., transportation and replenishment. Each problem is itemized, with a list of possible causes of the problems. The causes are usually separated into common causes and less frequent causes of a problem. Table 19–1 demonstrates a troubleshooting chart for the replenishment system.

Notice that Table 19–1 refers to the components of the replenishment system (section A), a list of problems (section C) and a list of causes (sections B, D, and E). To use the chart, a specific problem is located in section C. To determine the cause of the problem, record the numbers (sections D and E) referencing the possible reasons for the problem and refer to section B to identify the specific cause. For example, if the problem is "chemical volume low" (see section C), common causes are listed as numbers 6–8 (see section D). In section B, causes 6–8 are pump setting, pump accuracy and pump reproducibility, respectively. Less common causes are identified as 1–5 and 9–24 (see section E). As for the common causes, less frequent causes are specifically identified in section B.

LABORATORY EXPERIENCE

The *Concepts in Medical Radiographic Imaging: Laboratory Manual* contains two laboratories relating to this chapter: Laboratories 30, Processor Inspection, and 29, Processor Parts and Function. Additional related laboratories are 34, Sensitometry, and 35, Silver Recovery. It is recommended that the related laboratories be performed in conjunction with Chapters 21 and 22, respectively.

The Processor Parts and Function laboratory is designed to familiarize the learner with the components of an automatic processor. This laboratory consists of three experiments. In the first experiment, the learner is introduced to the various racks and their parts. The researcher removes the various racks of the processor and draws a diagram of each rack. The second experiment requires the learner to develop a film with the lid of the processor off. Thus, the student observes the transportation system and the processing effect on the film. Lastly, the experimenter observes the effect of the developer and fixer solution by submerging part of a green film in the each respective solution.

The Processor Inspection laboratory enables the experimenter to perform preventive maintenance checks of the processor. Checks are performed on the transportation, circulation/filtration, replenishment and dryer systems. The checks performed on the transportation system include inspection of the gears of all the racks for wear, the feed tray for cleanness, tension of the belts or chains on all racks,

Table 19–1. TROUBLESHOOTING CHART FOR REPLENISHMENT SYSTEM

Section A: Components

Detector switch (microswitch)
Detector assembly–airflow, rollers
Main switch
Fuses relays
Pump—head, motor, gearbox
Lines—tubing, fittings
Gauges—flow indicator, meters
Tanks—outside processor
Check valves
Needle valves
Filters

Section B: Location of Causes of Replenishment Problems

1. Detector switch malfunction
2. Detector switch adjustment
3. Detector assembly malfunction
4. Cleanliness of detector assembly, switch
5. Electrical supply
6. Pump setting
7. Pump accuracy
8. Pump reproducibility
9. Pump leak
10. Pump malfunction
11. Lines kinked, blocked
12. Lines—air lead, air block
13. Lines solution leak
14. Lines—fittings damaged
15. Gauges not calibrated
16. Filters or strainer clogged
17. Tanks not calibrated
18. Check valves stuck
19. Check valves deteriorated
20. Check valves installed incorrectly
21. Adjustment valve failure
22. Replenishment tanks empty
23. Frequency of mix
24. Absence of floating lid
25. Water supply problems

Section C: Replenishment Problems	Section D: Common Causes	Section E: Less Common Problems
Chemical volume low	6–8	1–5, 9–24
Chemical volume high	6–8, 18	1, 2, 4, 15, 17, 19, 20, 23
Chemical activity low	6–8	1–5, 9–24
Chemical activity high	6–8, 18	1, 2, 15, 17, 19, 20, 23
Increased density	6–8	1–4, 15, 17–21, 23
Unclear films	6–8	1–5, 9–24
Unwashed film	6–8	1–5, 9–24
Undry films	25	1–24
Scratches, abrasions	6–8	1–5, 9–24
Film jams	6–8	1–5, 9–24
Decreased density	6–8	1–5, 9–24
Chemical breakdown	6–8	1–5, 9–24
High consumption	6, 24	1–5, 9–24
Leaks	13, 14	9, 11, 12, 16, 17–21
Variable sensitometry	7, 8	1, 4, 17

From E.I. DuPont de Nemours & Co., Inc.

position of the deflector plates and the detector system (bell and safelight function). Circulation/filtration inspections include checks of the tubing, developer filter and pump function. Included in the replenishment checks are observation of the replenishment rate and flow level. The dryer inspection include checks of the function of the thermostat, blower, heater and tension of the belt on the motor.

Bibliography

Bushong, SC. Radiologic science for technologists (4th edition). St. Louis: Mosby, 1988.

Carroll, QB. Fuchs's Principles of radiographic exposure, processing and quality control (3rd edition). Springfield, IL: Thomas, 1985.

Chesney, DN and Chesney, MO. X-ray equipment for student radiographers (3rd edition). Boston: Blackwell Scientific Publications, 1984.

Cullinan, AM. Producing quality radiographs. New York: Lippincott, 1987.

E.I. DuPont de Nemours & Co., Inc. Darkroom technique for better radiographs. (reference number A-28545.) Wilmington, DE: E.I. DuPont de Nemours & Co., Inc.

Eastman Kodak Co. Kodak RP X-omat standby control model M6A-N. (Publication print number 639751.) Rochester, NY: Eastman Kodak Co., May 1972.

Fuji Photo Film Co., LTD. Control of the photographic properties of medical x-ray films processed in automatic processors. (Medical x-ray products technical handbook reference number XM3-34E.-74.4-OB.3-1.)

Fuji Photo Film Co., LTD. The fundamentals of automatic processors for medical x-ray films. (Medical x-ray products technical handbook reference number XM3-35E.-74.5-OB.3-1.)

Fuji Photo Film Co., LTD. Processing and handling of medical x-ray films. (Medical x-ray products technical handbook reference number XM3-3E.-73.11-OT.b3-3.)

General Electric. A look at x-ray film processing. (Publication 8A-3371C.) Milwaukee, WI: General Electric Technical Services.

Gevaert. Processing of medical x-ray films. (Reference number 21.3856 [264A].) New York: Low X-ray Corporation.

Gray, J, et al. Quality control in diagnostic imaging. Baltimore: University Park Press, 1983.

Hendee, WR, Chaney, EL and Rossi, RP. Radiologic physics, equipment and quality control. Chicago: Year Book Medical, 1976.

Hiss, SS. Understanding radiography. Springfield, IL: Thomas, 1980.

McKinney, WEJ. Radiographic processing and quality control. Philadelphia: Lippincott, 1988.

McLemore, J. Quality assurance in diagnostic radiology. Chicago: Year Book Medical, 1981.

Selman, J. The fundamentals of x-ray and radium physics (7th edition). Springfield, IL: Thomas, 1985.

Thompson, TT. Cahoon's Formulating x-ray techniques (9th edition). Durham, NC: Duke University Press, 1979.

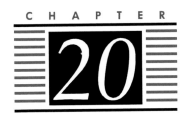

FILM, FILM PROCESSING AND PHOTOGRAPHIC TECHNIQUES

JOAN K. MacDONALD

INTRODUCTION

Photography is the process of producing a permanent image by the action of light (electromagnetic radiation) on a photosensitive material (film) after proper chemical treatment (processing). During conventional photography, light is reflected from the surface of an object in proportion to the brightness of various parts of that object. The brighter the part, the greater the reflection. Conversely, more light is absorbed within darker areas, thereby decreasing the amount of reflection. The design of a camera's lens enables this reflected light to converge on a sensitive film surface, producing a hidden (latent) image of numerous shades or tones corresponding to the various degrees of brightness of the object.

Some film materials react to light by producing darker shades from brighter areas and lighter shades from darker areas. This reversal of shades is referred to as a photographic negative. Cameras used to produce color or black and white prints employ negative film (Figure 20–1). If the photographic negative is further exposed to a source of light while in direct contact with an unexposed negative film, there is a reversal of the shades. This process results in positive prints or images, demonstrating the object's true shades (Figure 20–2). Films with a direct response to light (lighter shades from bright objects and darker shades from dark objects) are referred to as photographic positives. An example of a photographic positive is the film used in a Polaroid camera.

Radiographic imaging is similar to photographic imaging in that a permanent record on a photosensitive material is obtained by the action of electromagnetic radiation (x-rays and/or light) on an object. The radiation in this case, however, passes through a subject rather than being reflected by the subject. The more radiation passing through the object (remnant radiation) and striking the film, the darker the recorded image.

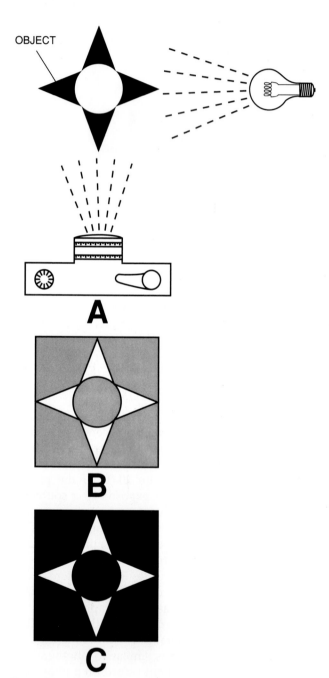

Figure 20—1. Producing photographic negatives. Light reflected from an object as in A goes through the lens of a camera to form the latent image on a film (B). After development, the film (C) shows opposite densities than the object (negative reproduction).

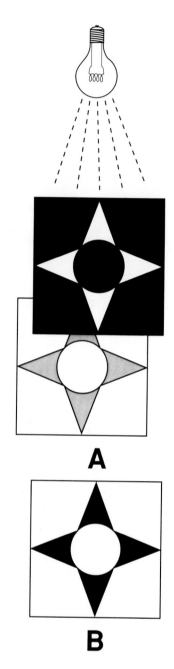

Figure 20—2. Photographic positive film. If a photographic negative film is placed on top of an unexposed film and exposed to light (A), the result is a reversal of the negative, or a positive reproduction of the image (B).

Remnant radiation is primarily determined by the atomic number of the part, the composition of the object, the thickness of the subject matter and the penetrating ability of the radiation (kilovolt peak). If all other factors are held constant, subject matter of high atomic number, dense tissue and thick body parts absorb more radiation (resulting in less remnant radiation) than their opposites. Also, relatively low energy x-rays (low kilovolt peak) are more apt to be absorbed in the subject matter than high energy radiation, limiting the radiation transmitted to the film (less remnant radiation).

Negative and positive films are available in radiography. Subject matter that allows greater radiation transmission to the film appears dark on negative and light on positive recording materials. By convention, however, almost all radiographic images are recorded on negative film.

The content of this chapter approaches film from three aspects: film structure, radiographic film processing and photographic techniques. The film structure segment concentrates on the composition and function of film parts. The radiographic film processing section is a brief discussion of the formation of the latent image in both manual and automatic processing. The photographic techniques portion is a discussion of subtraction, stereoradiography and film duplication. In all sections, reference to film assumes it is a negative unless otherwise specified.

TYPES OF FILM

Two main types of film are commonly employed for radiographic procedures: those that are affected by x-rays alone or by x-rays in combination with light (simply called x-ray film) and those that are affected only by light (cineradiographic, duplication and subtraction film).

Within the x-ray film group, two subgroups exist to accommodate the different exposure techniques available in radiography. The two exposure methods are x-rays and x-rays in combination with light. In the former method, the film is wrapped in a light-tight envelope and is referred to as nonscreen, or direct exposure, film. The latter exposure technique uses a film (called screen film) sandwiched between two intensifying screens in a cassette. Both subgroups are similar in that they usually consist of two layers of sensitive emulsion. Such films are said to be duplitized. The subgroups differ primarily in the thickness of the emulsion layers, with nonscreen film having thicker emulsions (see under Emulsion Layer).

Images produced solely by light, such as in cineradiography, duplication or subtraction require only one layer of photosensitive emulsion. These films are, therefore, called single emulsion films.

FILM STRUCTURE

All double emulsion films have four common features. These include a support (base), two layers of photosensitive emulsion, a gluelike adhesive to connect the emulsion to the base (substratum layer) and an outer protective coating (supercoat) (Figure 20–3A). Single emulsion films have the same features as double emulsion film with the exception that single emulsion film has only one emulsion layer. Regardless of whether found in duplitized (double emulsion) or in single emulsion film, each layer has basically the same composition (see below). In addition to the common features, single emulsion film may add an anti-curl and/or an anti-halation layer (Figure 20–3B).

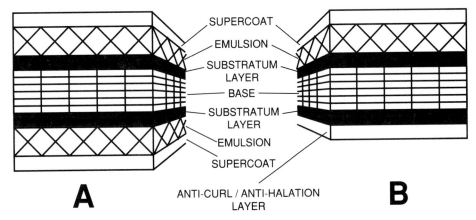

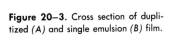
Figure 20–3. Cross section of duplitized (A) and single emulsion (B) film.

SUPERCOAT
EMULSION
SUBSTRATUM LAYER
BASE
SUBSTRATUM LAYER
EMULSION
SUPERCOAT
ANTI-CURL / ANTI-HALATION LAYER

A

B

BASE

The base is the thickest part of the film (0.2–0.4 mm). An ideal base must be consistent in thickness to ensure uniformity of the emulsion layers and be uniform in its ability to transmit light (transparency). The base must also have sufficient flexibility to allow for transportation through an automatic processor and yet be rigid enough to avoid kinking and bending. Other important characteristics include being strong enough to prevent tearing or accidental destruction, flat enough for good handling and storage, stable enough to provide permanence in its dimensions and relatively nonhygroscopic (resistant to water absorption) to prevent swelling during processing.

The film base was originally manufactured from cellulose nitrate. This material was undesirable because the physical properties of cellulose nitrate were safety hazards. These hazards included cellulose nitrate's ability to burn readily, combust as easily as paper and emit noxious fumes when burning. Safety bases of cellulose acetate, cellulose triacetate or a similar material were developed to eliminate the problems associated with cellulose nitrate. The material currently used is a polyester base (polyethylene terphthalate). A polyester base is preferred because it meets safety and radiographic requirements. Traditionally, both acetate and polyester bases have been tinted blue to reduce eyestrain caused by reading numerous radiographs.

SUBSTRATUM LAYER

Physical differences exist between the base and the emulsion. The primary difference occurs during processing when the emulsion tends to swell and shrink with temperature changes to a much greater degree than the base. To avoid having the emulsion and the base separate during film processing, the emulsion should be attached to the base. The substratum layer provides for such a means of adhesion. This is achieved by applying a thin layer, primarily of gelatin and cellulose ester, to the emulsion layer(s). In single emulsion films, the substratum layer also serves to fix the anti-curl layer to the base.

EMULSION LAYER

The portion of a film sensitive to light and/or radiation is called the emulsion. It consists of innumerable microcrystals of silver halide (silver and bromine, iodine or chlorine) suspended in gelatin.

Gelatin serves as a good medium in which to form, suspend and keep the silver halide crystals well dispersed. Because it is relatively stable, it also provides relative permanency to the emulsion both before and after processing. Additionally, it is easily penetrated by various solutions, thereby allowing rapid processing.

Silver, when combined with one of the halogen elements (bromine, iodine or chlorine) forms a salt, which on exposure to light or x-rays changes physically. This change enables a latent image to be formed. The crystals used in the majority of x-ray films are silver bromide in combination with iodide, ranging in size from 0.0005 to 0.002 mm.

The size and distribution of the crystals within the gelatin help determine two important film characteristics, namely speed and contrast. In general, the larger the grains, the faster the film. This translates to less light and/or x-ray exposure necessary to produce a similar image when compared with another film of less speed. The distribution of crystal size within the gelatin affects contrast. Emulsions consisting primarily of the same sized crystals, whether large or small, show greater contrast (higher contrast or shorter scale) than those with a wide range of crystal sizes.

Placing the emulsion on both sides of the base (duplitized films) is beneficial for several important reasons. Because x-rays and/or light from the intensifying screens activates both emulsion layers simultaneously, nearly twice the amount of silver is deposited than in a single emulsion film exposure. With this doubling of efficiency, shorter exposure times are required, resulting in the following benefits: radiographs with less blurring, as the risk of patient movement is reduced; less radiation exposure to the patient; longer life for the x-ray tube. Also, because contrast decreases with increased tube voltages, the doubling of silver deposits in duplitized films produces higher contrast than in single emulsion films at high tube voltages.

The latent image formed in nonscreen film is produced entirely by x-rays, whereas the majority of the latent image of screen film is produced by light photons after x-ray stimulation of the intensifying screen. The emulsion layers in direct exposure film are thicker than those in screen film. If this were not the case, many of the higher energy x-rays would pass through the film without interacting with the emulsion layer, thereby producing a low quality film.

SUPERCOAT LAYER

Silver compounds, owing to their superiority in photosensitivity, stability and reproducibility, have been the photosensitive substances of first choice since 1939. Their high photosensitivity, however, makes them extremely susceptible to pressure and friction, common forces associated with normal film handling. Crystals damaged by either force appear as artifacts on the finished radiograph. To prevent this occurrence, a supercoat of anti-abrasion gelatin is applied to each layer of emulsion.

ANTI-CURL LAYER

As mentioned above, the base and emulsion react differently during processing. The base does not allow for much water absorption, whereas the emulsion swells and shrinks depending on the processing chemicals and the temperature. It can readily be seen that, if left untreated, the emulsion layer would have a tendency to curl or shrink away from the base. The tendency to curl is significant in single emulsion films. A method of equalizing this curl on the nonemulsion side is accomplished by applying a thin, prehardened gelatin layer to the substratum layer opposite the emulsion side, forming an anti-curl layer. Anti-curl layers are unnecessary in duplitized films, as the emulsion layers tend to shrink equally on both sides of the base.

ANTI-HALATION LAYER

Ideally, all electromagnetic photons pass directly to the silver halide crystals and become completely absorbed. Unfortunately, the nature of radiation is such that it has a tendency to scatter after interacting with various materials. The scattered radiation is capable of exposing the photosensitive crystals, as is primary radiation. The unwanted evil of this scatter is that crystals not in the original radiation path are exposed, leading to the formation of an image with untrue borders (unsharpness). In general, larger crystals and thicker emulsions create more scattered radiation. Therefore, the best way to limit this phenomenon is to use thin emulsions with fine grained crystals.

Radiation that has scattered and not been absorbed in the crystals may pass completely through the remaining layers of the film or may strike the bottom layer and be reflected back to the emulsion (depending on the angle of impact). If this occurs, another untrue image results, generally in the form of a halo, or a ring around the image proper. To prevent this halation effect, a carefully chosen dye capable of absorbing scatter radiation is added to the backing of the film; this is referred to as the anti-halation layer. Although the dye can be added to any film backing, it is more often incorporated in single emulsion film.

RADIOGRAPHIC FILM PROCESSING

The purpose of film processing is to produce a permanent, visible (manifest) image from the latent (invisible) image originally created by x-rays and/or light exposure. Before one considers processing techniques, it is necessary to have a basic understanding of the chemistry involved in latent image formation.

FORMATION OF THE LATENT IMAGE

As mentioned above, the interaction between electromagnetic radiation and the silver halide crystals enables the formation of a latent image. Although not completely verified, a currently accepted hypothesis explaining this formation has been provided by two scientists named Gurney and Mott. The steps involved in latent and subsequent visible image formation are as follows (refer to Figure 20–4 for a pictorial analysis):

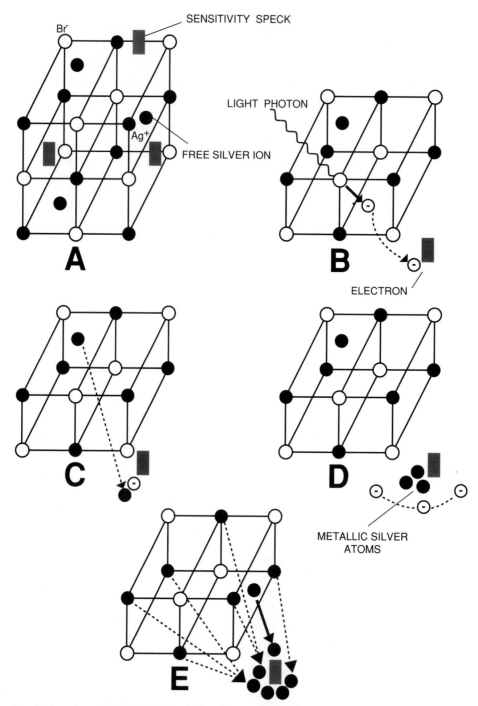

Figure 20—4. Formation of a latent image into a visible image. *A,* Crystal lattice structure showing bromide ions (Br⁻) alternating with silver ions (Ag⁺), free silver ions and sensitivity specks. *B,* Light striking a Br⁻ ion releases an electron, which is attracted by the sensitivity speck. *C,* Free Ag⁺ ions are then pulled to the sensitivity speck, creating metallic silver atoms. *D,* On development, additional electrons are added to the sensitivity speck. *E,* Owing to the negativity of the speck, all remaining free Ag⁺ ions, as well as those incorporated in the crystal, travel to the speck, thereby transforming the entire crystal(s) into metallic silver.

1. The greatest majority of silver halide crystals are octagonally shaped. It is assumed that the silver and the halide (primarily bromide) are arranged in an alternating geometric cuboidal pattern. Also present, but not integrated within the crystal lattice structure, are free silver ions and special compounds forming sensitivity specks (Figure 20–4A).

2. When an electromagnetic photon strikes a crystal, an electron is released from the bromide particle. This electron moves freely within the lattice structure until it is eventually captured by a sensitivity speck. The speck subsequently becomes negatively charged (Figure 20–4B).

3. A free, nonintegrated silver ion, being positively charged, is in turn attracted to the sensitivity speck and one neutral silver metallic atom is created (Figure 20–4C).

4. If the process were to end after the creation of one metallic silver atom, a latent image would never be formed, as the silver atom would quickly revert back to an electron and a silver ion. Special properties within the crystal structure, however, enable the silver atom to attract other free electrons, thereby enhancing the trapping mechanism of the sensitivity speck. Stability of the speck occurs when three or more metallic silver atoms are formed. The speck is now called a development center. Several clusters of metallic silver are actually formed in each crystal, thus creating the latent image. The image remains invisible to the human eye unless the radiographic exposure is increased by a factor of millions (both impractical and unsafe for patients) or unless the development center is greatly enlarged by the action of certain chemicals during processing.

5. From this point on, in medical radiography, further build-up of metallic silver and the creation of the visible image occur only after the film is submerged in a developing solution. Developers supply enough electrons to make the development centers negatively charged (Figure 20–4D).

6. The development centers are so negatively charged that all the remaining free silver ions, as well as those incorporated within the crystal lattice structures, are drawn to the centers. This results in a transformation of the crystals from silver halide to metallic silver (Figure 20–4E).

PROCESSING SOLUTIONS

Film processing consists of four basic operations, regardless of whether it is accomplished automatically or manually. These include developing, fixing, washing and drying. It is not the intent of this section to provide detailed information on chemical reactions but rather to present the rationale behind each operation and the most common solutions employed. Differences between automatic and manual processing are described when necessary.

Development and Developers

Development is the process of changing a latent image into a visible image by further reduction of exposed silver halide crystals to metallic silver. In other words, it is the darkening of those areas on a film that have become sensitive owing to the absorption of electromagnetic radiation. Although simply termed the developer, this solution actually contains several chemicals as described in the following:

Developers. Mixtures of compounds (organic reducing agents) such as metol (elon) and hydroquinone (Phenidone) are responsible for converting silver halide crystals to metallic silver. Metol produces the basic gray image early in the development, whereas hydroquinone builds up density and contrast in the later stages. Neither chemical has any significant effect on the unexposed silver halide crystals.

Preservatives. Antioxidants such as sodium or potassium sulfite serve two primary purposes. They protect the developers from wasteful oxidation by air, thus extending the life of the developers, and they help prevent discoloration of the developers, protecting against unwanted staining of the emulsion.

Accelerators. Compounds (alkali) such as sodium or potassium carbonate and sodium or potassium hydroxide speed up the action of the developers. Hydroquinone remains quite inactive unless dissolved in an alkaline medium, so accelerators essentially serve as activators for the developers. They also cause the emulsion to swell slightly, enabling the developers to penetrate the emulsion more efficiently.

Restrainers. Compounds (antifoggers) such as potassium bromide and potassium iodide essentially prevent development of the unexposed silver halide crystals, minimizing fog. The restrainers have little effect on the exposed crystals.

Hardeners. Hardening compounds (aldehydes) are used only in automatic processors and prevent excessive swelling of the emulsion. Too much swelling causes greater absorption of developer in the emulsion, which may not be entirely removed before the film reaches the fixer tank. This may result in contamination of the processing chemicals. Additionally, a soft emulsion may stick to the rollers, thus damaging the film and jamming the processor.

Solvents. Solvent compounds, primarily water, dissolve and ionize developing chemicals. Water additionally causes the emulsion to swell, allowing the developers to reach the silver halide crystals.

Miscellaneous additives. Compounds such as water softening agents, wetting solutions, anti-swelling agents for tropical climate processing and special silver halide solvents may be added to improve development.

Rinse Bath

Rinsing removes excess developing agents from the film before fixing by submersion and agitation in clean circulating water. If too much alkali is carried from the developer, some of the acid in the fixer is neutralized, leading to decreased film quality with possible staining. This step is important only in manual processing, as the roller assemblies in automatic processors act as squeegees to remove excessive developer.

Stop Bath

Stop baths provide a more efficient way of ensuring that excessive developer is not carried into the fixing unit. It replaces the rinse bath stage of manual processing. Rather than simply rinsing with water, the film is placed in an acidic solution (128 ml of 28% acetic acid to 1 L of water) and the alkaline developer is literally neutralized before the film proceeds to the fixing stage.

Fixer

As mentioned above, developers convert the exposed silver halide crystals to metallic silver while leaving the unexposed crystals virtually untouched. Without some method of removing (clearing) the unexposed crystals and completely stopping the action of the developer, the film would be subject to eventual discoloration and darkening on exposure to light after processing. Fixation accomplishes these important tasks without damaging the silver image. It also helps the film to resist abrasion by hardening the emulsion. The fixing solution consists of several chemicals, as described in the following:

Fixing (clearing) agents. Either sodium thiosulfate (liquid) or ammonium thiosulfate (powder) removes the unexposed, undeveloped silver halide from the emulsion, allowing these areas to become transparent rather than milky in appearance. These agents are commonly known as hypo. Without proper clearing, the image becomes obscure, as the remaining unexposed crystals darken on exposure to electromagnetic radiation.

Preservative. A compound of sodium sulfite is added to prevent decomposition of the fixing agents.

Hardener. An aluminum salt (either chrome or potassium alum) prevents excessive swelling and softening of the emulsion. The hardening process "tans" the gelatin in the emulsion and protects it against abrasion. It also prevents excessive softening, which damages the emulsion during washing or drying with warm air. Lastly, drying time is shortened with harder emulsions.

Acidifier. Acidic compounds, either sulfuric or acetic acid, neutralize any remaining alkaline developer and also accelerate the action of other chemicals by providing an optimum working medium.

Solvent water. The primary solvent serves several important functions. It dissolves the other fixing ingredients, helps to transport the clearing agent into the emulsion and removes silver thiosulfate complexes from the film. If not removed, these complexes cause the film to turn yellowish brown in time.

Wash

To ensure permanence of the film without further discoloration or fading, it is necessary to remove all processing chemicals. The desired result is a radiograph that contains only developed metallic silver masses suspended in gelatin. Washing must be accomplished in a manner that exposes both film surfaces to constant agitation and recirculation of fresh running water.

During manual processing, it is recommended that the films be placed in a special fixer neutralizing bath to remove any fixer left in the emulsion. This drastically reduces the washing time.

Dryer

This final step of processing is basically accomplished in automatic processors by allowing warm air to blow across the film during its transportation through the rollers. Drying films that are manually processed is accomplished either by hanging them on racks or by placing them in special film dryers. Keeping films well separated is of utmost importance, for they tend to stick together if wet, making it impossible to separate them later. By immersing manually processed films in a wetting agent (liquid detergent) after washing, drying time can be reduced by 50%. This agent improves drainage and helps to prevent teardrop marks from forming during the drying process.

DEVELOPMENT FACTORS

The degree of development depends on two critical factors, time and temperature. Without the correct combination of these factors, even a properly exposed radiograph will not be of diagnostic quality. Standardized formulas and charts, available through various film manufacturers, are useful in determining development times and temperatures necessary to produce optimum values of density, contrast and fog. Generally speaking, the higher the temperature, the more active the developer. In other words, higher temperatures necessitate less development time, and conversely, lower temperatures necessitate more time. Extremes, at either end, can produce unacceptable results. Manual developers in low temperatures are virtually inactive (hydroquinone becomes inactive below 60° F). High manual developer temperatures (above 75° F) can cause extreme fogging, as well as separating the emulsion from the base. Optimal manual temperatures for development range between 68 and 72° F. Most manual development is based on the combination of 5 minutes at 68° F.

Development time depends not only on temperature but also on the type of film used, the nature of the developer and the degree of agitation during development. The rate at which various film types develop is more thoroughly discussed in Chapter 21, Sensitometry and Processor Quality Control; however, the thinner the emulsion, the faster the developing time.

Certain developers are inherently more active than others. Therefore, when using a different developer, the time and temperature chart indicators may have to be adjusted to achieve the desired contrast. With continued use and age, any developer solution becomes exhausted. Exhausted developer demonstrates an alkalinity decrease, accumulation of restraining products and oxidation by air. Owing to these variations in the composition of the developer, the time required to reach a certain contrast increases. To help control the diminished efficiency of exhausted solutions, replenishment solutions are continually added.

Lastly, development time is affected by the degree of agitation employed. Generally speaking, the more vigorous the agitation, the shorter the development time. Bromide ions are released from the emulsion after development. These waste products stick to the emulsion if they are not removed and inhibit development. Film agitation removes these particles and provides for more uniform development.

FIXING FACTORS

Two steps are involved in fixation, clearing and hardening the film. After the unexposed and undeveloped crystals become transparent, clearing is completed. In manual processing, hardening of the emulsion necessitates that the film remain immersed in the solution for about twice as long as for developing. Total fixing time depends primarily on the following five factors: type and thickness of emulsion, nature of the fixing solution, temperature, degree of agitation and degree of radiographic exposure.

Relative to the first factor affecting fixing time, nonscreen film generally requires longer fixing than screen film owing to its thicker emulsion. Fine grained emulsions require less fixing than do coarse grained emulsions simply because of their smaller size.

The second factor affecting the length of fixing is the nature of the fixer solution. When sodium thiosulfate and ammonium thiosulfate are used at the same concentration, ammonium thiosulfate has the faster fixation rate. Generally, the higher the concentration of the fixer, the faster the clearing time. Also, as in the case of the developer, fixing agents also become exhausted with age and use, thus increasing clearing time. Again, replenishers are added to increase the life of the fixer and the rate of clearing.

Another factor affecting fixing time is temperature. Higher temperatures yield faster clearing times. As the gelatin becomes more permeable with higher temperatures, diffusion of the solution into the gelatin is enhanced. The control of temperature is not as strict as in developing, but there should not be a great difference between temperatures for these two stages of processing.

Agitation also affects fixing time. Because the fixing process is primarily controlled by diffusion, agitation decreases the clearing time. It also ensures that fresh fixing solutions contact the film and displace any exhausted fixer adhering to the film surface.

The last factor affecting fixing time is radiographic exposure. Generally stated, the greater the radiographic exposure, the faster the rate of fixation for the same size films. This occurs because fewer unexposed crystals remain from heavier exposures; thus fewer crystals need clearing.

REPLENISHING AGENTS

Each time a film is processed, either manually or automatically, a certain quantity of both developer and fixer solution is lost from the system. The chemistries of both solutions also change with age, leaving them less active. To avoid the necessity of constantly refilling the tanks with fresh solutions, specially formulated replenishers are added to help keep the original solutions close to their initial state of activity.

Developer replenisher differs from the original solution in that it is more alkaline (higher pH) and it contains no restrainers (bromides). Bromides within the crystal structure dissociate from the emulsion during development, lowering the pH of the developer. The main ingredient in the original restrainer is also bromide. It can be seen, then, that these two sources of halogen ions (bromide) drastically increase the restraining effect of the developer. The increased alkalinity and the lack of restraining solution in the replenisher effectively counteract the undesired chemical changes of the developer. Replenisher is generally added only a couple of times a day during manual processing simply to return the fluid level to its original state. With automatic processing, however, a continuous feed system is employed, which ensures appropriate replenishment of the developer after the passage of each film.

Fixer replenisher contains the same ingredients as the original fixer solution. Automatic processors provide for continual fixer replacement through feeding mechanisms similar to those used for developer replacement. In manual processing, fixer replenisher is added as the solution level falls.

MANUAL PROCESSING AND EQUIPMENT

Because the use of automated processors is so widespread, this section discusses only the basic equipment necessary for manual processing and the average times and temperatures of each stage.

Equipment

Manual processing can be accomplished with a minimum of equipment, including two stirring paddles (one for the developer and one for the fixer), one thermometer (to check various temperatures), several processing tanks and a drying device. Because the materials are either immersed in or contain corrosive chemicals, they must be noncorrosible and unbreakable. Most are made from hard rubber, enamel, plastic or a stainless steel alloy. It is important to state that mercury thermometers should not be used, as mercury can contaminate the processing solutions if the thermometer breaks.

Numerous types and arrangements of processing tanks are available, but the most common system consists of one large tank, evenly separated into two compartments. Individual developer and fixer tanks are then inserted and separated in one of the main compartments. Both compartments are filled with water. The area between the developer and fixer inserts is used for the rinse bath, while the other compartment serves as the wash area (Figure 20–5). The size of all tanks is relative to the volume of films processed, keeping in mind that the films must be completely submerged in all processing solutions. Proportionately, the fixer tank is twice the size of the developer tank and the wash tank is twice the size of the fixer tank. This is because it generally takes twice as long to fix a film as it does to develop it and twice as long to wash it as to fix it. Not only is circulating water in the compartments important for rinsing and washing, but it also provides a means of temperature control for all the solutions. Optimum temperatures are usually maintained through thermostatically controlled warm and cold water outlets.

Drying can be accomplished by hanging the films in special racks, but this is extremely slow and subject to varying climatical factors (humidity, heat, etc.). Numerous drying devices are available to speed up the process and offer a more controlled environment. These are basically simple cabinets in which air is heated and circulated (by fan) around the hanging films.

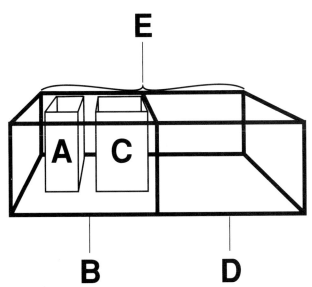

Figure 20–5. Manual processing tank. A, Developing tank; B, rinse bath; C, fixing tank insert (twice the size of A); D, washing tank (twice the size of C); E, double compartment tank.

Processing Time

Processing time, as noted above, depends on a variety of factors, such as the temperature, nature and concentration of the solutions, the film type, the degree of agitation, the degree of exposure, the use of a fixer neutralizer, and the use of wetting agents. The following is an example of processing times assuming that the developer, fixer and wash solutions are maintained at 68° F while the drying temperature is between 90 and 110° F:
1. Developing time: 5 minutes
2. Rinse time: 30 seconds
3. Fixing time: 10 minutes
4. Washing time: 20 minutes (this can be shortened to 5 minutes by using a fixer neutralizer bath)
5. Drying time: 30–60 minutes (drying time can be reduced by 50% if a wetting agent is used).

Adding up the times for the various processing stages reveals that the time required to manually process one film can be well over 1 hour. Standardization of this process is also difficult, as it is highly unlikely that identical techniques are employed by each individual involved in the process.

AUTOMATIC PROCESSING AND EQUIPMENT

There are several advantages of automatic processing. Of greatest importance to any imaging department is the drastic increase in the number of studies that can be performed daily and the great improvement in radiographic quality control. Depending on the particular type of unit, chemicals and film type used and the temperature of the solutions, processing time can be decreased to as little as 90 seconds. An example of processing times based on a developer temperature of 103.5° F, a fixer temperature of 90–95° F, a wash temperature of 98° F, and a drying temperature of 135–150° F follows:
1. Developing time: 25 seconds
2. Fixing time: 21 seconds
3. Washing time: 9 seconds
4. Drying time: 20 seconds.

As discussed above, the chemicals used in automatic processors differ from those employed during manual processing. This is primarily because films must be able to withstand the higher temperatures and rapid processing without swelling excessively or becoming sticky or slippery during travel through the unit.

Equipment

Although the construction of automatic processors may vary, they all include some means of providing strict control over the temperature of solutions; addition of replenishers; developer and fixer recirculation; water circulation; agitation; and transportation of the film through the developer, fixer, washing and drying areas. An in-depth discussion of the components of an automatic processor is located in Chapter 19, Automatic Processor and Preventive Maintenance.

Temperature Control

The opportunity to continually alter developing and/or fixing times to compensate for temperature or radiographic exposure variations is no longer possible with automatic processors. Although processors that operate on cold water wash and relatively low developer temperatures are being manufactured today, most continue to function on warm temperatures of all solutions. Accurate temperature control can be achieved in a variety of ways. Some processors allow thermostatically controlled water to flow under the developer and fixer tanks on its way to the wash, thereby heating these solutions through the simple process of conduction. Some processors use thermostatically controlled heating elements placed at the bottom of the tanks, whereas others may use a more sophisticated device such as a heat exchanger to control temperature. Recall from a previous discussion that the developer temperature is much more critical than that of the other solutions.

Replenishment

Without accurate replenishment of developer and fixer solutions, radiographic film quality suffers, as the original chemicals become less active and full of waste products. Most systems consist of two external reservoirs and a replenishment pump. The size of the replenishing reservoirs (developing and fixing agents) depends on the number and size of the processors they feed as well as the volume of radiographs processed. The reservoirs should never be allowed to become empty, as ensuing air bubbles can effectively block the continued flow of solutions, even after they have been refilled. In-line pumps transport replenisher from the reservoirs to the processing tanks in quantities relative to the area of the films and to the average density of the radiographic examinations performed. Replenishment rates are generally recommended by the manufacturer.

Recirculation

Constant recirculation of the developer and fixer solutions, as well as the replenishers, keeps the solutions well mixed, filters particulate matter from the solutions before their reentry into the tanks, helps maintain thermal control of the solutions and increases agitation of the solutions. The solutions are pumped from their processing tanks, heated, filtered and then returned under pressure. The usual recirculation rate is such that a solution travels through a tank approximately six times per minute.

Water Circulation

The most important function of the water circulatory system in an automatic processor is to provide adequate washing of the films. This necessitates a continual supply of clean running water under a sustained pressure. The water flows through the system and is eventually drained out. As can be imagined, water consumption can be astronomical. To help lessen the cost, many processors incorporate an electronic water saving device, which reduces the flow during inactive times. As mentioned above, the water system may also serve as a means of temperature control for the developer and the fixer.

Agitation and Film Transportation

The film transportation system is important not only for conveying films through the processing unit but also for providing the primary mechanism of agitation through constant and vigorous movement of the rollers. Although films can travel horizontally through processors, the most common method is by way of a vertical transport system. All vertical models must incorporate a main drive motor, entrance rollers, racks, turnarounds, crossovers and a squeegee assembly.

The main drive is usually made to electronically sense the entry of a film and automatically set the roller assemblies and other electrical components into action. It also senses a film's exit from the dryer and switches the processor to a standby mode. This prevents the motor and other electrical components from operating during inactive periods.

The normal sequence of film transport is as follows:

1. The film is placed on the feed tray and inserted until it is sensed by the detector. The drive system is thus enabled.
2. It then proceeds to the developer tank via a crossover assembly.
3. Next, it travels down the rollers, completes a 180 degree turn at the bottom (via a turnaround assembly) and returns up the opposite side of the developer tank.
4. Transportation through the fixer and wash tanks is accomplished in the same manner as in steps 2 and 3.
5. From the wash tank, the film proceeds through a special crossover rack that contains squeegee-type rollers (to remove excessive water and chemicals) to the dryer.
6. The roller assembly in the dryer routes the film straight into the film receiving bin and film processing is completed.

Although all roller assemblies have the same function and essentially the same design, the arrangement of the rollers may differ slightly. Some processors use a face to face type, whereas others use a zigzag type. Face to face models provide for greater agitation of the solutions and greater stability of film travel, but they are more likely to cause uneven processing than the zigzag type. Also, because the two opposing rollers create greater pressure on the film, harder emulsions should be used with face to face rollers. Rollers in the processing tanks are generally assembled as a single unit, or rack, so that they may be easily removed for cleaning.

PHOTOGRAPHIC TECHNIQUES

The remainder of this chapter addresses the basic details and procedures for three photographic techniques used in imaging departments, namely subtraction, stereoradiography and duplication.

SUBTRACTION

Radiographic subtraction, a technique employed primarily in angiographic procedures, removes unwanted or hindering structures so that areas of interest may be more clearly delineated. Small vessels tend to run through or around various bony structures, making their visualization in these areas quite difficult. Subtraction effectively removes most or all of the interfering bone, thus enhancing small vessel detail. Many modern angiographic departments currently have computer systems capable of performing digital subtraction automatically. (Digital subtraction is beyond the scope of this text. However, a brief introduction to the concept is found in Chapter 16, Digital Imaging Overview.) If these are unavailable, manual techniques are employed. There are three different methods of subtraction: first order, second order and third order. Second order is not discussed, as this method is rarely used.

First Order Subtraction

Two radiographs must be obtained before performing subtraction; a scout film, or base, taken before the introduction of contrast medium, and an angiographic film, or angiogram, taken after the injection of contrast medium (Figure 20–6A and B, respectively). First order subtraction is accomplished in the following manner:

1. A mask of the base film is made by placing the emulsion side of the subtraction film in contact with the base film and exposing both to light. The mask is a negative of the base film in which the images are reversed (diapositive), or the dark areas of the base appear as light areas on the mask and vice versa (Figure 20–6C). If the mask and the base are superimposed, no images are visible.
2. The mask, when carefully placed over the angiographic film, effectively subtracts all structures common to the base and the angiogram, leaving only the vascular detail or contrast medium image.
3. A final print of this information is made by placing the emulsion side of a subtraction film against the mask and the angiogram and then exposing them to light (Figure 20–6D). The print, being a negative film, shows reversed densities

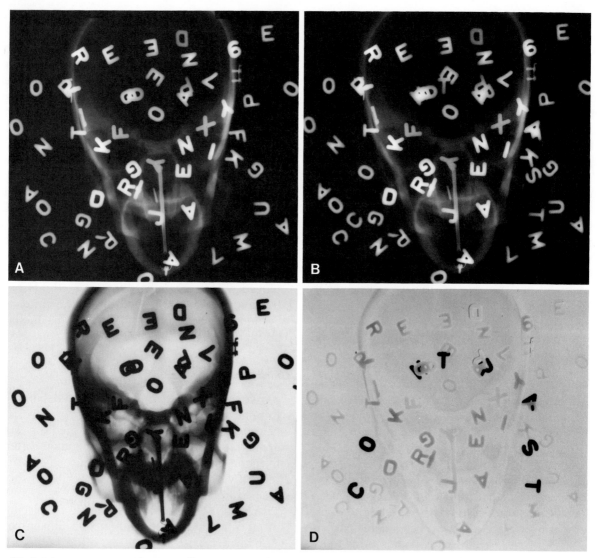

Figure 20–6. Subtraction process. *A,* Base (scout) film; *B,* contrast media (angiogram) film; *C,* mask of base film; *D,* print (mask, angiogram and subtraction film). Refer to text for explanation of process.

and eliminates superimposed structures. After the bony detail is subtracted, the contrast medium filled vessels are easier to visualize.

The preceding steps can be completed using a subtraction machine (Figure 20–7). Commercial subtraction units are available and can also be used to duplicate film (see under Duplication). Directions are supplied with the equipment and are employed to determine the operation of the unit.

The most important consideration, regardless of whether the subtraction films are produced with commercial units or by homemade devices, is that

the light source must pass through the base, the angiogram or the superimposed films before striking the subtraction film. In other words, the subtraction film is farthest from the light source.

Third Order Subtraction

To obtain better detail of contrast medium filled vessels, an additional print is added to the first order subtraction process. This is, however, more involved and more care must be taken to ensure that the films are superimposed exactly before mak-

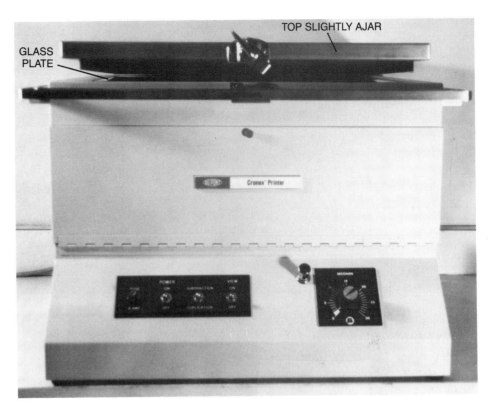

GLASS PLATE

TOP SLIGHTLY AJAR

Figure 20–7. Subtraction/duplication unit.

ing the subtraction films. The addition of an intermediate subtraction print is called third order subtraction. The procedure is as follows:

1. An additional mask film is made of the angiographic film by placing the emulsion side of the subtraction film in contact with the angiographic film and exposing it to light.

2. The angiographic mask is superimposed on the scout film. If done properly, all structures common to both films appear black and the contrasted vessels also appear dark. An intermediate subtraction print is made by placing the emulsion side of the subtraction film against the superimposed angiographic mask and base film and exposing them to light. The most visible object in this print is now light (white) colored vessels.

3. A final subtraction print is made by superimposing the intermediate subtraction print, the original angiogram and the base mask. These films are placed against the emulsion side of a subtraction film and exposed. This literally adds two sets of contrast medium filled vessels; thus the third order print enhances the first order print.

STEREORADIOGRAPHY

It is well known that radiographs show only two dimensions, length and width, whereas all objects have a third dimension of depth. To enable the radiologist to perceive depth, lateral or oblique views are typically taken along with anterior or posterior views. The ability to see depth provides better localization of lesions or foreign bodies as well as more clearly demonstrating their true relationship to adjacent anatomical areas. A sophisticated radiographic method of incorporating all three dimensions into one image is called stereoradiography.

Simply stated, stereoradiography involves a duplication of how the human eyes see depth. The eyes, individually, do not have the ability to see three dimensions. Each eye actually views an object from a slightly different angle and forms this image on the retina. A fusion of the two slightly different images, as seen from both eyes, occurs within visual centers of the brain, thus creating three dimensional perception.

In stereoradiography, the x-ray tube represents one eye. If two radiographs from slightly different projections are taken of a stationary object, these images are equivalent to the impressions formed on the retinas of both eyes. The only other item necessary to produce a three dimensional image is a means of fusing the two radiographs into one. This is accomplished in a variety of ways, as explained below.

Procedures for Obtaining a Stereoradiograph

Two factors must be considered before obtaining the two radiographs, namely the amount and the direction of tube shift. It has been determined that the ideal viewing distance for a stereoscopic image is 25 inches. Also, the average interpupillary (between the pupils) distance is 2.5 inches. As can be seen, these specific distances represent a ratio of 1:10. This same ratio can be applied to tube shift (representing the pupil distance) versus source-image distance (SID) (corresponding to the viewing distance). Thus, the total tube shift is one-tenth of the SID. For example, if the SID is 40 inches, the tube shift is 4 inches. Stereoscopic radiographs taken at 72 inches employs a tube shift of approximately 7 inches. Keep in mind that these figures apply only when the viewing distance is 25 inches and the interpupillary distance is 2.5 inches. If a change in either the viewing distance or interpupillary distance occurs, the tube shift or SID also changes respectively.

The direction of tube shift is perpendicular, or at right angles, to the predominant lines of the body part being radiographed. For example, the ribs form the dominant lines in the chest. Therefore, the tube is shifted in the same direction as the vertebral column, or at right angles to the ribs during chest stereoscopy. For evaluation of a long bone, the tube is shifted across the bone. It is extremely important to remember that if a high ratio grid is used, tube shift must remain parallel to the lead strips of the grid or the two radiographs display unequal densities (grid cutoff).

The steps involved in stereoradiography are:

1. Accurately center the part to be radiographed to the film. (Make sure that the long axis or predominant lines of the part are placed perpendicular to the lead strips of the grid. This allows proper tube shift to avoid grid cutoff.)

2. Immobilize the part so that it maintains the identical position during both radiographs.
3. Determine the direction of tube shift (perpendicular to the long axis of the part).
4. Determine the total tube shift distance, positioning the tube one-half of this distance from the center of the part. For example, if a 72 inch SID is used (total shift of 7 inches), position the tube 3.5 inches to the left of center.
5. Use lead markers to properly identify the correct side of the patient and the correct stereoradiograph side (see under Marking Stereoradiographs) and take the first exposure.
6. Without moving the patient, change the cassette.
7. Shift the tube the entire distance as determined in step 4 to the opposite side. In this example, move the tube 7 inches to the right (this is the same as moving it 3.5 inches to the right of center). This step as well as step 6 is performed either automatically by the equipment or quickly by the technologist. This helps avoid movement of the part.
8. Use lead markers to properly identify the correct side of the patient and the correct stereoradiograph side (see under Marking Stereoradiographs) and take the second exposure, making sure that all factors remain constant. When obtaining radiographs of voluntary moving organs, e.g., lungs, to maintain the same part position the patient must *not* breathe between exposures. In other words, the patient must hold his/her breath during steps 5 through 8.

Marking Stereoradiographs

To ensure that the radiographs are properly placed on the illuminator, it is important to mark the films correctly. In addition to the usual R and L markers, stereo R and stereo L markers should be placed on the films. If the radiographs are either improperly marked or improperly displayed on the illuminator, transposition of the object and/or reversal of the projection occurs. For example, in a correctly displayed anterior-posterior stereoradiograph of the pelvis, the pubic symphysis should appear closer to the observer than the sacrum does. If the films are reversed around their axis, the projection appears as a posterior-anterior view, with the sacrum closer than the symphysis. Also, if the radiograph intended for viewing from the right eye is placed on the left side of the illuminator, an original anterior-posterior projection of the left femur would appear as a posterior-anterior projection of the right femur. As can be imagined, either situation could be disastrous.

Viewing Stereoradiographs

It is important to know how and where each radiograph is to be placed before viewing. In general, the films are placed on the illuminator in the position as if seen by the tube, the left stereoradiograph on the viewer's left and the right on the viewer's right with the tube side of the film facing the observer. Films taken with a transverse (side to side) shift of the tube, e.g., of long bones, are displayed on the illuminator relative to the anatomical position. Those films employing a longitudinal shift, e.g., of the chest, are placed in a horizontal position on the illuminator (it should look as though the patient was lying on his/her side).

There are several ways to view stereoradiographs, including direct vision, stereomonoculars, stereobinoculars and more sophisticated stereoscopes. Direct vision viewing requires no equipment. The radiographs are placed side by side in the conventional manner and the observer simply crosses his/her eyes until the two images appear to fuse into one. Considerable practice is necessary before successful viewing can be accomplished. For those who are unable to perform this maneuver, other devices are available at relatively little expense.

The stereomonocular, a 30 or 40 degree glass prism, is the simplest and least expensive device for viewing stereoradiographs. When the thinner portion is placed close to the nose, in front of one eye, the light rays from one radiograph are bent in such a way as to make it appear as if they are coming from the other radiograph. This effectively fuses the images and provides the perception of depth.

Stereobinoculars basically consist of two monoculars. The simplest method of binocular viewing is using two 20 degree glass prisms, one for each eye. They may also be manufactured in the shape of simple opera glasses or in large, sophisticated assemblies of mirrors, glass and prisms. Viewing instructions need to be followed carefully when utilizing the more sophisticated models, as some radiographs will be viewed in the conventional manner and others must be flipped around their vertical axis before being viewed.

DUPLICATION

Duplication, as the name implies, is a method of copying or making a facsimile of an existing radiograph. The need for copying films arises on numerous occasions, such as for teaching or other academic endeavors, for a patient to take to outside referrals or specialists, for library references and for the patient's file.

In general, a copy is made by exposing a duplicating film, which is in direct contact with the radiograph to be copied, to a source of light. As already learned, regular x-ray film has a negative response to exposure in that the darker areas represent greater exposure than the lighter areas do. Duplicating film shows a reversal in this response in that darker areas represent less light exposure, whereas lighter areas represent greater exposure. As can be seen in Figure 20–8, the higher density areas on the original radiograph limit the transmission of light to the duplicating film, and conversely, the lower densities allow the light to pass through.

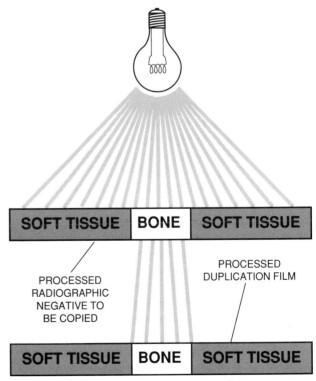

Figure 20–8. Duplication or facsimile production. The darker areas (soft tissue) of a processed radiograph limit or restrict light transmission to the duplication film, resulting in corresponding dark areas on the processed duplication film. Lighter areas (bone) show the opposite response.

If duplicating film had the same response as x-ray film, the result would be a reversal of the negative. However, because their responses are opposite, the duplicating film shows the same densities as in the original radiograph.

The two most important considerations in producing a high quality copy are ensuring that the radiograph and the duplicating film are in close, uniform contact during exposure and determining the correct exposure time. Commercial printers are available for accomplishing both tasks simultaneously. They basically consist of a box with a light source (or sources) in the bottom, a glass platform onto which to place the films, and a lid heavy enough to ensure that the films maintain close contact when the box is closed. Homemade printers can be just as effective as the commercial ones. A piece of hardwood covered with a thin layer of polyfoam (as large as the largest film used) can serve as a base on which the films are placed. A heavy, clear plate of glass can serve as the cover to allow for light transmission as well as to apply even pressure over both films.

Regardless of the type of printer, the films and the light source must maintain certain relationships to each other. The emulsion side of the duplicating film must be in close contact with the radiograph to be copied and the light source must be facing the original radiograph. Therefore, when using a commercial printer with the light source on the bottom, the original radiograph is placed on the glass facing the light. The emulsion side of the duplicating film is then placed against the radiograph. If the light source is above the working bench, the emulsion side of the duplicating film is placed face up on the hardwood platform with the radiograph on top, also face up, toward the light.

For commercial printers, charts published by the manufacturer are used to determine the exposure time necessary to duplicate the original radiographic density and contrast. A trial and error method is normally used with homemade printers. In this case, it is essential to remember that duplicating film has the opposite response to exposure than does the original negative film. If the density appears too light, it can be darkened by lowering the exposure. Conversely, if the density of the copy is too dark, it can be lightened by increasing the exposure.

Duplicating films designed for use in most imaging departments are sensitive to the same color spectrum as x-ray film (blue light). They are, therefore, suitable for use under the same darkroom safelight filter. They can also be processed under the same conditions as x-ray film, either automatically or manually.

LABORATORY EXPERIENCE

Laboratories 31, Subtraction; 32, Stereoradiography; and 33, Film Duplication, are associated with this chapter. For laboratory experience related to automatic processing or sensitometry, the researcher is referred to Laboratories 29, 30 and 34.

The Subtraction laboratory enables the researcher to perform first and third order subtraction. This provides the learner with the opportunity to compare the quality of first and third order subtraction techniques. The subtraction may be performed with a commercial machine or by manual methods.

In the Stereoradiography laboratory, the researcher performs stereoradiography at a 40 inch SID. This provides the student the opportunity to produce and view stereoradiographs.

The Film Duplication laboratory experiment allows the experimenter to copy radiographs.

Bibliography

Bushong, SC. Radiologic science for technologists (4th edition). St. Louis: Mosby, 1988.

Chesney, DN and Chesney, MO. Radiographic imaging (4th edition). Boston: Blackwell Scientific Publications, 1981.

Curry, TS, Dowdey, JE and Murry, RC. Christensen's Introduction to the physics of diagnostic radiology (3rd edition). Philadelphia: Lea & Febiger, 1984.

Eastman Kodak Company. Fundamentals of radiography (12th edition). Rochester, NY: Eastman Kodak Company, 1980.

E. I. du Pont de Nemours & Co., Inc. Principles of subtraction in radiology. Wilmington, DE: E. I. du Pont de Nemours & Co., Inc., 1974.

Freeman, M. The Amphoto photography workshop series. New York: Amphoto, 1988.

Fuji Photo Film Co., Ltd. Fundamentals of photography. Tokyo: Fuji Photo Film Co., Ltd., 1978.

Fuji Photo Film Co., Ltd. Fundamentals of sensitized materials for radiography. Tokyo: Fuji Photo Film Co., Ltd., 1982.

Jacobson, R, Ray, S and Attridge, G. The manual of photography (8th edition). Boston: Focal Press, 1988.

Jenkins, D. Radiographic photography and imaging processes. Baltimore: University Park Press, 1980.

Principles of radiographic exposure. San Antonio, TX: Fort Sam Houston, Department of the Army, Academy of Health Sciences, 1977.

Tortorici, MR. Fundamentals of angiography. St. Louis: Mosby, 1982.

United States Department of Health, Education and Welfare. Course manual for x-ray measurements. Rockville, MD: U.S. Government Printing Office, 1973.

Walls, HJ and Attridge, GG. Basic photo science. New York: Focal Press, 1977.

Williams, J. Image clarity. Boston: Focal Press, 1990.

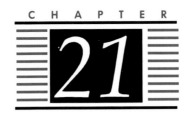

SENSITOMETRY AND PROCESSOR QUALITY CONTROL

JOAN K. MacDONALD

INTRODUCTION

To make accurate diagnoses, the radiologist needs to be presented with a film that provides the best possible detail and information. Major changes in radiographic contrast or density during specific examinations are unacceptable, as significant detail may be lost, possibly resulting in either a need for a repeated examination or a misdiagnosis. As will be learned in following chapters, radiographic density and contrast are primarily controlled by the kilovoltage, milliamperage and time settings on the x-ray machine. However, even if these technical factors remain constant, different types of film and different processing conditions may produce extreme fluctuations in density and contrast.

This chapter focuses on the relationship between radiation exposure and film response during certain processing conditions. The study and measurement of these relationships is referred to as sensitometry. By having adequate knowledge of sensitometric properties of films, the radiographer is able to determine how density and contrast are altered with a change in film types, radiographic techniques or processing conditions.

Sensitometry is also used as a daily method of automatic processor quality control. This may be the most important reason for performing sensitometric measurements, as inferior processing conditions can be responsible for the production of inferior quality images, even if the exposure techniques are ideal. Because the response of film varies with different processing conditions, sensitometry allows the radiographer to determine major or minor changes of the processor on a day to day basis. This chapter explains how sensitometric factors affect the characteristic curve and processor quality control.

CHARACTERISTIC CURVES

DESIGN

The most common method of expressing the response of film to exposure is by the use of a characteristic curve. It is also referred to as a sensitometric, H and D (Hurter and Driffield) or D-log E curve. By plotting a series of known exposures against their resulting densities, several fundamental factors affecting photographic quality can be evaluated. The most important factors investigated are speed (sensitivity), contrast and fog.

By convention, characteristic curves are generally structured to express exposure in relative terms rather than in real, or absolute, numbers. Only during certain applications in research, radiation therapy and monitoring (via film badges) are absolute values necessary. The logarithmic scale is used as an expression of relative exposure for two primary reasons: the graph is easier to produce and understand, as a greater range of values can be recorded along the customary horizontal axis (abscissa), and exposures whose ratios are constant are separated by equal increments along the axis regardless of their absolute values.

Photographic density (see Chapter 27, Photographic Image Quality) is a logarithmic value. This quantitative measurement of film blackening is actually the logarithm of the intensity of light falling on a particular area of a processed film divided by the intensity of that light transmitted through the film. Logarithms are used to measure density because the human eye perceives light intensity logarithmically. In other words, when light intensity is increased by 100% (intensity × 2), the eye perceives this not as a doubling of the density but rather as an increase by a factor of approximately 0.3 (log 2 = 0.301).

The characteristic curve is, therefore, a graph of the relationship between two logarithmic values, density on the vertical axis (ordinate) and relative exposure on the horizontal axis (Figure 21–1A). Figure 21–1 also shows how the actual or absolute exposure (milliampere-seconds) corresponds to the log of relative exposures and how density corresponds to the percentage of light transmission (transmission is the reciprocal of density, expressed as a percentage).

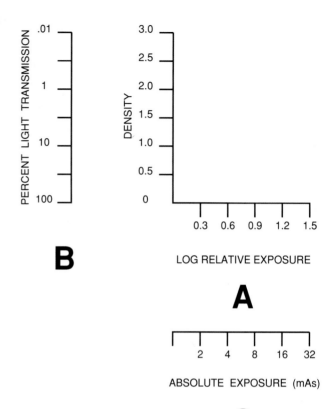

Figure 21–1. Characteristic curve axes design showing the relationship between log density and log exposure (A). The figure also demonstrates how the percentage of light transmitted through the film correlates with log density (B) and how the absolute exposure (or mAs) (C) correlates with the log of the relative exposure.

METHODS OF MAKING CHARACTERISTIC CURVES

Characteristic curves can be made for any type of film, using a variety of radiations (x-rays, x-rays in combination with light or light only). A curve is made by simply presenting the film material to a series of stepwise exposures. Stated another way, the film is exposed to a range of exposures from low to high. The steps must be designed so that the exposures of two adjacent steps are related to each other by some constant factor, called the wedge constant. If x-ray equipment is used to create a curve, the stepwise exposures can be obtained either by varying the time scale (milliampere-seconds) or by varying the intensity (using a penetrometer, or stepwedge). If light photons generate the curve, a device called a sensitometer is used.

TYPICAL AREAS REPRESENTED ON CHARACTERISTIC CURVES

A typical curve demonstrates that density does not respond to uniform rates of exposure in a uniform manner. The plotted responses to a series of stepped exposures generally yield an elongated S shaped curve rather than a continual straight line. The actual shape varies with different film types and processing conditions. Figure 21–2 shows three well-defined portions that are visible on most characteristic curves, the toe, straight line and shoulder portions, representing regions of underexposure, correct exposure and overexposure, respectively. A fourth portion, called the region of solarization, is generally not evident on diagnostic radiographs, as high exposure levels are necessary to produce this phenomenon.

It is logical to assume that areas of a radiograph receiving no exposure produce areas of zero density. However, after processing, the film base always produces some density. The amount of density varies slightly depending on the type of material used, its inherent transparency, its thickness and the color of the dye. Base density is usually about 0.1. Some degree of fog (usually 0.1) is also present on all processed films. Thus, the base plus fog generally relates to a density of about 0.2. This area, called the base plus fog, gross fog or minimum density (D_{min}) portion, is represented by the lower part of the characteristic curve, which is parallel to the abscissa.

The point of a characteristic curve where the lower end ceases to be parallel to the abscissa is called the threshold. This represents the first reaction of the film to actual radiographic exposure. The corresponding density, from 0.2 to 0.25, represents the first observable density above base plus fog.

The first area to respond to exposure by demonstrating an increase in density is the toe portion. It includes that portion above threshold up to a density of about 0.5. Radiographically, this relates to those areas on the film receiving the least exposure, e.g., dense bone, thick body organs and lead markers.

A relatively linear relationship between exposure and density is usually observed in the straight line portion of the curve. This implies that, as exposure increases, density increases in a fairly direct manner. In this area of the curve, the most useful radiographic densities are encountered (from gross fog plus 0.25 through gross fog plus 2). This is the most important area of the curve for comparing radiographic contrast (see Film Contrast, later).

From the upper end of the straight line portion to the point where density ceases to increase with increased exposure is the shoulder portion of the curve. The density corresponding to the top of the shoulder is called maximum density (D_{max}). This expresses the maximum density achievable under certain exposure and processing conditions. Although considered to be in the range of overexposure, this area can contribute radiographic information. Most illuminators, however, do not allow light to penetrate these dark areas, thereby making it difficult to interpret the images without the use of a spotlight.

In the solarization region, density actually decreases with increased exposure. As mentioned above, this occurs only at exposure levels much higher than those normally encountered in diagnostic radiology.

INFORMATION OBTAINED FROM CHARACTERISTIC CURVES

It is not unusual for radiographers to question how the curve applies to the everyday practice of imaging. Recall that there are many different types of film: fast, slow, high contrast, low contrast, direct x-ray exposure (cardboard holder), intensifying

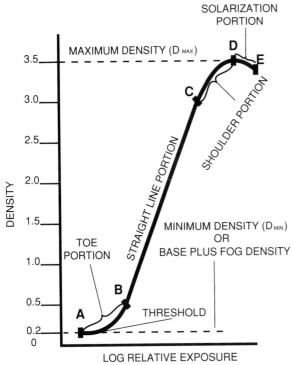

Figure 21–2. Portions of the characteristic curve.

screen combination film, etc. Each type of film, as well as different batches of the same film, may produce different densities (and therefore contrast) when exposed to identical radiographic techniques. By referring to characteristic curves, either ones produced by the radiographer or those furnished by particular film manufacturers, one can answer the following questions:

1. How does film speed affect exposure rates?
2. Which film yields higher (or lower) contrast for the same exposure rate?
3. Which film allows more latitude in the setting of x-ray intensities and yet still produces a satisfactory radiograph?
4. Which film type produces a higher level of fog and what are the consequences?
5. Is the processor functioning properly?

FILM SPEED

Film speed, or sensitivity, is a measurement of the exposure required to produce a particular radiographic effect. It identifies silver halide crystal sensitivity to radiation, regardless of the source. Film speed is inversely proportional to exposure. In other words, faster films require less exposure to produce a desired effect than do slower films. Conversely, slower films require more exposure to produce the same effect.

Because the abscissa of a characteristic curve expresses exposure and because film speed is a measurement of exposure, it is logical to assume that the speed of a film can be identified by the location of its curve along the x axis. Note that, in Figure 21–3, the plot of film A lies to the left of that of film B and that the curves do not cross at any point. Also, note that less relative exposure is required to produce any given density for film A. Film A is, therefore, faster than film B throughout the entire range of relative exposures.

Relative quantitative information relating to differences in speed can be obtained from these graphs. In Figure 21–3, it is evident that, for each relative exposure, the position of the curve changes. Stated another way, film speed changes with varying exposures and it can actually be measured anywhere along the curve. It is generally customary, however, to define speed by the exposures necessary to produce a film density of 1 above base

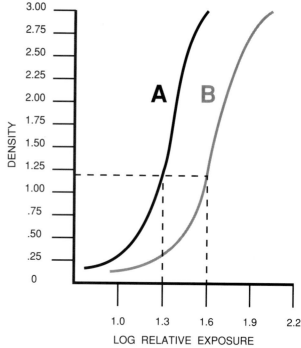

Figure 21–3. Film speed (sensitivity). Film A is faster than film B throughout the entire range of exposures. Refer to text for further explanation.

plus fog or gross fog. Assuming a gross fog of 0.2, the reference point on the density axis is then 1.2. A horizontal line from this reference point is drawn through the characteristic curves. Vertical lines are then dropped from the curve's point of intersection with the horizontal line to the exposure axis. It can be seen that, in producing a density of 1.2, films A and B required 1.3 and 1.6 log units of relative exposure, respectively. Recall that logarithmic values, when separated by the same increment, correspond to constant exposure ratios. In this example, the log of 20 equals 1.3 (this is determined by using a log table) and the log of 40 equals 1.6. A constant ratio of 2 exists in this situation, as 20 × 2 = 40, or 40 is twice 20. This means, in relative terms, that film A is twice as fast as film B in producing a density of 1.2, or conversely, film B is twice as slow as film A.

Although these relative speeds can be defined numerically, it is beyond the scope of this text to illustrate the necessary computations. The reader is referred to sensitometry pamphlets furnished by the various film manufacturers for additional information.

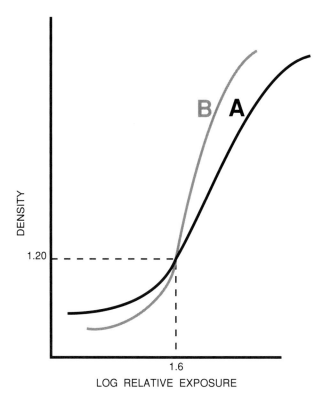

Figure 21–4. Variable film speed. Both films require the same exposure to produce a density of 1.20 (same speed). Film A is faster in producing densities below 1.20 but slower for densities above 1.20.

Sometimes, the curves of two different films may cross over each other. In this instance, speed is determined in the manner illustrated above, but the density reference points may be different. In Figure 21–4, both films require the same exposure to produce a density of 1.2 and, therefore, are the same speed at that point. Film A, however, is faster than B below this density level and slower above it. However, these two films generate curves of different slopes and, hence, exhibit different degrees of contrast. The following discusses how the slope of the curves relates to the degree of film contrast.

FILM CONTRAST

The concept of contrast can be confusing for the beginning radiographer, especially when considering that the word contrast can have three different uses: radiographic contrast, subject contrast and film contrast. Briefly, radiographic contrast is the difference between the densities of two areas on a radiograph. When the density difference is small,

radiographic contrast is low (many shades of gray). When the difference is large, radiographic contrast is high (black and white). Both subject and film contrast influence radiographic contrast.

Subject contrast relates to the absorption of x-rays within different regions of a subject and, therefore, is an expression of the ratio of x-ray intensities exiting the subject to those striking the film. It is dependent on the nature of the subject (bone, soft tissue, fat or thin patient, etc.), the quality of the radiation (kilovolts) and the degree of scattered radiation. These two types of contrast are discussed more thoroughly in Chapters 11, Kilovoltage and Quality Control, and 27, Photographic Image Quality.

Film contrast, or that contrast identified on characteristic curves, is an expression of how exposure relates to the various densities displayed on a radiograph. It is measured by determining the slope or steepness of the characteristic curve. This can be accomplished qualitatively, as the steeper the curve, the higher the contrast, or conversely, the less steep the curve, the lower the contrast. Quantitatively, the slope is measured and expressed as a gradient or an average gradient, contrast index or gamma constant. The most commonly used value in medical radiography is the average gradient (Figure 21–5).

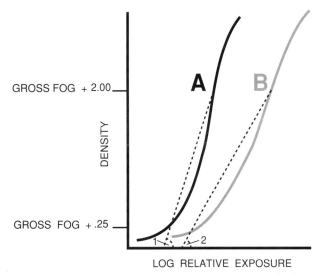

Figure 21–5. Contrast and the characteristic curve. A numerical value is determined by drawing a straight line from the curve's points of intersection with the minimum and maximum useful densities to the exposure axis. The tangent of these angles represents the average gradient. The angle formed with film A (1) is greater than that for film B (2), proving that film A has a higher contrast than B.

As mentioned above, the most useful radiographic densities are represented by the straight line portion of the curve. This may be somewhat misleading in diagnostic x-ray films, as the straight line portion may be relatively short, not extended throughout the entire useful density area (gross fog + 0.25, or D_{min}, to gross fog + 2, or D_{max}). To define the slope, in this case, a line is usually drawn through these two specified densities to establish an average gradient. Although the actual computations are beyond the scope of this text, Figure 21–5 demonstrates the manner in which the lines are drawn. Note that the line drawn for film A is steeper than that for film B (the angle is greater). Therefore, film A has a higher average gradient value and, consequently, displays a higher contrast.

LATITUDE AND ITS RELATIONSHIP TO CONTRAST

Latitude may be defined as the range of x-ray exposures that allows structures within a subject to be satisfactorily imaged. The factor that relates most to the ability to separate structures is contrast. Generally, the higher the contrast, the better the detail. As seen on characteristic curves, however, high contrast films cover a lower range of relative exposures than do low contrast films. This means that, to achieve a satisfactory radiograph of high contrast, less latitude in exposure settings is allowed. Latitude is therefore inversely or reciprocally related to contrast.

As can be seen in Figure 21–6, film A has a higher contrast and less latitude than film B. However, a smaller relative exposure range is necessary to keep the straight line portion of the curve within a chosen diagnostic density range (D_{min} to D_{max}). It must be remembered that both films are of diagnostic quality; however, film A should demonstrate greater detail. The technologist must be more accurate in setting the exposure conditions for film A than for film B.

Latitude is divided into two categories: film latitude and exposure latitude. Film latitude is determined by film contrast and exposure latitude is determined by subject contrast. Because both types of contrast may produce identical appearances on a characteristic curve, no further distinction is made between these two types of latitude.

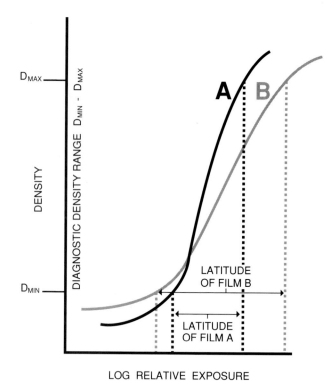

Figure 21–6. Demonstration of reciprocal relationship between contrast and latitude. Film A has a higher contrast and less latitude than film B.

FILM FOG LEVEL

As mentioned above, any processed film shows some degree of density even if it has received no radiographic exposure. This is due to the base material and to fog. Normal film fog comes from the development of silver halide crystals that have received no exposure or such a small amount of exposure as to produce no latent image. Although fog is inherent in all films, fog levels are a function of numerous variables, many of which can be controlled through proper quality control programs. Increases in fog occur with film age, high processing temperatures, long development times, overactive developer (too much replenisher), high speed films, improper film handling and improper film storage (close to certain chemicals, hot and humid environment, etc.).

The main radiographic effect of fog is to decrease contrast. This occurs because greater density is added in the lower relative exposure ranges, which causes the toe portion of the curve to be pulled out

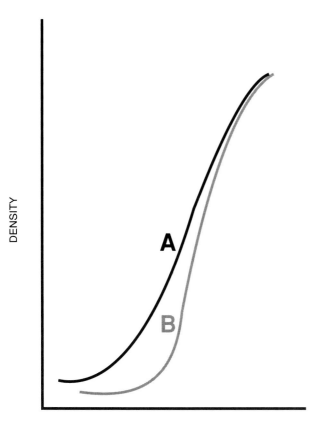

Figure 21–7. Film fog and its effect on the characteristic curve. Film A exhibits a higher level of fog than film B, causing the toe portion of the curve to be pulled out and resulting in a flatter curve and less contrast.

(Figure 21–7). The shape of the curve becomes flatter, indicating lowered contrast.

FACTORS AFFECTING THE CHARACTERISTIC CURVE

Numerous factors affect the shape and the location of characteristic curves. The following identifies these factors and provides a brief discussion of how they influence the characteristic curve.

FILM TYPE

The emulsion ingredients, emulsion thickness and treatment during film manufacturing affect both film speed and contrast. In general, speed is directly related to the size and number of crystals in the emulsion. There is an increase in film speed as the number and size of the crystals increase.

Film contrast is directly related to the distribution of crystal sizes within the emulsion and to crystal sensitivity. Films with a wide range of crystal sizes have the lowest contrast. Those with a small range display medium contrast and those with only one size of crystal have the highest contrast. Because duplitized films contain more crystals than single emulsion films do, they are considerably more sensitive, thus revealing higher contrast.

EXPOSURE TYPE

The speed and contrast of screen-type films are also affected by the type of exposure, either x-rays alone or x-rays and light combined in intensifying screens. Because direct x-ray exposure film is rarely used in medical radiography, little is mentioned here regarding its characteristic curve. Suffice it to say that a relatively larger exposure is necessary before the straight line portion of the curve is reached, and the shoulder portion is not reached until high densities are achieved.

Less exposure is necessary to produce a diagnostic radiograph on screen-type film when using intensifying screens as compared with using direct x-ray exposure. The screen-film combination is, therefore, faster than the film by itself. The speed of screen-films is dependent on the wavelength, hence color, of the exposing or fluorescent light originating in the cassette. For example, blue-sensitive x-ray film is more sensitive to ultraviolet, violet and blue light than it is to green, amber or red. Green-sensitive film, on the other hand, responds to the same colors as blue-sensitive film plus green but not to amber or red. The films chosen for cassette use must therefore be sensitive to those colors emitted by the intensifying screens. In the previous example, it would not be appropriate to use blue-sensitive film with screens that emit green light. Because neither the green nor the blue films are sensitive to red, red safelight filters are effectively used in the developing section of the processing area.

Contrast is decreased in direct x-ray screen-type film exposures as opposed to that in screen-film combinations. The slope becomes less steep and the toe portion is pulled out (Figure 21–8).

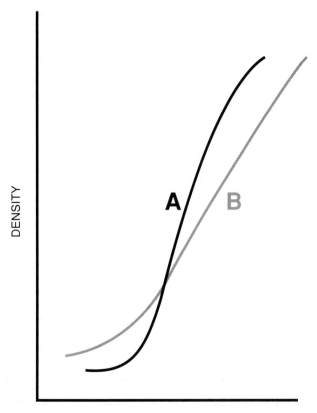

Figure 21–8. Characteristic curves of screen film exposed to intensifying screens (film A) and to direct x-rays (film B). Note how direct x-ray exposure lowers the contrast.

FOG

As mentioned above, increases in film fog decrease film contrast. To prevent fog from affecting the film's sensitivity and contrast, films must be protected from all sources of unwanted radiation (x-ray machines, synthetic or naturally occurring radioactive materials and light). Also, old films or those stored in hot, humid places may have increased fog levels.

RECIPROCITY LAW FAILURE

The foregoing discussion has been based on the assumption that a film's response to radiation exposure is the same regardless of the milliamperage and time settings, as long as the product of these factors (milliampere-seconds) remains constant and as long as the quality (kilovoltage) is unchanged.

This is known as the reciprocity law. It implies that a shorter than normal exposure time can be used to produce a specific radiographic exposure, provided the milliamperage is increased in a proportional manner. This law holds true for direct x-ray exposures, but it is not exactly accurate for exposures to light from intensifying screens. However, the milliamperage or the time must be changed by a factor of about 8 before this reciprocity law failure is noticed radiographically. Because this rarely occurs, it is assumed that any change of lesser degree is insignificant.

PROCESSING CONDITIONS

Processing conditions play the most important role in determining a film's response to radiation. Those components of processing that have the greatest impact are developing times, developing temperatures, quality of the developer and time and quality of fixation. The time and temperature examples indicated in the following two sections refer to manual processing.

Developing Times

Figure 21–9 shows several hypothetical films developed for various times at a fixed temperature. As evidenced, speed increases with developing times, rapidly at first and more slowly after approximately 5 minutes (for manual processing). Speed may decrease if extensive developing times are used. Contrast also increases rapidly at first but may actually decrease in films that have been immersed too long in the developing agents. This is due to an increase in fog with developing time as seen by the higher minimum density level of the 12 minute film.

Developing Temperatures

Figure 21–10 shows several hypothetical films developed for a fixed time at various temperatures. Note that the response to increased temperatures is similar to that observed with increased developing times. Speed increases throughout the temperature range, rapidly at first and then more slowly. Contrast also increases rapidly up to 68° F but then begins to increase more slowly or may even decrease with the addition of more film fog. Because

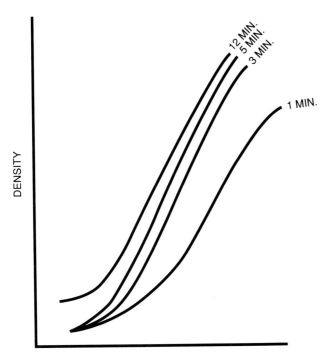

Figure 21–9. Characteristic curves of hypothetical films developed for different lengths of time at a fixed temperature (see text for explanation).

alterations in developing times and temperatures produce similar film characteristics, an increase in temperature could be compensated for by decreasing the developing time. Conversely, a decrease in temperature could be compensated for by increasing the developing time. This is the basic principle used for automatic processing.

Quality of Developer

Recall from Chapter 20, Film, Film Processing and Photographic Techniques, that developer solutions greatly enhance the process of reducing exposed silver halide crystals to metallic silver. They are responsible for darkening those areas of a film that have been made sensitive through the absorption of radiation. If the developer solution becomes too concentrated or too diluted, density levels are artificially enhanced or diminished, respectively.

Fixation Time and Quality of Fixing Solutions

Fixers remove the unexposed crystals and stop the action of the developer. If a film is left in the

fixer solution for a long period of time, these chemicals may actually begin to remove some of the exposed crystals, thus lowering the density on the film. This is more of a potential problem than a real one, as it is highly unlikely for a film to accidentally be left in the fixer solution for such a long time. Weak fixer solutions or inadequate replenishment may cause increased densities on films, as unexposed crystals are not properly cleared and may even undergo some degree of development.

PROCESSOR QUALITY CONTROL

Considering that processing conditions have such a dramatic effect on a film's response to exposure, it is mandatory that a daily sensitometric monitoring system of all automatic processors in an imaging

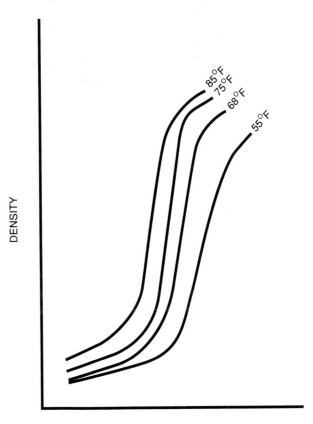

Figure 21–10. Effect of development temperature on characteristic curve. Both speed and contrast increase rapidly as developing temperature increases from 55° F to 68° F, and at greater temperatures the speed and contrast increase at a slower rate. Fog increases slowly from developing temperatures of 55° F to 68° F but more rapidly at temperatures greater than 68° F.

department be established. Radiographers must have confidence that these processors consistently produce high quality diagnostic radiographs from day to day. This can be accomplished by exposing strips of film to a series of stepped exposures, processing them, analyzing them and finally recording the data.

STEPPED EXPOSURES

Recall that each exposure step must be related to its adjacent step by a constant, or wedge, factor. The number of exposure steps may vary, depending on the device or the method of testing. However, the two most acceptable numbers are 11 and 21. The use of 21 steps is more exact in that 21 different densities and, therefore, 20 density differences can be evaluated. Likewise an 11 step device can measure 11 different densities and 10 density differences. Regardless of the number of steps, any testing method should be able to evaluate densities in the diagnostic range from 0.25 to 2. The ranges of densities produced are referred to as gray scales.

Wedge factors are generally either $\sqrt{2}$ (1.414) or 2, depending on the method of testing and/or the device utilized. If it is 2, each step is related to its adjacent step by a factor of 2. To be represented on a characteristic curve as the log of relative exposure, however, the x-axis would be incrementally increased in units of 0.3 (log 2 = 0.301). If the factor is $\sqrt{2}$, the log of relative exposure axis would be incrementally increased in units of 0.15 (log $\sqrt{2}$ = 0.149).

A series of stepped exposures may be performed in several ways, through time scale variation tests, intensity scale variation tests and sensitometers. The first two methods relate to films exposed to x-rays only, or x-rays and light as in screen-film combinations, and the third method is used for films exposed to light only.

TIME SCALE VARIATION STEPPED TEST

No special equipment is necessary to perform the time scale variation stepped test. It is, however, probably the least used method, as it is time consuming and the least reproducible from day to day.

One particular x-ray machine should be chosen to provide each day's exposures. All factors, except the milliampere-seconds setting, should remain constant (kilovoltage, source-image distance, the cassette to be used and the batch of film).

After the cassette is properly placed and marked off to allow for a number of different exposures (at least five), lead shielding is placed over all areas except the one being exposed. If a wedge constant of 2 is used, the first area should be exposed at 1 mAs. This area should then be covered with lead and the next step exposed at 2 mAs. This process would continue by doubling the milliampere-seconds (4, 8, 16, 32, etc.) until all areas of the cassette have been exposed. The film is then processed and evaluated.

INTENSITY SCALE VARIATION STEPPED TEST

The intensity scale variation stepped method uses a specialized device called a stepwedge or penetrometer. For general radiographic work, the wedge is usually made of aluminum and cast to look like a metal staircase and usually has either 11 or 21 steps. As in the time scale method, as many variables as possible need to remain constant from day to day. In this case, the same x-ray machine, technical factors (kilovoltage and milliampere-seconds), source-image distance, cassette, film and stepwedge should be used.

The procedure is simple, as it requires only one exposure of the stepwedge for each processor to be evaluated. It is referred to as an intensity scale variation test because the stepwedge is designed so that known amounts of radiation are transmitted through each step (wedge factor of $\sqrt{2}$ or 2). The thicker step allows less radiation to be transmitted to the film, thereby producing the lowest density.

Although this test is more precise than the time scale method, it is not completely reproducible, as x-ray machines do not produce monoenergetic rays. Therefore, consistency of x-ray output cannot be ensured even when all other factors are held constant. There are also inherent problems with the metal wedge. Although the same intensity of radiation is used, the radiation striking the film does not maintain a constant relationship from step to step. This occurs because the thicker steps act as filters, thereby changing the quality and the intensity of the beam in these areas. Adding a thin filter of copper under the wedge helps alleviate this problem to some degree.

SENSITOMETERS

Sensitometers are special devices designed for exposing film strips to a highly controlled light source. Recall that the majority of exposure in a cassette comes from light within the intensifying screens and that some films, such as duplication and subtraction, are exposed only to light. It is therefore logical to assume that film strips exposed directly to light closely simulate most radiographic practices, especially if the light source emits a color compatible with radiographic film. Most sensitometers may be adjusted to emit either a blue or a green light to be compatible with the respective type of x-ray film.

Sensitometers operate on the same principle as the intensity scale test in that a stepwedge, of sorts, is utilized. However, in this case, the stepwedge is actually an internal light attenuating device that allows either 11 or 21 different intensities of light to strike the film. The wedge constants are either $\sqrt{2}$ or 2. The primary advantage in using a sensitometer instead of the other two methods is that, when the sensitometer is properly calibrated, the exposures it produces are more reproducible from day to day.

CAUTIONS IN OBTAINING THE TEST STRIPS

When obtaining the test strip exposures with the time scale test, the metal stepwedge or the sensitometer, at least one area of the film needs to remain shielded so that base plus fog level can later be determined. Because the purpose of these tests is to evaluate automatic processors, all other variables need to remain constant. A few of these factors are listed below:

1. A control box of film should be set aside and used solely for testing purposes. Before a new control box is needed, a crossover check must be performed between the old and the new film so that new control values can be established if necessary.

2. Sensitometric measurements need to be made for each sensitive side of the film. In duplitized film, for example, expose one side, turn the film over and expose the other side (make sure that the two exposures do not overlap).
3. One film strip exposure needs to be taken for each processor in the imaging department.
4. Film strips should be processed as soon as possible after exposure, as latent images tend to fade with time. For example, if two processors are to be evaluated, take one exposure, send it through the first processor, take the second exposure and then process it in the second unit.
5. Ensure that each processor has had sufficient time to warm up properly before processing any strips.
6. Ensure that the sensitometer and densitometer are properly calibrated, warmed up and zeroed if necessary.
7. Again, ensure the following factors are held constant (except when using the sensitometry method): kilovoltage, milliampere-seconds (except for time scale test), source-image distance, x-ray machine and cassette.

UTILIZING THE INFORMATION OBTAINED FROM STEPPED TESTS

Because the characteristic curve is an expression of density differences in relation to various exposures, the most logical manner of evaluating automatic processors is to measure the density of each step on the test film strips (recall that each step relates to a known exposure). If all factors used to obtain the test strips were constant and the density of each step remained the same from one day to the next, one could assume the processor to be in good working order. If, however, step 10 had a density of 2.3 one day and 3 the next day, one would be alerted that the processor was adding artificial density and that some adjustment was necessary. Measuring the density of each step, especially in a 21 stepped tool, could be quite time consuming in a department with three or four processors. Because film speed, contrast and fog are the three variables most readily affected by processing conditions, these can be evaluated by simply measuring the density levels of three different steps (see below).

It is possible to analyze density subjectively by simply comparing the densities visually. The preferred way, however, is to actually measure density with a densitometer. This removes the element of human variability and allows for a more objective evaluation. The results can also be more easily recorded.

Measuring Speed

Recall that speed can be dramatically affected by changes in the developing time, temperature or quality of chemical solutions. It is, therefore, the best indicator of processing conditions. Speed can be evaluated quite easily by simply measuring and graphing the density of one particular step each day and comparing it with a control strip. A step revealing density in the lower end of the straight line portion of the characteristic curve should be chosen. A commonly accepted step shows a density value of 1 above gross fog. This step may be referred to as the control step or point.

Variability exists even with the best of conditions. It is not reasonable to expect exact comparisons from day to day. A 15% range of error is, therefore, generally accepted when measuring speed. Figure 21–11 shows how to graph the daily results of film speed (density) measurements. In this example,

step 8 (control point) on the control strip has a density of 1.02. This becomes the center point of the graph. Values within plus or minus 15% of 1.02 are then calculated and identified on the graph.

A value of plus 15% represents the maximum upper limit, whereas a value of minus 15% is the lower limit. In Figure 21–11, the upper limit is 1.17 (or $0.15 \times 1.02 = 0.15$ and $1.02 + 0.15 = 1.17$) and the lower limit is 0.87 (or $1.02 - 0.15 = 0.87$).

Daily density values of step 8 are then plotted. If the density remains within the established limits, processing conditions are considered adequate. However, if the density is outside of these limits, a problem exists (as for day 10 in Figure 21–11). Values below the lower border signal loss of speed, whereas those above indicate gain in speed.

The attentive technologist should notice that in Figure 21–11 an upward trend begins to develop at approximately the sixth or seventh day. By paying close attention to developing trends, it may be possible to take corrective action before encountering serious problems. Some departments monitor their processors at the beginning of each shift rather than just in the morning. This makes it easier to notice trends, as more data points are available for evaluation.

Measuring Contrast

Contrast is measured by subtracting the density value of one step from another. It is common to use the speed point value of density (1 above gross fog) as the lower reading and a density of two steps higher for the upper reading. Again, a margin of error is allowed from one day to another. This is most often plus or minus 10% of the control strip contrast value.

Figure 12–12 shows a typical daily graph of contrast. The control strip, as revealed by day 1, shows a contrast of 1. This is based on the eighth step reading of 1.2 and the tenth step density of 2.2 ($2.2 - 1.2 = 1$). Contrast remains within the allowable limits until day 10, at which point it is reduced to unacceptable limits. If this information were added to the results shown in Figure 12–11, which identified an unacceptable value of speed, the technologist could be quite confident that this is not just random error; there is truly a problem with the processing conditions. It must be remembered that the previous examples assume that all other varia-

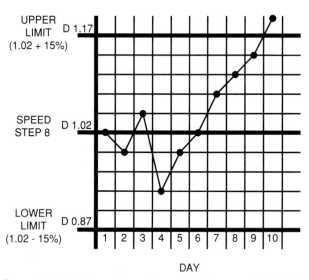

Figure 21–11. Daily speed chart. Acceptable density range of 0.87–1.17 with a control point of 1.02. The density on day 10 is outside the upper boundary.

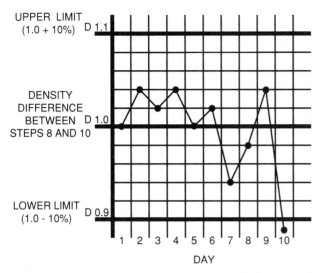

Figure 21–12. Daily contrast chart. Control strip resulted in a control point difference between steps 8 and 10 of 1.0. The daily contrast readings are within normal limits for all days except day 10, which demonstrates an unacceptably low contrast.

bles have remained constant and that the problem must lie in the processor.

Measuring Fog

Film fog is measured in a manner similar to that of speed and contrast. Rather than density being measured on a particular step of the stepwedge, however, it is measured on that area of the film that was shielded during exposure. Any density on that portion of the film receiving no exposure represents gross fog (base plus fog). The daily charting of gross fog is performed in the same manner as speed and contrast charting. The usual range (limits) of fog is 0.12 to 0.2.

Of the three variables mentioned (speed, contrast and fog), fog is the least sensitive indicator of processor conditions. As discussed above, considerable changes must occur in the developing times or temperatures for fog to significantly affect the film quality.

Charts

Film manufacturers provide comprehensive charts for daily quality control of the processor. These incorporate graphs for speed, contrast and fog and provide areas to record information such as the initials of the technologist performing the test, the developing temperature, developer and fixer replenishment rates, and water temperature.

LABORATORY EXPERIENCE

Laboratory 34, Sensitometry, is associated with this chapter. This laboratory is designed to allow the experimenter to determine if the automatic processor is functioning properly. The laboratory is performed over several class sessions. The first session is dedicated to obtaining the standard (control points) for speed, contrast and fog. The remaining sessions are designed to allow the experimenter laboratory experience in performing sensitometry and evaluating a sensitometry strip.

Bibliography

Bushong, S. Radiologic science for technologists (4th edition). St. Louis: Mosby, 1988.

Chesney, DN and Chesney, MO. Radiographic imaging (4th edition). Boston: Blackwell Scientific Publications, 1981.

Curry, T, Dowdey, R and Murry, R. Christensen's Introduction to the physics of diagnostic radiology (3rd edition). Philadelphia: Lee & Febiger, 1984.

Eastman Kodak Company. Sensitometric properties of x-ray films. Rochester, NY: Eastman Kodak Co., 1974.

Eastman Kodak Co. The fundamentals of radiography (12th edition). Rochester, NY: Eastman Kodak Co., 1980.

Fuji Photo Film Co., Ltd. Fundamentals of photography. Tokyo: Fuji Photo Film Co., Ltd., 1978.

Fuji Photo Film Co., Ltd. X-ray sensitometry. Tokyo: Fuji Photo Film Co., Ltd., 1978.

Fuji Photo Film Co., Ltd. Fundamentals of sensitized materials for radiography. Tokyo: Fuji Photo Film Co., Ltd., 1982.

Hendee, W, Chaney, E and Rossi, R. Radiologic physics, equipment and quality control. Chicago: Year Book Medical, 1977.

McKinney, WEJ. Radiographic processing and quality control. Philadelphia: Lippincott, 1988.

Stroebel, L. View camera techniques (5th edition). Boston: Focal Press, 1986.

Williams, J. Image clarity. Boston: Focal Press, 1990.

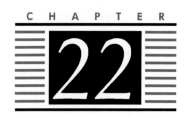

SILVER RECOVERY

BARBARA L. BARKER and JACKLYNN SCOTT DARLING

INTRODUCTION

In the late 1970s the price of silver skyrocketed, substantially increasing the moneys expended by imaging departments on film. Also, the U.S. government began to pass laws prohibiting the disposal of heavy metals, such as silver, into sewers and waterways. Consequently, a need developed to find a way to decrease costs and comply with government regulations. The solution was to implement a system to recover the silver from x-ray films and processor solutions. This decreased expenditures by using the income obtained from the sale of silver to defer department costs. Also, filtering the silver out of the fixer before it entered the sewer system prevented toxic waste from entering the waterways, enabling departments to comply with government laws. This chapter discusses the advantages of silver recovery and compares silver recovery systems.

GOVERNMENT REGULATIONS

Government regulations regarding the polluting of public water supplies are demonstrated in several acts of Congress. Four specific acts apply to imaging departments. They are the Water Control Act (1972), the Resources Conservation–Hazardous Waste Act (1976), the Clear Water Act (1987) and the Resource Conservation and Recovery Act (1976). The Water Control Act prohibited the depositing of toxic substances in public waterways or sewer systems. The Resources Conservation–Hazardous Waste Act required that some type of mechanism

be used to remove toxic wastes before allowing the liquid to flow to the sewer lines. The Clear Water Act mandated that the best equipment available be used to remove the toxic substances. The Resource Conservation and Recovery Act established the amount of silver waste being deposited by fixer solutions to be no more than 5 parts per million (ppm) or 5 mg per L.

Some states and cities have passed laws more stringent than the federal regulations. Consequently, the amount of waste allowed in the water system may vary from one geographical area to another. Thus, it is recommended that technologists check their respective state and local laws to ensure that their disposal of waste is in compliance with the law.

To meet even the most liberal regulations, it is critical that the fixer be desilvered (silver removed from the solution) before it is permitted to escape into the drain. Therefore, to be in compliance with federal and state regulations, some sort of silver recovery system is necessary.

MONETARY RETURN

During the late 1970s and early 1980s, the price of silver increased from $4.50 per troy ounce (1 troy ounce is equal to about 1.09 U.S. ounces) to $50.00 a troy ounce. The high cost of silver served as a strong impetus for facilities to find a way to cut expenses. This resulted in the implementation of silver recovery systems. Since 1980, the price of silver has decreased and, as of the printing of this text, it remains below $10.00 a troy ounce. The lessons of the 1970s made a deep and long-lasting impression on imaging departments. Most institutions recognize the value of silver recovery for monetary gain. Currently, it is estimated that 60–70% of hospitals have some type of silver recovery system.

The source of the silver recovered by imaging departments is the emulsion of the x-ray film. It is estimated that the emulsion from 500 sheets of 14 × 17 inch (35.6 × 43.2 cm) film contain about 10–12 troy ounces of silver. Assuming the price of silver to be $10 per troy ounce, the average value of silver in 500 sheets of 14 × 17 inch film is $110 ($10 per troy ounce × the average troy ounce value of 11 = $110). If each sheet of film costs about $2, the total cost for 500 sheets (one case of film) is $1000. As can be seen from this example, silver represents about 11% of the original cost of the film (110/1000 = 0.11).

Roughly 45% of the silver available for recovery is located in the fixer solution and 50% remains on the discarded films. Assuming that 500 sheets of 14 × 17 film contains an average of 11 troy ounces, the fixer contains 4.9 troy ounces (0.45 × 11 = 4.9) and another 5.5 troy ounces (0.50 × 11 = 5.5) is located in discarded film. The remaining 5% is found in the wash water and is rarely reclaimed.

It is possible to recover as much as 97% of the silver located in the fixer. Thus, 4.75 troy ounces (0.97 × 4.9 = 4.75) can be reclaimed from 500 sheets of 14 × 17 inch film. At $10 per troy ounce, this amounts to $47.50. One hundred percent of the silver in discarded film is recoverable. However, the cost of separating the silver from the film absorbs 70% of the silver value. Thus, the actual profit on recycled film is 30%, or approximately 1.7 troy ounces (0.30 × 5.5 = 1.7) for 500 sheets of 14 × 17 inch film. It can readily be seen that the combined recovery money of $47.50 from the fixer and $17.00 (1.7 troy ounces × $10 per troy ounce = $17) from scrap film is $64.50. This is 58.64% of the original value of the silver ($110) and 6.45% of the original cost of the 500 sheets ($1000). Although 6.45% seems low, an imaging department in an average sized hospital (about 200 beds) can easily expend $200,000 on film annually. A return rate of 6.45% on $200,000 represents $12,900.

The total amount of recoverable silver and its purity varies according to the efficiency of the reclamation methods. Some factors influencing the exact amount of revenue obtained from silver recovery are the cost of recovering the silver from fixer solution, film price, the current market value of silver and other overhead expenses, e.g., refining costs. An imaging department can minimize outgoing expenses by taking the following steps:

1. Ensure that the silver recovery unit is appropriate for the department's workload.
2. Ensure that the recovery unit is operating at its maximum efficiency.
3. Sell discarded film in large quantities.
4. Process green waste film to reclaim the silver via the fixer.
5. Purchase the lowest priced film meeting the department's standards.
6. Watch the market value of silver and sell when the rate is high.

SILVER CONSERVATION

Silver is a natural resource that may soon be depleted. Currently, approximately 60% of the silver used is mined. The remaining silver comes from reclamation efforts. The total amount of silver available depends on the amount of ore in the earth and reclamation. When all the ore has been mined, the natural source for silver will be depleted. Thus, the amount of silver available will be solely dependent on reclamation efforts. It is estimated that if the demand for silver continues to increase at its current rate and if the world continues to mine ore while reclaiming only a small percentage, then silver ore will be depleted within the first decade of the twenty-first century.

A problem contributing to the depletion of silver is that mining, refinement and reclamation costs have increased while the value of silver has decreased. Thus, it is less profitable to mine silver now than in the past. This trend seems to be positive because more ore remains in the earth. However, because silver's price is low, people do not seem to appreciate its value and tend to disregard protecting it. As the price of silver decreases and refining costs increase, there is a corresponding decrease in the revenue earned from recovered silver. Thus, there is less incentive for departments to continue the reclamation process. The end result is a continuing increase in silver use and a decline in its availability by either reclamation or mining.

Industries that produce x-ray and photographic film have found no other element that can match the light sensitive properties of silver. Because of these unique properties of photosensitivity as well as a decline in the amounts of silver mined and reclaimed, it is critical to conserve as much of this natural resource as possible.

SOURCES CONTAINING SILVER

PROCESSOR SOLUTIONS

A prime source from which to recover silver is processor solutions. The processor solutions containing silver are the wash water and the fixer. Most departments find that an effective squeegee rack removes enough fixer to limit the quantity of silver deposited in the wash water. Consequently, the silver in the wash water is so small (approximately 3–5%) that the recovery of this silver is not economically practical. The exception is manual processing. In this case, the amount of silver in the wash water increases (usually 12–15%), making the recovery of silver more significant. The more profitable processor solution silver source is the fixer.

Silver is recovered from the fixer by attaching a silver recovery unit to the line draining the fixer. Locating the silver recovery system before the drain provides a means to collect the silver before it enters the sewer system. The amounts of silver collected and the purity of the silver depend on the following factors:

The method used to recover the silver. Some methods are more efficient in their recovery of silver.

The type of examination, the subject being radiographed and the size of film necessary for the procedure. These factors determine the amount of unexposed or partially exposed silver halide crystals on the film, which are removed by the fixer.

The kind of film utilized. Double emulsion film leaves more undeveloped silver halide crystals in the fixer solution than does single emulsion film.

Efficiency of the squeegee action of the transport system to remove fixer before the film enters the wash tank. The more efficient the action is, the less silver is lost to the wash water.

DISCARDED FILM

Besides collecting silver from the fixer, another method of reclaiming silver is refining discarded films. Discarded films consist of archival films (patient radiographs that may be disposed of legally) and waste film. The amount of money obtained from the discarded film depends on the weight of the film. The price quoted to a department by a dealer for scrap film is based on how much expense the dealer expects to incur from shipping costs, assay costs and refining costs and how much profit the dealer expects to make relative to the current market price of silver. Because it is more economical for a dealer to refine 100 pounds of film than 20 pounds, the more likely a dealer is to quote the department a higher rate for a greater weight of scrap film. Consequently, it is most economical to sell discarded film when a substantial amount of film is collected.

The value of waste film varies according to the amount of silver in the film. The most valuable waste film is green film. This film contains the largest volume of silver. The second most valuable films are the pre-1974 archival films. These films were manufactured before the large increase in silver prices and contain 20% more silver than film manufactured after 1974. The least valuable films are post-1974 archival films and current reject films. Because of the differences in silver quantities, the rate paid for discarded films reflects their respective silver content. Thus, discarded films should be separated and sold relative to their silver content.

METHODS OF FIXER SILVER RECOVERY

METALLIC CARTRIDGE

Design

Metallic replacement cartridges operate on the principle of ion exchange. A typical cartridge is a sealed plastic bucket and contains an inlet line (tube), an outlet line (tube), a plastic spacer, a bypass and a base metal filter (Figure 22–1). The inlet tubing serves as a means of transporting the fixer to the cartridge. Desilvered solution exits the cartridge via the outlet line. The bypass tube is used

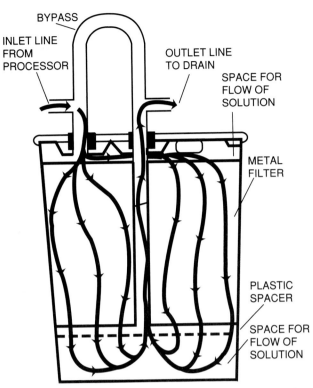

Figure 22–1. Flow of fixer solution through metallic replacement cartridge. (© Eastman Kodak Company. Reprinted courtesy of Eastman Kodak Company.)

to provide a passage for solution (overflow) in case the interior part of the cartridge becomes obstructed. A base metal filter is located inside the plastic bucket and is where the chemical reaction for silver recovery occurs. The plastic spacer is used to support the base metal. Most cartridges are sealed at the factory (Figure 22–2) and must be replaced when exhausted.

Function

Recall that metallic replacement operates on the principle of ion exchange. The exchange of ions takes place in a solution between the base metal and silver. Base metals may be steel wool, copper, iron, zinc or aluminum. The most commonly used base metal is steel wool. Although copper is more efficient, the units are more expensive, thus fewer departments use them. Iron impregnated foam has a larger surface area (increases silver recovery) and a longer life span than other materials. Regardless of the type of metal employed, it is available in one of three forms: cut-up screen, wound screen and fiber. They may also be coarse or fine.

Ion exchange occurs when silver-laden fixer flows through the inlet, comes in contact with the base metal (where it is desilvered) and then exits through the outlet. The ions of the base metal react with the acid in the fixer, emitting electrons (negative charge) used by the silver (positive charge) to form metallic silver. The metallic silver attaches itself to the base metal or settles to the bottom of the cartridge as silver sludge.

Efficiency

Metallic replacement cartridges can be used alone or as a back-up unit for another recovery system. Attaching a cartridge as a back-up to another cartridge or an electrolytic unit is called tailing (Figure 22–3). A tailing unit serves as a back-up unit, increasing the efficiency of silver removal. It also serves as a safety precaution in case the first unit permits an unacceptable amount of silver to flow through the outlet line. The amount of silver gathered by a tailing unit is usually too small to be economically beneficial to the department. However, it is often needed to meet stringent government regulations.

Six variables affecting the efficiency of metallic replacement are as follows:

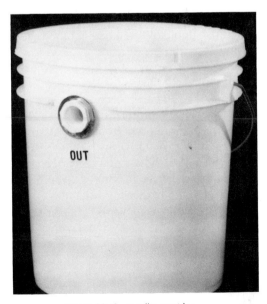

Figure 22–2. Metallic cartridge.

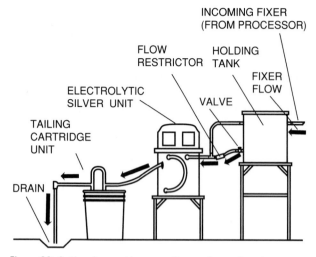

Figure 22–3. Use of a cartridge as a tailing unit for an electrolytic system. (From IMG Photo Products.)

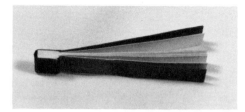

Figure 22–4. Silver estimating papers.

1. Rate of fixer flow
2. Length of time used
3. Proper monitoring
4. Amount of time the fixer is in the cartridge
5. Cartridge size
6. Base metal content.

The maximum amount of silver is recovered when there is a continuous flow of fixer. Consequently, care needs to be taken to avoid attaching a cartridge to a low volume or infrequently used processor.

A cartridge is most efficient when it is initially installed. With proper fixer flow, a newly installed cartridge can recover 100% of the silver. However, continued use depletes (or exhausts) the base metal, decreasing the amount of silver recovered. This is accompanied by an increase in the amount of silver leaving via the outlet line.

Assessing the efficiency level of a cartridge is achieved by proper monitoring practices. The silver content can be monitored by inserting silver estimating paper (Figure 22–4) in the fixer exiting the outlet line of the cartridge. The cartridge should be replaced when the fixer leaving via the outlet line contains 40–100 mg of silver per L.

Proper ion exchange requires time for the atoms to interact. Thus, the fixer must remain in the cartridge long enough for ion exchange to occur. This time is often referred to as dwell, or residency, time. The optimum residency time varies with fixer concentration, the cartridge size and the type of base metal.

Cartridges are available in a variety of sizes (Figure 22–5). The cartridge capacity should match the workload of the department and the pH of the fixer. There is no absolute method of determining proper capacity. However, commercial companies are helpful in assessing an imaging department's needs relative to cartridge size. In general, the greater the workload, the larger the cartridge required.

Previous discussion indicated that the type of base metal used, e.g., copper, affects the amount of silver removed. The type of metal should be matched with the manner in which the metal is constructed, e.g., coarse or fine. Silver is removed most efficiently in fixers with a high pH value by using a coarse base metal. Low pH fixers function best with a fine filter base metal. The acceptable pH fixer range is 4 to 6.5, with an optimum pH of 5.5.

Problems

Three problems can occur with metallic cartridges. They are channeling, rusting and precipitation.

Channeling occurs when small volumes of fixer enter the cartridge. The fixer drops onto the base

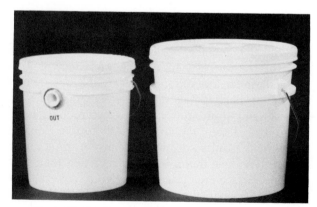

Figure 22–5. Different sizes of chemical recovery cartridges.

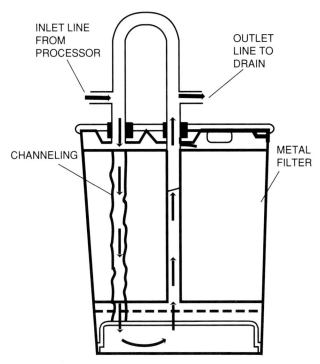

Figure 22—6. Channeling in a metallic replacement cartridge. (From IMG Photo Products.)

metal, causing the metal to erode in a path through the base metal (Figure 22–6). Future solution entering the unit follows the erosion path. Consequently, there is no ion exchange and little silver recovered.

Rusting is common with infrequently used cartridges. Because the cartridge is designed for a continuous fixer flow, fixer that remains static in the cartridge rusts (oxidizes) the base metal.

Precipitation occurs when there is a gradual build-up of precipitates or gelatin material. These materials may plug up the unit, preventing the normal flow of fixer. Rather than circulating through the cartridge, the silver-laden fixer flows through the bypass tube. Another type of precipitate is formed when exiting fixer combines with exiting developer. This results in iron hydroxide precipitation, which may plug the drain. The drain may be cleared by using an acid-type drain cleaner.

ELECTROLYTIC METHOD

Function

An electrolytic unit operates on the principle of electrolysis. A typical electrolytic unit consists of a desilvering tank, anode, cathode, transformer, motor and rectifier (Figure 22–7). Electrolysis is the chemical change produced in a solution with the application of a direct electrical current. An electrolytic silver recovery system removes silver from the fixer by sending a small electrical direct current between two electrodes (a cathode and an anode) suspended in a solution or an electrolyte. This produces a negative charge at the cathode and a positive charge at the anode. The positively charged silver ions located in the solution migrate toward the negatively charged cathode. After reaching the cathode, the silver ions plate the cathode. The cathode is removed from the unit periodically. This permits the silver to be stripped off and sold.

Efficiency

Good cathode plating depends on the type of cathode, agitation and amperage. Cathodes are available in a variety of designs. These include flat plate, multiple flat plates and circular discs. As long as the electrolytic unit is properly managed, no one cathode design has an advantage over another relative to the amount or level of purity of the silver recovered.

Although all cathodes are equally efficient, the type of agitation employed is important in silver recovery efficiency. The better the interface between the cathode and the silver-rich fixer solution, the more efficient the silver plating. There are three

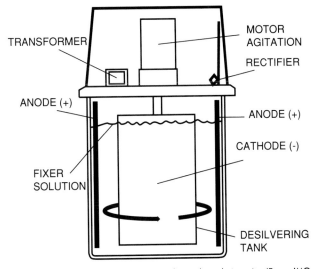

Figure 22—7. Common components of an electrolytic unit. (From IMG Photo Products.)

methods of agitation: a rotating cathode, a rotating anode and an external pump. The most efficient method of agitation is the rotating cathode. Recall that silver plates on the cathode. As more and more silver attaches to the cathode, the cathode's weight increases. Thus, if a rotating cathode is used, care must be taken to avoid increasing the weight of the cathode to a point at which it adversely affects the bearings of the motor or normal operation of the motor. A rotating anode eliminates the problem of weight at the cathode and possible motor damage. However, it is not as efficient as a rotating cathode. The advantage of the pump agitation method is that there is no need to attach a motor to the electrodes. However, there is a need for a high capacity pump and a motor to run it.

Besides the type of agitation, the correct amperage settings are important to obtain optimum silver recovery with an electrolytic unit. Correct settings maximize the amount of silver recovered. For example, high amperage settings create more negative charges, attracting more positively charged silver to the cathode for plating. If silver is recovered at too high a rate, the silver is depleted from the solution too quickly, decreasing the efficiency of the unit. As a result, the thiosulfate in the fixer breaks down to produce sulfide ions and silver sulfide. If a significant amount of sulfurization occurs, there is a deposit of yellow-brown sulfur in the unit. This deposit is often accompanied by a rotten egg–type odor.

Another cause of sulfur is a reduction in the concentration of silver in the fixer. The reduction in the percentage of concentration may be caused by a change in workload. For example, it is common for the number of procedures performed in the morning to be higher than that in the afternoon. This is attributed to the high number of patients being evaluated by fluoroscopy. Consequently, the concentration of silver in the fixer is high in the morning because of the large quantity of films processed. Later in the workday as the workload decreases, the fixer's concentration of silver diminishes. Fluctuation in the silver concentration requires corresponding amperage adjustments in electrolytic units.

It is impractical to have a technologist continually available to adjust the amperage of an electrolytic unit. Many units have the ability to attach an automatic timer to the unit's electrical cord. The timer is set to turn on the unit during high volume periods and shut off the unit when the workload is low. Another, more advanced apparatus involves a mechanism built into the processor that detects when a film enters the processor. The entering film activates the mechanism, which turns on the recovery unit. Consequently, the silver recovery unit functions only when films are being processed. The most sophisticated apparatus uses a sensor probe located in the fixer that measures the amount of silver concentration. The probe automatically controls the amount of amperage to correspond to the concentration of the silver.

Setup

Electrolytic units may be attached to the processor as a terminal setup or as a recirculating system (Figure 22–8). In the terminal system, the fixer flows from the processor through the silver recovery unit, where it is desilvered, and exits to the drain. In the recirculating system, the fixer flows through the unit, is desilvered and is recirculated back to the processor for use. Thus, a higher percentage of silver can be recovered (99%) and the fixer can be reused. However, many manufacturers do not recommend this method because of the possible problems. A risk of this method is that the preservative in the fixer (sodium sulfite) can be destroyed in the

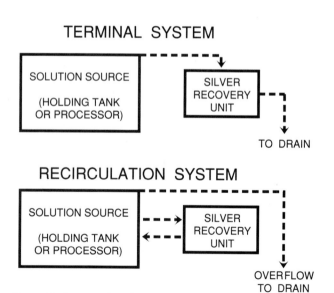

Figure 22–8. Terminal and recirculation fixer flow. (© Eastman Kodak Company. Reprinted courtesy of Eastman Kodak Company.)

electrolysis process, thereby causing improper fixing of the films. Installing a recirculating unit to save money on fixer solution is usually discouraged because the fixer is one of the least expensive solutions to purchase.

CENTRALIZED FIXER SILVER RECOVERY SYSTEM DESIGN

A centralized silver recovery system is designed so that several processors are attached to one recovery unit. This type of system is particularly advantageous in departments with large workload fluctuations or low volume workloads. The centralized system often employs a holding tank.

The holding tank functions by having the fixer solution enter the tank by being either poured in or pumped directly from the processor (batching). When the tank is full, the fixer is pumped at a constant rate into the silver recovery unit (Figure 22–9). The silver recovery unit may be terminal or recirculating. Recirculating units provide a means of ensuring that the maximum amount of silver is recovered. In a recirculating unit, the solution is recirculated through the recovery unit but not the processor. Consequently, the concerns regarding possible changes in fixer chemistry do not apply in this type of system.

DECENTRALIZED FIXER SILVER RECOVERY SYSTEM DESIGN

A decentralized design has a recovery unit attached to each processor. Many institutions prefer this design. These recovery units do not have a holding tank. The silver recovery unit may be terminal or recirculating. Two disadvantages of a decentralized design are the increased equipment costs and the decreased space available in the processing area.

ASSESSING SILVER CONTENT

SILVER ESTIMATING PAPER

Recall that the efficiency of a silver recovery unit can be evaluated by silver estimating papers. These test papers are the most economical method for an imaging department to assess the efficiency of the unit. Several commercial types of silver estimating papers are available. Instructions on their use may vary with different companies. It is important to follow the manufacturer's instructions carefully. For example, instructions often require the reading of the test papers under an incandescent light rather than with fluorescent lighting. Any variation from the instructions increases the probability of invalid test results.

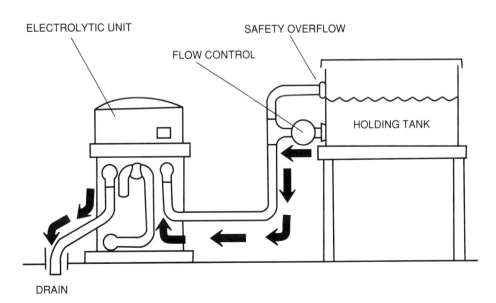

Figure 22–9. Batching system. (From IMG Photo Products.)

A common trait to all types of paper is that the paper undergoes a color change when it is submerged in the fixer. The color is matched to a color chart supplied by the company. The chart is used to estimate the silver concentration. The validity of the test results increases in the middle ranges of silver concentration. If there are high or low concentrations of silver, the accuracy diminishes.

METAL REPLACEMENT

Another method used to determine the presence of silver is the metal replacement or copper method. This method identifies the presence of silver but not the quantity. The copper or metal replacement method uses a copper penny or wire instead of test papers. Silver chemically plates a clean copper surface, providing a quick, inexpensive method to determine the presence of silver. To use this method, a clean copper wire or penny is dipped into the fixer solution for approximately 5 seconds, removed and examined. A silver or grayish cast on the copper indicates the presence of silver. This type of testing is subjective because it is difficult to clarify the amount of silver in the fixer by the amount of gray shading on the copper. Therefore, test papers are a far better method for assessing the quantity of silver in the fixer solution.

LABORATORY METHODS

Other methods utilized to evaluate efficiency of units are titration and atomic absorption. However, these methods are expensive and require an outside laboratory with highly skilled personnel.

TROUBLESHOOTING

There are many reasons for a unit to stop working or not to collect silver to its maximum potential. Before retaining a service person, it is best to check potential problem areas that can be corrected by someone with minimum knowledge of the unit, e.g., a technologist. Such assessments often correct the problem, saving the department money that would have otherwise been spent on service personnel, travel costs and professional fees. Numer-

ous problems can occur with silver recovery units. Table 22–1 presents some common problems and possible causes. Referencing all possible problems is beyond the scope of this text.

The best way to limit problems is to prevent them from happening. Thus, it is critical to follow the manufacturer's maintenance schedule for silver recovery units. Because a cartridge requires no electricity and has no moving parts, it is almost maintenance free. However, electrolytic units require routine maintenance. Most manufacturers recommend a daily and yearly maintenance program for electrolytic systems.

Daily maintenance includes cleaning the outside of the unit, checking for leaks, ensuring a free flow of fixer, verifying that the amperage setting is correct and observing all tube and electrical cords for

Table 22–1. TROUBLESHOOTING SILVER RECOVERY UNITS

Problem	Possible Cause
Fixer not flowing	Cartridge is higher than fixer in processor, prohibiting flow to inlet line
	Cartridge too low relative to drain, prohibiting flow of fixer to outlet line
	Clogged drain or line
Restricted fixer flow	Tubing too long, too small, kinked or bent
	Inlet and outlet line connections on unit reversed
Not collecting silver	Capacity and rate of unit do not match processor use
Amperage fluctuation	Loose cathode
	Loose connection in wiring
No amperage reading	Meter stuck
	Loose cathode
	Loose wire
	Failed diode
	Failed transformer
Blown fuse	Improper fuse size
	Loose fuse connection
	Failed transformer
	Failed diode
Cathode does not rotate	Loose connection
	Blown fuse
	Defective motor
	Jammed fan blade
	No power source
Silver falling	Cathode may be contaminated with grease or oil
Sulfuric odor (rotten egg smell)	Recovery is taking place at too high rate or cathode is not rotating

proper connections. Most of these tasks are performed several times a day. For example, manually operated amperage is adjusted as the workload changes.

Yearly checks usually include lubricating the unit; checking the bearings, motor and wiring; and cleaning the inside of the unit. It is important to check these items, even though the motor is sealed and away from the fixer tank, because the fumes from the fixer can cause corrosive deposits.

Units should be monitored on a regular basis by a trained individual. There is no substitute for experience, careful observation and a preventive maintenance plan to increase the efficiency of the unit and prolong its life.

SELLING SILVER

Several methods are used by dealers to buy silver. A wise administrator will investigate all potential dealers and select the best offer. Silver recovery from the fixer is performed by using either a cartridge or an electrolytic unit.

CARTRIDGE

Cartridge units are sealed and the silver content is unknown until it is refined. Consequently, payment usually occurs after refinement. Because the cartridge must be replaced, the dealer often deducts the shipping charges, refining costs and personal fees from the sale. After a department patronizes the same dealer for a significant time, it is possible to determine the average silver return. Thus, the dealer may agree to pay the imaging department when the cartridge is recovered rather than wait for the refinement. The payment is based on previous silver yields. This system may be adjusted if there is any substantial change in silver costs or the amount of silver recovered.

ELECTROLYTIC

A properly operating electrolytic unit can recover silver that is 97% pure. Thus, it is possible to be paid by the dealer at the time the silver is collected.

The dealer usually offers a price of 90–95% of the market value of silver.

There are two sources commonly used to determine the value of silver. One is the various stock market listings, such as Comex, Handy and Harmon, and Engelhard, and the other is the value cited in the Wall Street Journal. The stock market value of silver varies during the day. However, the price cited in the Wall Street Journal is constant for a given day. Most dealers use the market value quoted by the Wall Street Journal. It is advisable that the administrator ask the dealer which market is being used for silver quotes.

Dealers use three methods to buy silver. They are the percentage of the market price of silver, the percentage of a percent and the times market price. The simplest to understand is the percentage of market value. In this method, the dealer offers to pay the department a percentage of the market value of silver. For example, if a dealer offers to buy 10 troy ounces of silver for 90% of the market value and the market value is $6.25, the department receives $56.25 ($0.90 \times 6.25 \times 10 = 56.25$).

The percentage of a percent method is a little more confusing than the straight percentage method. In this method, a dealer estimates the purity of the silver and determines the price per troy ounce by multiplying the silver purity by the market value. For example, if the silver is 90% pure and the silver value is $6.25, the price is approximately $5.63 per troy ounce ($0.90 \times 6.25 = 5.63$). Next, the dealer deducts the costs for refinement, shipping (if applicable) and profit. If this amounts to another 5%, the offer to the department is 85% ($90 - 5 = 85$) of the $5.63, or $4.79 per troy ounce. If the department's silver is between 85 and 90% pure, this type of price quote is acceptable. However, if the purity of the silver is 95%, there is a significant loss of income and the department should elect to use another method of payment.

The last method of payment is a times market price for 1 pound of silver. In this method, if the market value of silver is $6.25 and the dealer offers to pay 10 times the market value, this amounts to $62.50 per pound. However, there are 14.583 troy ounces in 1 U.S. pound. Consequently, the real price of 1 U.S. pound of silver is $91.14 ($14.583 \times 6.25 = 91.14$). Thus, the department is getting about 68.6% of the market value ($62.50/91.14 = 0.686$).

SECURITY

Obtaining reclaimed silver can add thousands of dollars to a department's budget. Because of the potentially large monetary return, a security system to protect the silver should be implemented. This is often achieved by appointing a reliable person to be responsible for silver security.

One source needing security is the discarded film. Discarded films should be stored in a lockable well-ventilated area. Most departments have a box located in the processing area to collect reject films. All reject films collected during the day should be removed from the processing area and placed with the other secured discarded films.

To prevent the unnecessary waste of good green film, the security person should make sure that storage conditions for good green film meet the manufacturer's recommendations and that the film stock is rotated correctly (the oldest film is used first). Even though green film has the highest silver content among the various types of discarded film, the economical gain is only about 1% of the original silver value. Thus, there should be minimum green film discarded for silver recovery.

The other area needing security is the silver recovery unit. A centralized design has the advantage of providing an environment conducive to security. In a centralized design, the holding tank can be located in its own room. The room can be locked for security reasons. Recall that a decentralized design has one silver recovery unit per processor. This type of system makes it difficult to lock up the recovery unit. However, it is possible to put locks on the unit. A double key lock is effective as a security measure, because two keys are needed to open the lock (similar to a safety deposit box security system). The silver reclaiming agency has one key, and the imaging department has the other key. Thus, both parties must be present when opening the lock. Another security system is a lock with a numbered seal. Because opening the lock requires the seal to be broken, visual inspection of the condition of the seal is useful in determining if anyone has entered the unit.

LABORATORY EXPERIENCE

Laboratory 35, Silver Recovery, supports the silver recovery concept. This experiment is simple and requires little time to perform. The objective is to provide the researcher with the opportunity to investigate the method of fixer silver recovery employed by his/her department. The experimenter also determines the method of discarded film storage. In both the fixer and the discarded film silver recovery systems, the experimenter is asked to assess and evaluate the type of security system used to protect the silver. Lastly, the question section of the laboratory requires the researcher to perform mathematical calculations to determine an estimated silver recovery income.

Bibliography

Adams, J. Personal research entitled "Overview of silver recovery." Danville, KY.

Chesney, DN and Chesney, MD. Radiographic imaging (3rd edition). Boston: Blackwell Scientific Publications, 1981.

Eastman Kodak Company. Recovering silver from photographic materials. (Standard book number 0-87985-227-5.) New York: Eastman Kodak Company, 1979.

IMG Photo Products. How to manage your silver recovery system to meet silver discharge regulations. CPAC, Inc., Leicester, NY, 1988.

McKinney, WE. Radiographic processing and quality control. Philadelphia: Lippincott, 1988.

McLemore, J. Quality assurance in diagnostic radiology. Chicago: Year Book Medical, 1981.

Thompson, TT. Cahoon's Formulating x-ray techniques (9th edition). Durham, NC: Duke University Press, 1979.

X-Rite Co. Electrolyte silver recovery. Grandville, MI: X-Rite Co. (P/N 301-10 Rev. C-8745.)

FACTORS AFFECTING

FILM QUALITY

Numerous factors influence the quality of a radiograph. Generally speaking, these factors may be divided into photographic factors (density and contrast) and geometric factors (distortion and magnification). Radiographers have attempted to develop a system or form that enables the technologist to look at a radiograph and determine the factor responsible for the inferiority of the film. These systems have some success, but using the specific primary factor to correct the film is not always the best choice. For example, if a film is too light, the assessment form suggests that the operator should increase the milliampere-seconds (mAs). However, although mAs is the primary factor controlling density, in practice it is not unusual to have to adjust the kilovolts peak (kVp). Increasing the kVp to obtain a darker radiograph is especially important when exposure time must be minimal, e.g., when the patient has trouble holding his/her breath. In these cases, it is better to alter density by adjusting the kVp rather than the mAs.

I believe it is important to determine the specific technical changes needed to correct a poor quality film by correlating the radiographic image with the clinical environment. There are too many variables from one patient to the next to allow the radiographer to look at a radiograph and determine the factor to adjust without giving any consideration to the patient factors. Consequently, this section is designed to provide the learner with a solid understanding of the factors affecting the photographic and geometric quality of an image. This knowledge must be applied to the clinical environment and correlated with the patient's condition, the type of procedure, and so forth, when determining the best factor(s) to change in order to improve the quality of inferior radiographs.

Unlike other texts this includes information on quality control (QC), and specific chapters that discuss QC or chapters in which learning is reinforced by practical laboratory experience contain cross-references to laboratory experiments in the laboratory manual, *Concepts in Medical Radiographic Imaging*.

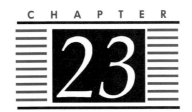

C H A P T E R

23

FILM HOLDERS AND INTENSIFYING SCREENS

INTRODUCTION

Most conventional radiographic machines use film to record images permanently. There are many types of film on the market (Chapter 20, Film, Film Processing and Photographic Techniques, provides an in-depth discussion about film). Regardless of the type of film employed, after a film box is opened, the film must be protected from light. Special equipment is used to protect film during transportation and development. Film transported from room to room for imaging is protected by placing it in a light-tight holder. Film used to replace exposed films (used to reload film holders) is stored in a light-tight bin located in the developing section of the processing area.

Images are recorded by exposing the film to radiation, blue-violet light or green light. Consequently, films are manufactured to be radiation or light sensitive. As the name indicates, radiation sensitive film produces an image by being exposed directly to radiation. An image created on light sensitive film is achieved by exposing the film to light emitted from an intensifying screen located in the film holder.

This chapter explains the types and uses of film

holders, with an in-depth discussion of intensifying screens. Specific information regarding film or film processing is found in Chapter 20.

FILM HOLDERS

Film holders are generally identified relative to the method of film exposure. Holders used to expose film primarily by radiation are termed direct exposure. Those using light as a means of film exposure are termed indirect film holders or cassettes.

DIRECT FILM HOLDERS

Direct film holders may be reusable or disposable. Reusable direct film holders are made of cardboard or plastic (Figure 23–1). These holders protect the film from light by wrapping the film in paper. There is a thin lead foil on the back of the paper to absorb scattered radiation (backscatter). Consequently, it is important to have the unleaded side (this side is labeled tube side) facing the x-ray tube. It is also important to wrap the film properly in the paper or

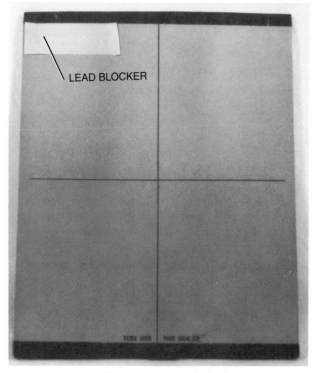

Figure 23–1. Direct film holder.

4. Short life span because reusable holders are not made of durable material
5. Limited to use with parts measuring 13 cm or less.

CASSETTES

Many types of cassettes are commercially available. Some of the more common types include curved, phototimer, grid, rapid film changer, multisectional, vacuum and conventional rectangular flat cassettes. Curved cassettes are arched or bent and are used to obtain an image of a curved anatomical part. Phototimer cassettes are used with automatic timing devices. They are characterized by having no lead in the back lid of the cassette. Grid cassettes have a grid constructed on the front cover and are used in place of a moving grid (see Chapter 24, Grids and Quality Control). Rapid film changer cassettes are used for serial filming, e.g., angiographic procedures. Multisectional cassettes are employed in tomography (see Chapter 14, Conven-

the image will be recorded incorrectly (Figures 23–2 and 23–3). The direct film holder usually contains a lead blocker in the corner to protect the film from radiation (see Figure 23–1). After the examination, this area is exposed with the patient information, e.g., name.

Disposable direct film holders are manufactured with film already wrapped in paper. Like the reusable film holders, the disposable holder contains a lead foil. Thus, care needs to be taken to face the correct side of the holder toward the x-ray tube.

The advantage of direct film holders is the high degree of image sharpness. The amount of sharpness varies with the resolution of the film. High resolution film produces the sharpest image. Sharp images are important in some radiographic procedures, such as mammography.

Direct film holders have several disadvantages.
1. Increased exposure to the patient.
2. Decreased image sharpness owing to long exposure times or involuntary organ movement
3. Decreased life span of the x-ray tube because of the need to use higher kilovoltage and milliampere-seconds than those used in cassettes.

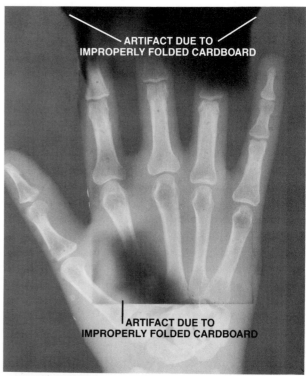

Figure 23–2. Radiograph of a phantom's hand taken on an improperly folded direct film holder.

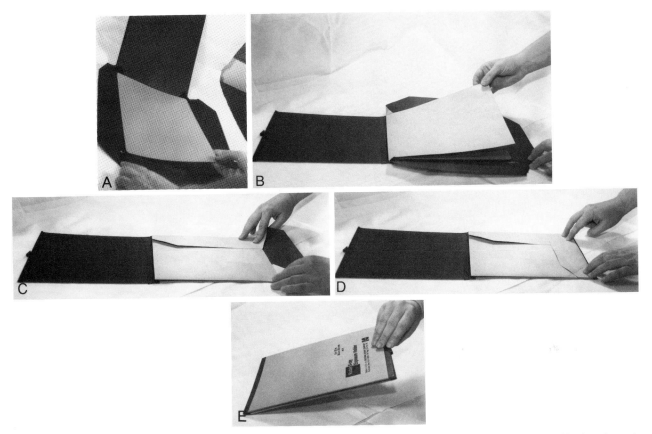

Figure 23–3. Proper film loading of a reusable direct film holder requires the film to be placed in the holder *(A)*. The film is wrapped by first placing the large paper flap on top of the film *(B)*. The side flaps are folded over the film *(C)*, and the bottom flap is positioned over the side flaps *(D)*. The film loading is completed by closing and locking the holder *(E)*.

tional Tomography and Quality Control). Vacuum cassettes are generally used with rapid film changers and angiographic procedures. They are also used in some mammography work. The conventional rectangular cassette is most commonly used and is discussed in detail.

Conventional flat cassettes are rectangular and are available in a variety of sizes. The following are desirable characteristics of a cassette:

1. Lightweight
2. Sturdy and durable
3. Easy to open and close
4. Capable of protecting film from light
5. Able to provide good film-screen contact when closed.

A cassette consists of two rigid plates, or covers (referred to as the front and back), which are attached at one end by a hinge. Some form of spring device is used to lock the cassette. Affixed to the inside of both covers is a backing material (felt, plastic foam or rubber). The backing material and spring are used as compression devices to maintain good screen-film contact when the cassette is closed. They are also helpful in preventing room light from entering the cassette.

Mounted on the backing material are intensifying screens (Figure 23–4). The intensifying screens are purchased separately from the cassette. The purpose of the intensifying screen is to expose the film with light emitted from the screen on irradiation (see under Intensifying Screens below).

The front plate, or cover, is identified as the front because it faces the x-ray tube. The front cover is designed to allow the radiation to pass through it without absorbing or altering the x-ray beam. Characteristics of the front cover material include

1. Thinness
2. Durability and sturdiness

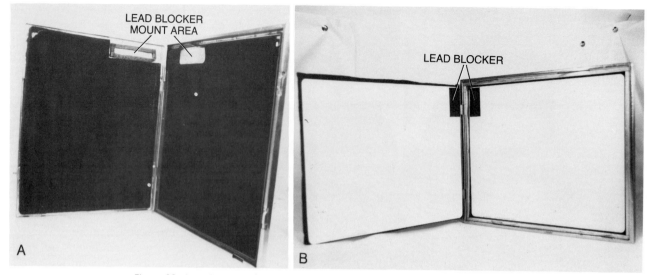

Figure 23—4. *A, Cassette without intensifying screens mounted. B, Cassette with intensifying screens.*

3. Inability to attenuate the x-ray beam
4. Low atomic number
5. Radiolucency.

Because cassettes are reused and the patient may rest on them, e.g., portable chest x-ray, they must be made of material that is durable and sturdy. Commonly used materials for front covers are Bakelite, cardboard, plastic and carbon fiber. Of these materials, carbon fiber is the best but is expensive. Some cassettes have a vinyl front cover. Vinyl is easy to keep clean and it feels warm to the touch. This is helpful when a cassette comes in contact with the patient.

The back cover is heavier than the front because it contains material to absorb scattered radiation (backscatter). Commonly used materials for back covers include aluminum, stainless steel and plastic. These materials may have a thin layer of lead to help absorb scattered radiation.

Although cassettes are durable and last for years, their life span may be increased with proper care. The most common problem is leakage of light into the cassette, exposing the film. Light leaks are often a result of loose hinges, warped cassette, torn backing material or loose springs. Consequently, to help prevent damage, it is important to handle cassettes gently. Another precaution is to inspect cassettes regularly for loose hinges, torn backing material, damaged intensifying screens or loose springs.

Cassette problems are often discovered when an artifact appears on a radiograph. If an artifact appears on a radiograph, it is necessary to identify the cassette used during film exposure. Cassette identification is made simple by placing an identification number in the corner or edge of the intensifying screen (the number is imaged on the radiograph during exposure). The same identification number is marked somewhere on the outside of the cassette. Thus, to determine the cassette used, match the number on the radiograph with the number on the outside of the cassette.

INTENSIFYING SCREENS

Producing an image using direct film holders requires a significant amount of radiation. Consequently, parts radiographed with this method are limited to those measuring 13 cm (about 5 inches) or less (about the size of an average knee). The length of exposure required to produce an image of thick parts using direct film holders is substantial. Intensifying screens significantly decrease the amount of radiation needed to produce a radiographic image, providing the opportunity to produce images of large organs. This is achieved when the intensifying screen fluoresces during irradiation, exposing the film with light rather than radiation. Before an explanation of the importance of film exposure by light, a discussion of intensifying screen construction is in order.

CONSTRUCTION

There are four layers to intensifying screens (Figure 23–5). They are (from the front of the screen to the back)
1. Protective layer
2. Phosphor, or active, layer
3. Undercoating, or reflective, layer
4. Base, or support.

The thickness of each layer is microscopic. The size of the layers varies with the manufacturer and the intensifying screen speed (see Intensifying Screen Speed section). The protective layer is the smallest and ranges from 0.5 mil (0.0127 mm) to 1 mil (0.025 mm). The second thickest layer is the phosphor layer ranging from 3 mils (0.076 mm) for slow speed screens to about 6 mils (0.152 mm) for high speed screens. The undercoating layer is approximately 1 mil (0.025 mm) thick. The thickest layer is the base, which ranges from 7 mils (0.178 mm) to 10 mils (0.254 mm).

The outermost layer of an intensifying screen is the protective layer. This layer is closest to the film and is made of plastic. It protects the phosphor from abrasion or damage, prevents static and provides a surface that can be cleaned without damage to the phosphor.

Located below the protective layer is the phosphor, or active, layer. This section contains crystals incorporated in a plastic suspension. The purpose of the crystals is to convert x-ray energy to light (crystals are explained in more depth under Phosphor). Characteristics of a good crystal include its ability to respond well to x-rays, to glow a color light to which film is sensitive (spectrum matching), to maintain stability when irradiated and to be manufactured with uniform consistency.

The third layer, an undercoating or reflective layer, is designed to direct the light emitted by the phosphor. When the crystals are irradiated, they emit light in all directions, including away from the film. The undercoating either reflects the light back toward the film or absorbs the light. Whether the undercoating reflects or absorbs is determined during its manufacture. Because this layer may be designed to reflect or absorb, undercoating is a more descriptive term than reflective layer.

The base serves as a support. It is made of cardboard or, more recently, plastic. The material used for its composition must have several characteristics. It is unable to react to the phosphor, is radiolucent, does not discolor with age or use, is flexible, does not curl and is moisture resistant.

The sides of all the intensifying screen layers are surrounded by an edge seal. The seal helps protect the screen from moisture or dust particles.

LUMINESCENCE

The process by which a material emits light when stimulated occurs with the conversion of energy. This process is called luminescence. The type of energy used as a stimulus varies. Some examples are electrical current, light and radiation. In radiography, the stimulus used for the emission of light by an intensifying screen is radiation.

The scientific explanation of luminescence is beyond the scope of this text. However, a simplified summary of the process is helpful in understanding other properties associated with intensifying screens. The basic process of luminescence occurs

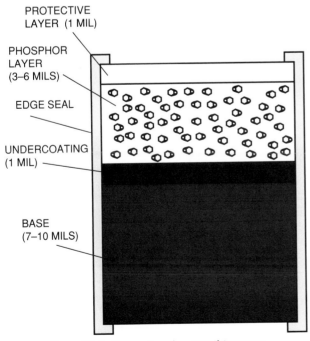

PROTECTIVE LAYER (1 MIL)

PHOSPHOR LAYER (3–6 MILS)

EDGE SEAL

UNDERCOATING (1 MIL)

BASE (7–10 MILS)

Figure 23–5. Cross section of an intensifying screen.

when a material (called phosphor) is stimulated by some form of energy. If the energy is high enough, the atom of the phosphor becomes excited and an electron is removed from an outer shell. This makes the atom unstable. To stabilize the atom, an electron from another shell must replace the lost electron. The movement of electrons from one shell to another results in the emission of electromagnetic energy (visible light). The amount of energy needed to remove an electron from the outer shell varies relative to the composition of the phosphor and is measured in electron volts. The length of the electromagnetic wave (and subsequent color of light) depends on the energy emitted when the atom becomes stable. There are two forms of luminescence. They are fluorescence and phosphorescence.

In fluorescence, a substance emits light only when stimulated. The atom returns to stability after 1 electron revolution or in less than 10^{-8} second. In phosphorescence, a substance continues to emit light after the stimulation has stopped. The atom returns to stability after several electron revolutions or in more than 10^{-8} second. In radiography, this delay is often referred to as screen lag or afterglow. It is desirable for intensifying screens to exhibit fluorescence rather than phosphorescence.

Many phosphors exhibit luminescence. Radiography requires phosphor that is pure and in a crystalline form. This limits the number of phosphors available for use in intensifying screens. Currently, the crystals used include
1. Calcium tungstate
2. Barium fluorochloride
3. Yttrium
4. Rare earths, gadolinium and lanthanum.
The characteristics of these crystals are discussed under Phosphor.

EFFICIENCY

The efficiency of an intensifying screen depends on its ability to absorb x-rays and convert the x-rays to light. These phenomena are referred to as absorption efficiency and conversion efficiency, respectively. The intensifying screen is more efficient as the x-ray absorption and conversion increases.

Absorption efficiency refers to the intensifying screen's ability to absorb x-rays. A high absorption is desired. Most absorption is a result of the photoelectric effect. Briefly, this effect occurs when the x-ray energy is high enough to remove an electron from the K shell of an atom. Figure 23–6 is a graph of the absorption for calcium tungstate. Observation of the chart reveals that, at low energies, there is a high degree of x-ray absorption. This is followed by a decrease in absorption until the x-ray energy equals the binding energy of the electrons in the K shell of the atom. When this occurs, the x-ray energy is able to remove the electron from the K shell (photoelectric effect). At this point, there is a maximum absorption of the x-ray energy seen as an increase in energy on the chart in Figure 23–6. This area is referred to as the K shell absorption edge, or K edge. The K edge is measured in kilo electron volts (keV). Table 23–1 is a summary of the K shell absorption edges for some intensifying screen crystals.

Conversion efficiency is the ratio of light energy emitted by the crystal to the x-ray energy absorbed by the atom. The conversion efficiency is expressed as a percentage. The percentage of x-ray energy converted to light is small. For example, calcium tungstate has a conversion efficiency of 5%. This means that only 5% of the x-ray energy is converted to light. The rare earth elements' conversion efficiency ranges from 15% to 20%. Unfortunately, 50%

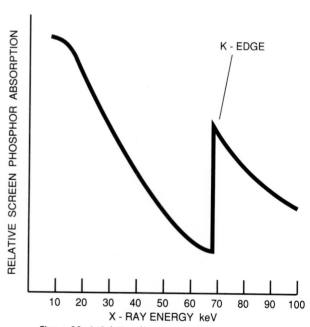

Figure 23–6. Relative absorption of calcium tungstate.

Table 23–1. APPROXIMATE K SHELL ABSORPTION ENERGY OF INTENSIFYING SCREEN CRYSTALS

Element	K Edge (keV)
Yttrium	17
Barium	37
Lanthanum	39
Gadolinium	50
Tungsten	70

of the converted light is absorbed by the intensifying screen. Consequently, only half of the light emitted reaches the film for exposure.

PHOSPHOR

As stated above, several types of phosphors can be used in intensifying screens. The most common phosphors employed are calcium tungstate, barium fluorochloride, yttrium (this element is often erroneously referred to as a rare earth, probably because it has characteristics similar to those of rare earth elements) and the rare earths gadolinium and lanthanum. These phosphors exhibit fluorescence when irradiated. An activator is often added to the phosphor (the exception being calcium tungstate) to help in the fluorescence process. The activators used are terbium, thulium and europium.

For years, the phosphor of choice was calcium tungstate. Although calcium tungstate does not enjoy the popularity it did in its earlier years, it is still found in many imaging departments. Calcium tungstate is desirable because it is inexpensive to produce, has an acceptable absorption efficiency, is able to convert x-rays to light in a short time and emits a color light to which x-ray film is sensitive.

In 1973, the rare earth phosphors began to emerge. The rare earth elements are located in group III of the periodic table and have atomic numbers between 57 and 71. The name rare earth implies that the elements are not found in abundance in the earth. In reality, these elements are relatively common. Unfortunately, they are expensive and difficult to refine. These phosphors are more desirable than calcium tungstate because they increase the rate of absorption three to five times

and convert x-rays to light much faster than does calcium tungstate. The rare earths are able to increase intensifying screen efficiency without adversely affecting the resolution (sharpness) of the image. Consequently, there is a decrease in the amount of radiation absorbed by the patient and an increase in the life span of the x-ray tube.

Figure 23–7 illustrates how rare earth elements increase the absorption rate. The graph in Figure 23–7 reveals that the absorption rate of the rare earth element is less than that of calcium tungstate in all kilovoltage ranges except those between the lanthanum oxybromide and calcium tungstate K edges. In this area, the rare earth element absorbs three to five times faster than calcium tungstate. Consequently, the rare earth element has a better absorption rate in the kilovoltage ranges between the two respective K edges.

Besides absorption and conversion efficiencies, another factor that needs to be considered is the

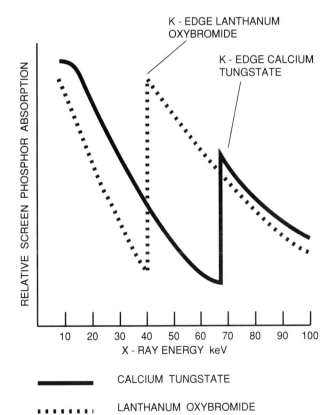

Figure 23–7. Comparison of calcium tungstate and lanthanum oxybromide absorption rates.

color of light the phosphor emits. The color of light emitted by the intensifying screen should be similar to the color required to expose the film. Correlating the color of the screen with that needed to expose the film is termed spectrum matching. The color of light is determined by the length of the electromagnetic wave. The following is a list of wavelengths (in angstroms and nanometers) associated with different colors.

3000 A (300 nm)—ultraviolet light
4000 A (400 nm)—blue light
5000 A (500 nm)—green light
6000 A (600 nm)—yellow light
7000 A (700 nm)—red light

X-ray film is manufactured to be either blue-violet (panchromatic) or green (orthochromatic) light sensitive. It is important to combine blue-violet sensitive film and green sensitive film with phosphor that emits the respective color. Calcium tungstate and barium fluorochloride phosphors emit blue light. The color emitted by the rare earth and yttrium depends on the activator added to the phosphor. The activator terbium emits a green light, whereas europium and thulium emit a blue color. In general, if the spectrum is mismatched, the speed of the screen decreases.

INTENSIFYING SCREEN SPEED

The amount of exposure needed to obtain a given amount of film density is referred to as screen speed. For example, given a film density of 1.5, the intensifying screen requiring the least amount of exposure to reach that density has the fastest speed. Screen speed may be expressed by a manufacturer's name or by number.

Most companies identify three intensifying screen speeds. Common names are detail, or slow; par, or medium; and high, or fast. Because manufacturers use different names to identify screen speed, this method can be confusing. However, expressing intensifying screen speed by a number is more specific and universal in its application to the meaning of intensifying screen speed. The screen speed is faster as the screen speed number increases. A screen speed of 200 requires 50% less exposure than a screen speed of 100.

In general, screens identified as slow have a corresponding speed number less than 100 (usual range of 40 to 60). Par speed screens are expressed as having a speed number of 100. Intensifying screens classified as fast have a wide range of speed numbers. They may be rated from 200 to 1200. Slow screens are employed if examinations require good detail and when motion is not a factor, e.g., for extremity work. Fast screens are useful in examinations needed to limit time or reduce radiation exposure to the patient, e.g., procedures evaluating trauma and examinations of children.

The speed number may be derived by calculating the intensification factor (IF). This factor is useful in determining the amount of dose decrease to the patient. It is the comparison of two radiographs taken at different exposures but approximately the same density. The IF is expressed mathematically as

$$IF = \frac{\text{exposure without screens}}{\text{exposure with screens}}$$

Because the numerator is always greater than the denominator, the intensification factor is always greater than 1. In practice, the technologist rarely uses the IF.

Several factors influence the speed of an intensifying screen. The technologist is able to control some and unable to influence other factors. Controllable factors are kilovoltage and room temperature. Factors that are not under the control of the technologist are emulsion thickness, size of phosphors, absorption efficiency, conversion efficiency and undercoating efficiency.

Room temperature can usually be controlled by the technologist. As room temperature increases, the speed of the intensifying screen decreases. However, as room temperature increases, the speed of the film increases. Consequently, there is no appreciable change in the image with temperature ranges between 20°F and 115°F. The effect of the other controllable factor, kilovoltage, varies with the type of phosphor. In intensifying screens employing calcium tungstate or barium fluorochloride, the amount of change in speed is minimal with any kilovoltage change. However, rare earth elements tend to be more kilovoltage dependent, especially above 70 kV. Rare earth screens have an increase in screen speed as the kilovoltage increases.

The factors not controlled by the technologist are those incorporated in the intensifying screen during its manufacture. Screens made with thick emulsions are faster than screens with thin emulsions. This is because thick emulsion screens emit more light. Screens manufactured with large crystals also emit more light and are faster than screens with small crystals. Another factor inherent in the screen that affects speed is the type of phosphor. Phosphors with a high rate of absorption and rapid x-ray to light convergence are employed in fast speed screens. The speed may be reduced by adding a dye to the screen. The dye absorbs the rays traveling the greatest distance (the divergent rays), decreasing the amount of light striking the film. The last inherent screen factor affecting screen speed is the efficiency of the undercoating. Screen speed is increased with an increase in the reflection of the undercoating.

IMAGE SHARPNESS

Intensifying screens affect the sharpness of the image. An intensifying screen's ability to produce a sharp image is often referred to as screen resolution. Screen resolution is measured with a resolution grid. A resolution grid has several sets of lead strips separated by a gap, or space (Figure 23–8). The number of lead strips and gaps per set varies. The number of lead strips and gaps in a set is

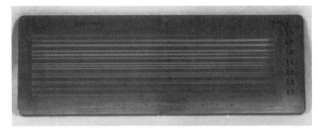

Figure 23–8. Resolution grid.

measured in line pairs (lp) per millimeter; 1 lp per mm has one lead strip and one gap in a 1 mm space. The higher the screen resolution, the more line pairs per millimeter that an intensifying screen can image with clarity. In general, a fast intensifying screen may resolve 7 lp per mm. A detail intensifying screen can resolve about 15 lp per mm. The difference in degree of image sharpness between an intensifying screen and direct film holder is significant (Figure 23–9). The direct film holder has the better resolution at approximately 100 lp per mm (assuming that a high resolution film is employed).

Four primary factors influence the image sharpness resulting from intensifying screens:
1. Screen speed
2. Crossover
3. Film-screen contact
4. Quantum mottle

Figure 23–9. Image sharpness. A, Direct film holder; B, intensifying screen.

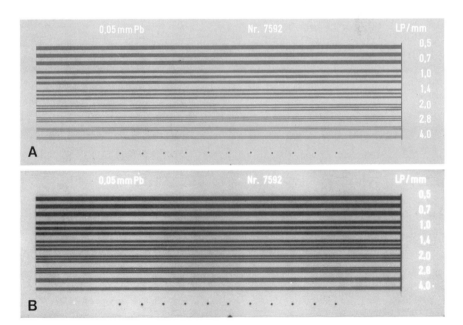

Generally, image sharpness decreases as the speed of the screen increases. Screen speed that is increased by increasing the thickness of the emulsion or the size of the phosphor results in a corresponding decrease in image sharpness. This occurs because an increase in diverging light rays striking the film creates more penumbra and decreases the sharpness of the image. Conversely, decreasing screen speed by adding a dye decreases the diverging light rays striking the film and increases image sharpness.

Divergent rays also play a role in decreasing image sharpness in crossover. Crossover is a term used when light emitted from one intensifying screen passes through the film, strikes the other intensifying screen and is reflected back to the film (Figure 23–10). Crossover occurs when double emulsion film and two intensifying screens are used. Some detail cassettes employ only one intensifying screen and single emulsion film to eliminate crossover.

To have good image sharpness, there must be a good film-screen contact. When there is a space (no matter how small) between the film and the screen, the light emitted from the screen diverges, creating a blurring effect on the film. This decreases image sharpness. Poor film-screen contact tends to be more common in large cassettes. Some causes of poor film-screen contact include foreign body in the cassette, loose springs or hinges and a twisted or warped frame. A procedure to determine if poor film-screen contact exists is the wire mesh test. In this test, a wire mesh (commercial wire meshes are available) embedded in plastic is placed over the cassette and exposed. The radiograph is reviewed for any area of the wire mesh that may appear blurred. Because the wire mesh is made of images of small squares (Figure 23–11), it is best to view the radiograph from a distance or from an oblique angle.

Quantum mottle, or noise, appears on a radiograph as irregular film densities, or blotches. Quantum mottle results because the random distribution of x-ray quanta to produce the image is too small. In general, quantum mottle increases as screen speed or kilovoltage increases. In laboratory expe-

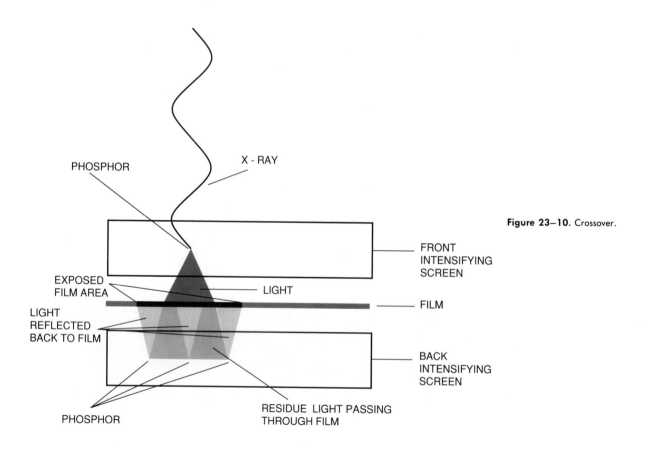

Figure 23–10. Crossover.

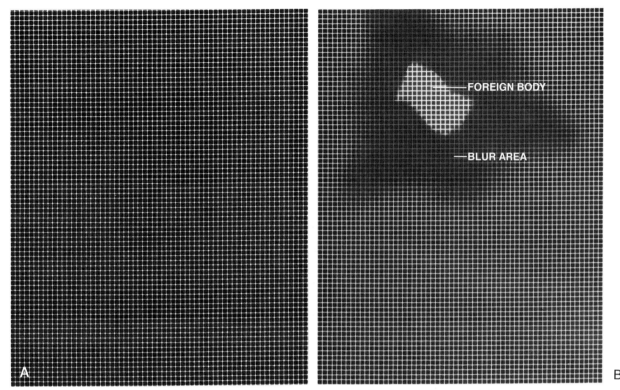

Figure 23–11. Wire mesh test for poor screen contact. *A*, Good contact; *B*, poor contact.

rience, quantum mottle is most apt to be a problem with extremely fast (1200 speed) intensifying screens.

INTENSIFYING SCREEN CARE

Intensifying screens are delicate. Consequently, they should be handled with care. Intensifying screen care involves mounting the screens with caution, loading and unloading x-ray film properly and regular cleaning.

As mentioned above, intensifying screens are purchased separately from cassettes. After screens have been purchased, they are mounted in the cassette. Mounting of intensifying screens is a simple process. However, care needs to be taken to avoid damaging the screens or mounting them incorrectly.

Intensifying screens are usually purchased in pairs—one front screen and one back screen. Some screen pairs are manufactured so that the front screen has a slower speed than the back. This is because x-rays are absorbed by the front cover, front intensifying screen and film before striking the back screen. Consequently, there is less radiation available to illuminate the back screen than the front screen. To compensate for the loss of radiation, the back screen speed is faster. Therefore, the person mounting these types of screens must read the label on the screen to determine which screen is front and which is back. The appropriate screen must be mounted on its respective cover. More recently, intensifying screen pairs are being manufactured so both have the same speed. This eliminates possible errors in mounting.

Other screen pairs may be manufactured with a graduated screen speed. In other words, one end of the screen is faster than the other end. These screens are usually large (about 3 feet) and are usually used for examinations of body parts with a significant variance in density, e.g., the leg. When these screens are mounted, it is important to have the fast parts of the screens opposite each other. Also, the outside of the cassette should be labeled as to which end has the faster speed.

In mounting intensifying screens, it is wise to read and follow the manufacturer's instructions. The following is a brief seven step method of mounting screens. This method is used as a guide and should not preclude the manufacturer's instructions.

1. Before mounting the screens, open the cassette and inspect the backing. Make sure it is clean.
2. Remove the protective cover from the adhesive on the screen to be mounted on the front lid of the cassette (Figure 23–12A).
3. Place the screen on the front cassette cover and center, being careful to position the lead blocker in the desired area (Figure 23–12B).
4. After the screen is centered properly, either use a lint-free soft cloth to gently press down around the edges (over the adhesive) with the palm of your hand or, to avoid touching the screen directly, proceed to steps 5–7. If steps 5–7 are not used, mount the back screen in the same manner as the front screen (steps 1–4).
5. Remove the protective cover from the adhesive on the screen to be mounted on the back lid of the cassette. Place the screen face down on top of the front screen. Position the screens so that the sides are even (Figure 23–12C) and the lead blocker is in the same position as that of the front screen.
6. Close and latch the cassette for about a minute (Figure 23–12D). Reopen the cassette to check that the screens are positioned properly. If the screen position is correct, close and latch the cassette.
7. Press along the edges on the outside of the cassette (over the screen adhesive area) with the palm of your hand (Figure 23–12E).

Some intensifying screens have an identification number imprinted on them during manufacturing. If the screen has a preprinted number, record that number on the outside of the cassette. If no number is on the screen, use some form of permanent marker to place a number on a part of the screen that will not interfere with the radiographic image. Use a marker that will not rub off on the film or on the screen or when a cleaning solution is used.

Another important factor in proper intensifying screen care is the loading and unloading of the x-ray film. When loading and unloading x-ray film it is important to protect the intensifying screen from abrasions or foreign objects that enter the cassette. To remove a film, unlatch the cassette (Figure 23–13) in an area free from possible chemical spills, e.g., developer, and where dirt is not apt to enter the cassette, e.g., away from a vent. While the cassette is unlatched but closed, turn the cassette over so that the front side is facing up (Figure 23–13B). Open the cassette and let the film drop out (Figure 23–13C). If the film does not fall out, rock the cassette slightly. Although this method is preferred, it is common for technologists to find this process too slow. An alternative method for unloading film is to open the cassette with the face down and pull the film out from the upper corner of the cassette using the tip of a finger (Figure 23–14). Many technologists use the lower corner to remove film. However, a technologist using the lower corner tends to dig fingernails in the intensifying screen, damaging the screen. Consequently, the upper corner method if preferred.

To load the cassette, place the cassette so that the front cover is facing down (Figure 23–15A). Open the cassette and place the film over the front intensifying screen (Figure 23–15B). Close and latch the cassette (Figure 23–15C).

It is almost impossible to keep an intensifying screen clean. One reason that screens commonly get dirty is that, when a cassette is first opened, there is an intake of outside air into the cassette. The room air may contain dust particles or other forms or dirt, e.g., moisture from a cough. Any dust or dirt on the screen creates an artifact on the radiograph. Consequently, it is important that intensifying screens be cleaned on a regular basis. The frequency of cleaning varies according to the workload of the department. Some imaging departments may need to clean intensifying screens once a month, whereas other departments may need to clean them only once every 2–3 months.

To clean intensifying screens, place the unloaded and opened cassette in a well-lighted area that is free from dirt and chemicals. Obtain a soft, clean lint-free cloth and the manufacturer's cleaning solution (a mild soap and water may be substituted for the manufacturer's solution). Although a manufacturer's solution tends to be expensive, it has the advantages of being antistatic and tends to evaporate readily. This helps prevent artifacts from appearing on the radiograph.

The process of cleaning is simple. Use the lint-free cloth and solution to wash the screens. Care

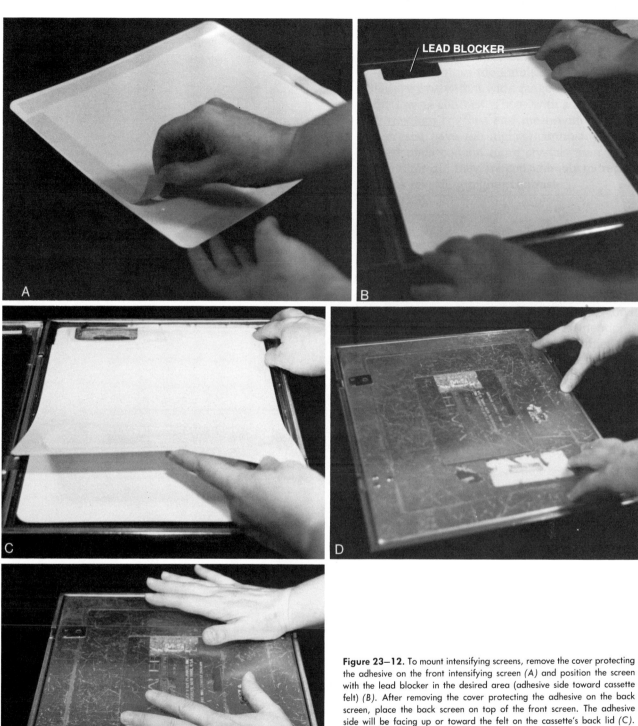

LEAD BLOCKER

Figure 23–12. To mount intensifying screens, remove the cover protecting the adhesive on the front intensifying screen *(A)* and position the screen with the lead blocker in the desired area (adhesive side toward cassette felt) *(B)*. After removing the cover protecting the adhesive on the back screen, place the back screen on top of the front screen. The adhesive side will be facing up or toward the felt on the cassette's back lid *(C)*. Close and latch the cassette *(D)*. To secure the screen to the cassette backing, press the palm of hand over the edges of the cassette *(E)*.

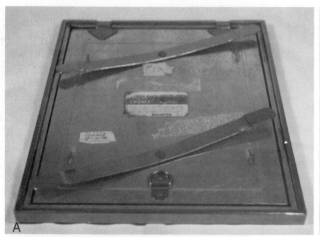

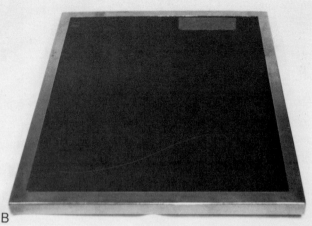

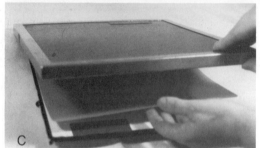

Figure 23–13. To unload a film from a cassette, unlatch the cassette *(A)* and place the cassette so the front cover of the cassette is face up *(B)*. Then open the cassette and let the film drop out *(C)*.

Figure 23–14. An alternative method of removing film from a cassette is to pull the film out from the upper corner.

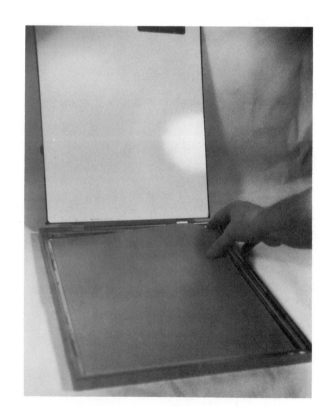

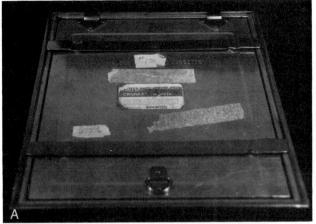

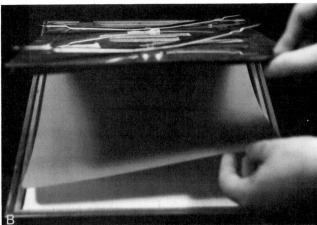

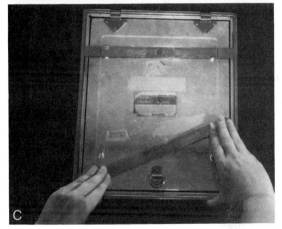

Figure 23–15. To load the cassette, place the cassette so the front cover is facing down *(A)*. Open the cassette and place the film over the front intensifying screen *(B)*. Close and latch the cassette *(C)*.

should be taken to avoid pressing too hard on the screen. There are several recommendations relative to the motion used to clean intensifying screen. Some professionals recommend circular motions, and others suggest figure eight movements. The primary objective is to remove all dirt without damaging the screen.

After the screens are washed, use another clean, dry lint-free cloth to wipe off the solution. After the solutions have been removed, the cassette should remain open for several minutes to ensure that it is completely dry. The length of time the cassette is open depends on the type of solution used. If the cassette remains open for more than 15 minutes, recheck to ensure that no dirt entered the cassette before closing the cassette. When the screens are dry, close the cassette. Remove any previous cleaning dates that may be attached to the outside of the cassette, then write the date on which the cassette was cleaned on a label and attach it to the outside

of the cassette. This helps to determine the next date for cleaning the cassette.

LABORATORY EXPERIENCE

Additional experience is available to individuals interested in practical applications of the theories presented in this chapter. *Concepts in Medical Radiographic Imaging: Laboratory Manual* contains three laboratory procedures on intensifying screens. They are Laboratories 36, Intensifying Screen Light Emission; 37, Intensifying Screen Resolution; and 38, Intensifying Screen Contact.

The Intensifying Screen Light Emission laboratory is designed to provide the experimenter with the opportunity to observe the color and level of intensity of light emitted when a screen is irradiated. This is achieved by irradiating several types of intensifying screens in a darkened room. Each screen is irradiated with several different kilovoltages. The experimenter records the color and brightness of the light emitted from each screen for each exposure.

The Intensifying Screen Resolution laboratory utilizes a resolution grid to determine the number of line pairs per millimeter. The numbers of line pairs per millimeter are compared among several different screen speeds and a direct film holder.

The Intensifying Screen Contact laboratory is performed as a quality control check of the intensifying screen. A wire mesh is used to assess film-screen contact.

Bibliography

Bushong, SC. Radiologic science for technologists (4th edition). St. Louis: Mosby, 1988.

Carroll, QB. Fuchs's Principles of radiographic exposure, processing and quality control (3rd edition). Springfield, IL: Thomas, 1985.

Chesney, DN and Chesney, MO. Radiographic imaging (4th edition). Boston: Blackwell Scientific Publications, 1981.

Cullinan, AM. Producing quality radiographs. New York: Lippincott, 1987.

Cullinan, JE and Cullinan, AM. Illustrated guide to x-ray technics (2nd edition). New York: Lippincott, 1980.

Curry, TS, Dowdey, JE and Murry, RC. Christensen's Introduction to the physics of diagnostic radiology (3rd edition). Philadelphia: Lea & Febiger, 1984.

Donohue, DP. An analysis of radiographic quality (2nd printing). Baltimore: University Park Press, 1982.

DuPont. Split-second exposure booklet. E. I. DuPont de Nemours & Co. (Inc.), Wilmington, DE. Publ number A-68927.

Fuji Photo Film. Intensifying screens. (Fuji film medical x-ray products technical handbook.) Tokyo: Fuji Photo Film Co., Ltd.

Gray, JE, et al. Quality control in diagnostic imaging. Baltimore: University Park Press, 1983.

Hendee, WR, Chaney, EL and Rossi, RP. Radiologic physics, equipment and quality control. Chicago: Year Book Medical, 1976.

Hiss, SS. Understanding radiography. Springfield, IL: Thomas, 1980.

Kelsey, CA. Essentials of radiology physics. St. Louis: Warren H. Green, 1985.

McLemore, J. Quality assurance in diagnostic radiology. Chicago: Year Book Medical, 1981.

Selman, J. The fundamentals of x-ray and radium physics (7th edition). Springfield, IL: Thomas, 1985.

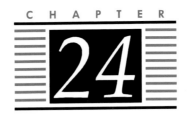

C H A P T E R

24

GRIDS AND QUALITY CONTROL

INTRODUCTION

Remnant radiation consists of radiation (Figure 24–1) from the primary x-ray beam and scatter radiation. Primary beam remnant radiation originates from the x-ray tube and passes through the body in a straight path. Scatter radiation is produced when the primary beam interacts (Compton effect) with the body. It is desirable to have the primary remnant radiation image the radiograph. Scatter radiation causes fog, which increases the radiographic density, creating a low contrast (many shades of gray) image. In a good diagnostic radiograph, there is a sharp demarcation between density differences (high contrast). Removing scatter radiation produces increased contrast (few shades of gray), improving the diagnostic quality of the radiograph.

In 1913, Dr. Gustave Bucky developed a grid to prevent scatter radiation from striking the film. His original grid contained two sets of a series of parallel lead strips. The sets were perpendicular to one another. The lead strips were about 2 cm apart. Today, Dr. Bucky's original principle of using lead strips separated by radiolucent interspaces is still used. This chapter discusses modern construction and proper use of grids.

GRID CONSTRUCTION

The difference between Bucky's original grid and modern grids is in their construction. Modern grids

use thinner lead strips, better interspace material and a sturdier support system (Figure 24–2).

INTERSPACE MATERIAL

The primary purpose of interspace material is to ensure a uniform distance between lead strips. The thickness of the interspace material (0.33 mm) is significantly greater than the thickness of the lead strips (0.05 mm). The interspace material is radiolucent and may be aluminum or plastic fiber. There is some disagreement as to which material is better. Aluminum has the following advantages over plastic fiber:

1. A higher atomic number to absorb some scatter radiation produced by the lead strips
2. Nonhygroscopic (does not absorb moisture)
3. Easier to manufacture.

However, aluminum increases the absorption of the primary beam. This is particularly critical at low kilovoltage ranges. For example, if two radiographs are taken of the same object at low kilovoltages, one exposed using a grid with aluminum interspaces and the other being exposed using a grid with plastic fiber interspaces (with all other technical factors remaining the same), the radiograph taken with the aluminum demonstrates a lighter radiographic image.

LEAD CONTENT

The amount of lead in a grid (lead content) is defined as the weight of the lead in a specific area.

277

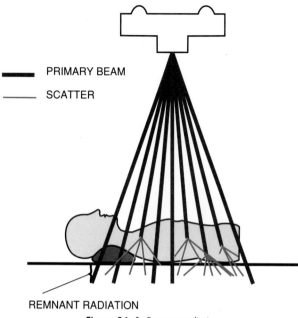

PRIMARY BEAM

SCATTER

REMNANT RADIATION

Figure 24–1. Remnant radiation.

GRID RATIO

Grid ratio is the ratio of the height of the lead strips to the distance between the lead strips (the interspace width). Grid ratio is usually expressed as two numbers. The first number is determined by dividing the height of the lead strip by the interspace width (the width of the lead strips is not considered when calculating the grid ratio). The second number is always 1. For example, if the height of the lead strip is 2 mm and the interspace width is 0.25 mm, the ratio is 8:1, or 2/0.25 = 8. There are seven grid ratios available. They are (from lowest to highest)

$$4:1, \ 5:1, \ 6:1, \ 8:1, \ 10:1, \ 12:1, \ 16:1$$

Generally, ratios between 8:1 and 12:1 are most commonly used in imaging departments. Low grid ratios are used for kilovoltages below 90 kV. High grid ratios are better for kilovoltages greater than 90 kV.

Grid ratio is increased by reducing the width of the interspace and/or increasing the height of the lead strips. Regardless of the method of increasing the grid ratio, the higher the ratio, the greater are the technical settings required to obtain a diagnostic film. This increase in technique causes an increase in patient exposure. To minimize the amount of radiation absorbed by the patient, it is best to increase the kilovoltage rather than the milliampere-seconds.

Generally speaking, the higher the grid ratio, the more effective (more absorption of scatter radiation) the grid. Table 24–1 demonstrates the percentage of scatter removed as the grid ratio increases. It can be seen from Table 24–1 that, as the ratio increases, more scatter is absorbed. However, there is a

The weight of lead is usually measured in milligrams and the area is measured in square centimeters. Grid content may be expressed mathematically in milligrams per square centimeter. A grid with a lead content of 600 mg per cm² contains the equivalent of 600 mg of lead for every 1 cm² area of the grid.

The higher the lead content, the more scatter radiation is absorbed, assuming that all other factors remain the same. The amount of lead in a grid is related to the grid ratio (see under Grid Ratio) and the number of lines per inch or centimeters (see under Grid Frequency). If the grid ratio is constant and the number of lines per inch or centimeter increases, the lead content decreases.

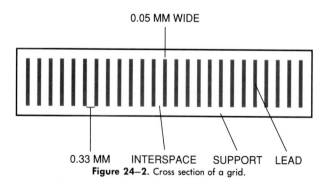

0.05 MM WIDE

0.33 MM   INTERSPACE   SUPPORT   LEAD

Figure 24–2. Cross section of a grid.

Table 24–1. AMOUNT OF SCATTER REMOVED PER GRID RATIO	
Grid Ratio	Scatter Removed
No grid	None
5:1	82.0%
8:1	90.0%
12:1	95.5%
16:1	96.0%

smaller difference in the amount of scatter removed at the higher ratio levels than at the lower ratio range. For example, changing from a 5:1 grid to a 8:1 grid increases the efficiency by 8%, whereas switching from a 12:1 to 16:1 grid has a 0.5% increase in efficiency. This is an important factor to consider when determining what grid ratio to use, because increasing the grid ratio increases patient exposure. Thus, there is a need to determine if the amount of image improvement outweighs the increase in patient exposure.

As stated above, high grid ratios are more effective than low grid ratios. This is because high grid ratios necessitate scatter radiation to pass through more lead strips before hitting the film than do low grid ratios (Figure 24–3). Because the scatter must penetrate more lead strips in higher ratio grids, the radiation is likely to be absorbed in the grid, never reaching the film. Regardless of how high the ratio is, some scatter radiation passes though the interspaces without striking a lead strip (is not absorbed by the grid).

However, the amount of scatter radiation passing through the grid unabsorbed is related to the grid ratio. The higher the grid ratio, the less scatter is allowed to pass uninterrupted through the grid (Figure 24–4). Figure 24–4B demonstrates that in a low ratio grid, scatter entering between the angles of 0 and 15 degrees (a 15 degree range) passes through the grid. The higher ratio grid in Figure 24–4A permits only the scatter entering within a 10 degree range (0 to 10 degrees) to penetrate the grid uninterrupted.

GRID FREQUENCY

Grid frequency is the number of lead lines per inch or centimeter. The range of grid frequency is 50 lines per inch (or 20 lines per cm) to 110 lines per inch (or 43 lines per cm). If a constant grid ratio and interspace width are maintained, the grid with the higher frequency is less efficient. This is because, to increase the number of lead lines per inch or centimeter, the lead must be thinner. Thinner lead lines are more easily penetrated and decrease the amount of scatter radiation absorbed, making the grid less efficient. Consequently, in this case, to maintain similar grid efficiency when using a grid with a higher grid frequency, the grid ratio should also be increased.

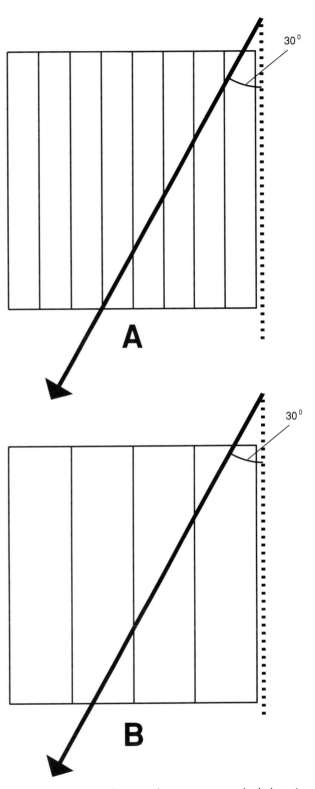

Figure 24–3. Scatter radiation needs to penetrate more lead when using a higher grid ratio (A) than when using a lower grid ratio (B).

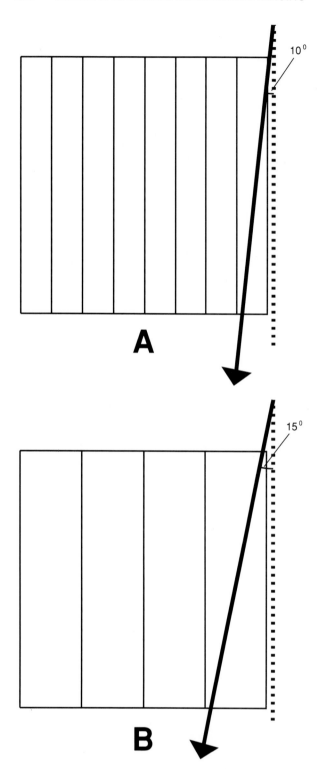

Figure 24–4. Angle needed for scatter to pass through grid without striking a lead strip is small for high ratio grids (A) and large for low ratio grids (B).

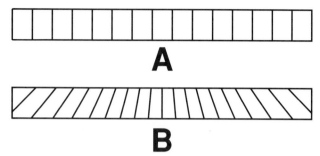

Figure 24–5. Cross section of a grid demonstrating the type of grid. A, Parallel; B, focused.

TYPES OF GRIDS

PARALLEL

As the name indicates, a parallel grid has all lead strips parallel to one another (Figure 24–5). A parallel grid is most efficient when used at a long source-image distance (at least 48 inches) and with a small film (8 × 10 inch) size. These limitations are a result of the characteristics of x-ray beam travel relative to the lead strips of the grid.

The primary x-ray beam originates from a point (focus of the x-ray tube) and travels in all directions (diverges) as it exits the x-ray tube. Because the lead strips in a parallel grid are vertical, the radiation must be almost perpendicular (straight) to pass through the grid and strike the film. The amount of straight (perpendicular) rays striking the film is determined by the source-image distance and the field size. The longer the source-image distance, the more perpendicular rays strike the film (Figure 24–6). Most radiographs are taken at a 40 inch source-image distance. At this distance, most of the straight radiation occurs about 4 inches from either side of the center of the film (or 8 inches total). Toward the periphery of the film, the radiation becomes more angled. Consequently, by using field sizes of 6–8 inches, the angled rays are essentially eliminated, leaving mostly perpendicular rays to expose the film.

When short source-image distances or large field sizes are used, the peripheral lead strips of a parallel grid demonstrate unwanted absorption of the primary beam. The unwanted absorption at the edges of the grid (grid cutoff) produces a radiographic image that is dark in the center and lighter toward the sides of the film.

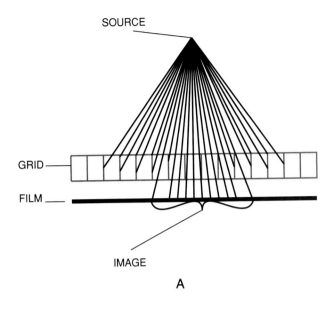

SOURCE

GRID ——

FILM ——

IMAGE

A

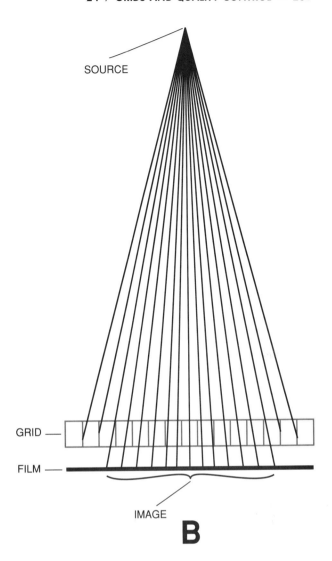

SOURCE

GRID ——

FILM ——

IMAGE

B

Figure 24–6. Relationship of source-image distance (SID) to the amount of perpendicular rays striking the film. Short SIDs have fewer perpendicular rays reaching the film *(A)* than do long SIDs *(B)*.

Because of the peripheral grid cutoff, parallel grids are most often used for spot filming devices employing small films.

FOCUSED

The lead strips in a focused grid are designed so that they point toward the center of the grid. Thus, there is an increase in the angle of the lead strip as one moves toward the periphery of the grid (see Figure 24–5). The difference between a parallel and a focused grid is demonstrated by extending an imaginary plane of the lead strips. On a focused grid, when imaginary planes are drawn, the planes meet at an imaginary point (convergence point) a specific distance from the grid (Figure 24–7A). The convergence point is where the focus of the x-ray tube should be located. The distance from the convergence point to the grid (*not* the film) is called the focusing distance. When imaginary planes of the lead strips are extended on a parallel grid, they never meet (Figure 24–7B). Thus, there is no convergence point.

In practice, there is some latitude as to the amount of distance the x-ray tube may be placed above or below the convergence point (focal distance range) to obtain a diagnostic radiograph. The amount of latitude is affected by the grid ratio. As the grid ratio is increased, the latitude is decreased.

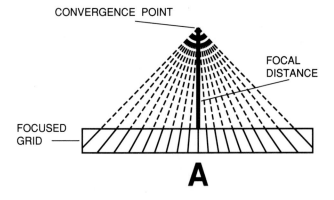

Figure 24–7. Effect of extending imaginary planes of lead strips on a focused grid *(A)* and a parallel grid *(B)*.

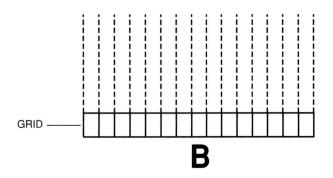

For example, if the focal distance for a 5:1 grid is 40 inches, it is possible to set the x-ray tube at any focal distance between 28 and 72 inches and still obtain a diagnostic film. However, for a 12:1 grid ratio employing a 40 inch focal distance, the focal distance range is decreased to 38 to 42 inches.

When a focused grid is used at the proper focal distance range, the angle of the primary beam coincides with the angle of the lead strips. This is useful in producing uniform density on the radiograph (Figure 24–8A).

Because the angle of the lead is constructed relative to the primary beam, it is essential for the grid to be positioned so that the lead lines point toward the x-ray tube. Thus, a focused grid has a specific side that must face the x-ray tube during exposure. If a radiograph is taken with the tube side down (inverted grid), the peripheral lead lines absorb almost all of the primary beam. The result is a radiograph that is exposed in the center and clear on the sides (Figure 24–9).

GRID CONFIGURATION

Grid configuration is the pattern of the length of the lead strips when viewed from above (looking down on the grid). There are two grid configuration patterns available: linear (Figure 24–10A) and cross-hatched (or cross-grid).

LINEAR

Grids with a linear configuration are constructed so that the lengths of all the lead strips are in the same direction. Linear grids may be parallel or focused. Parallel and focused linear grids should always be used within their respective limitations, e.g., proper focal distance and the correct side facing the tube. If the grid is used within its proper limits, the advantage of a linear configuration is the ability to angle the x-ray tube parallel to the length of the lead strips. This is a great advantage in

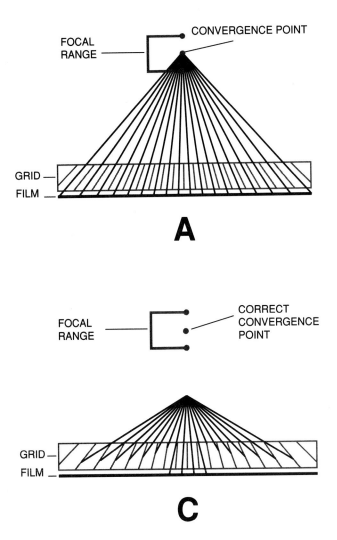

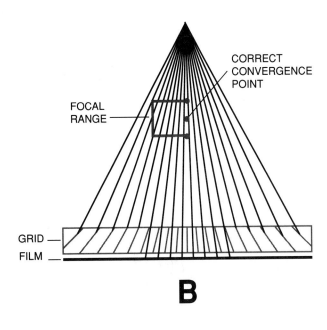

Figure 24–8. Peripheral grid cutoff is demonstrated when a radiograph is taken outside the focal range of a focused grid. *A,* Proper range; *B,* above the maximum focal range; *C,* below the minimum focal range.

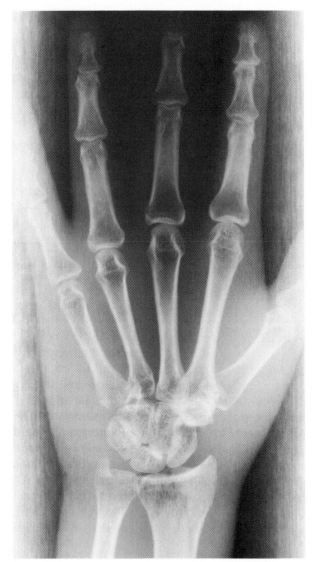

Figure 24–9. Radiograph obtained with an inverted focused grid, demonstrating the grid cutoff.

procedures that necessitate tube angulation, e.g., skull radiography.

CROSS-HATCHED

Cross-hatched grids are two linear grids positioned one on top of the other. They are positioned so that the length of the lead strips of the top grid is perpendicular to that of the lead strips of the lower grid (Figure 24–10B). If the lengths of the

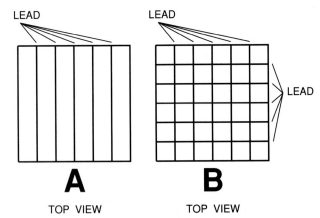

Figure 24–10. Grid configurations. *A,* Linear; *B,* grid plate.

lead strips of the grids are parallel to one another, a moiré pattern (Cullinan and Cullinan, 1980, p. 39) may occur (Figure 24–11). There are an infinite number of variations of the moiré pattern. This artifact occurs because it is essentially impossible for the lead strips of two linear grids to superimpose one another completely. Rather, they tend to be off-centered, forming a grid configuration that has a great deal of lead and only patches of radiolucent interspaces. Such a configuration absorbs much of the primary radiation, underexposing the radiograph.

As stated above, cross-hatched grids are made by placing two linear grids perpendicular to one another. Generally, the two linear grids are of the same type (parallel or focused). The efficiency of a cross-hatched grid is equivalent to adding the ratios of the two grids. For example, a cross-hatched grid consisting of two 8:1 grids has the efficiency of one 16:1 linear grid.

One advantage of using a cross-hatched grid of lower ratios is to increase the focal distance range. A cross-hatched grid consisting of two 8:1 linear grids has the efficiency of a 16:1 linear grid and a larger focal distance range than a single 16:1 linear grid. The increased focal distance range provides flexibility in performing difficult examinations when an efficient grid is necessary. Examples are radiography in the operating room, mobile radiography and examination of trauma patients.

Cross-hatched grids have two additional advantages. They allow an imaging department to salvage older linear grids and are able to absorb scatter

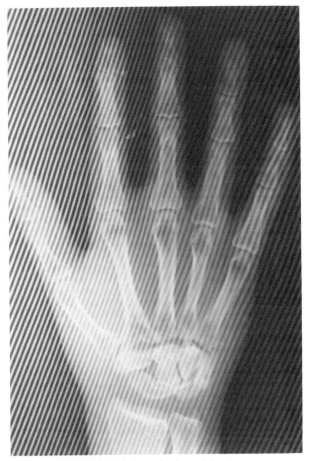

Figure 24–11. Example of a moiré pattern.

radiation in all directions. It is not unusual for grids to be damaged with use or age. Grids may be damaged several ways, e.g., radiolucent material may crack and lead may become misaligned. This damage appears as artifacts on the radiograph. The advantage of a cross-hatched grid is that grids with minor damage become usable because the overlapping of the lead from one grid tends to compensate for any minor damage that might exist in the other grid. Another advantage of the cross-hatched grid is its ability to absorb scatter radiation in all directions. Scatter radiation is absorbed in a direction that is parallel to the length of the lead strips. Because a cross-hatched grid has lead strips running crosswise and lengthwise, scatter radiation is absorbed in all directions. This is useful in procedures in which radiation is emitted from a variety of directions. One common use of the cross-hatched

grid is in angiographic examinations not necessitating tube angulation, e.g., lateral cerebral angiogram.

The primary disadvantage of a cross-hatched grid is that any angle of the x-ray tube causes grid cutoff. A cross-hatched grid has the lead strips running crosswise and lengthwise, making it impossible to angle the x-ray tube so that the primary beam is parallel to the length of the lead strips. A tube angled to be parallel to one grid is also at right angles to the lead strips of the other grid. Consequently, a 90 degree central ray is critical when employing a cross-hatched grid.

STATIONARY GRIDS

A stationary grid remains motionless (stationary) during the x-ray exposure. Stationary grids may be linear or cross-hatched. There are two types of stationary grids. One type is mounted in a cassette and is called a grid cassette (Figure 24–12A). The other is a grid plate (Figure 24–12B).

GRID CASSETTE

The grid cassette contains a grid attached to the tube side of a cassette. This type of grid tends to be sturdier and longer lasting than grid plates. Grid cassettes are usually stored near the other film holders. At first glance, a grid cassette looks similar to a regular cassette. However, the weight and the color of the grid make the grid cassette readily distinguishable from regular cassettes. The lead in the grid of a grid cassette makes it significantly heavier than a regular cassette. Even with the weight and color differences, grid cassettes are sometimes mistaken for regular cassettes. Care should be taken when selecting cassettes to ensure that the correct film holder is being used.

GRID PLATE

As the name implies, grid plates are grids in the form of flat plates. Grid plates are used on top of cassettes. They are delicate and should be stored flat to avoid damage to the lead strips or interspace

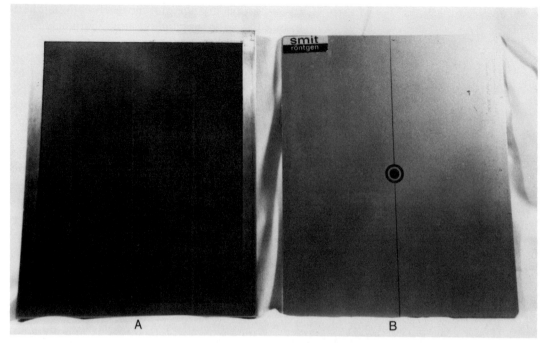

Figure 24–12. Stationary grids. *A,* Grid cassette; *B,* grid plate.

material. Care should be taken to avoid placing objects on top of stored grid plates. Any unnecessary weight or pressure on the grid may damage it. Grid plates are not as well protected as grid cassettes, making them more susceptible to damage.

GRID LINES

Both grid cassettes and grid plates create grid lines on the radiograph. Grid lines are white images produced by the lead in the grid (Figure 24–13). When these lines are wide, they tend to interfere with the radiologist's ability to determine a diagnosis. Modern high frequency grids have lead strips so thin that, when they are observed from a normal viewing distance, the grid lines are essentially invisible.

MOVING GRIDS

Seven years after Bucky invented the grid, Dr. Hollis Potter introduced the concept of moving the grid. The purpose of moving the grid was to remove the images of the lead (grid lines) from the radio-

graph by blurring them. The original mechanism of grid movement was called the Potter-Bucky diaphragm in honor of the inventors. Today, most practicing radiographers have shortened the name

Figure 24–13. Radiograph demonstrating grid lines.

to the Bucky diaphragm, which eliminates crediting Potter for his invention. The International Commission on Radiological Units and Measures (ICRU) recommends that the term Potter-Bucky diaphragm be used to refer to the mechanism and the term moving grid be reserved to describe a grid in motion.

A moving grid moves a short distance (1–3 cm) at right angles to the length of the lead strips. Long movement distances are avoided because the grid would become too far off-centered from the central ray, causing grid cutoff (see under Grid Cutoff). Even a minor 1–3 cm movement of the grid causes a 20% absorption of the primary x-ray beam. To compensate for the increase in radiation absorption of the primary beam, there must be an increase in the technical factors.

SINGLE STROKE

The oldest and simplest form of moving grid is the single stroke grid (Figure 24–14). The single stroke grid uses a spring mechanism to move the grid across the film. The grid is cocked to one side by pulling a string. The grid moves just before the x-ray exposure. The speed of the movement is adjustable. The single stroke grid is useful for an exposure range between 0.2 and 15 seconds. The advent of improved electronics and solid state technology has made the single stroke moving grid obsolete.

RECIPROCATING

The reciprocating grid is electronically operated and moves in a back and forth motion. It can be used with times as low as $\frac{1}{60}$ second without causing grid lines. After it reaches one side, it returns rapidly to the other side, limiting the lag time (time needed to change directions) to almost nothing. A lag time of essentially zero is vital in avoiding grid lines. If the grid hesitated before returning to the other side, a radiograph of the grid would occur, resulting in grid lines.

OSCILLATING

The most advanced grid movement is oscillating. The oscillating grid movement is circular. To achieve this type of movement, there are springs at all corners of the grid. While the anode is rotating (before x-ray exposure), an electromagnet pulls the grid to one side. On release from the electromagnet, the grid bounces from spring to spring, oscillating in a circular direction. After about 20–30 seconds, the grid stops all movement. Because of the circular movement, the tube cannot be angled or grid cutoff occurs.

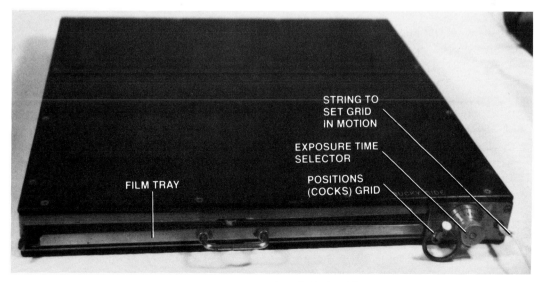

Figure 24–14. Single stroke Bucky grid.

PRECAUTIONS WHEN USING MOVING GRIDS

When using a moving grid, it is important to make sure that the grid moves fast enough so that several lead strips pass a given point on the film. Also, the speed of the grid should be out of sequence with the x-ray machine pulses.

It is important for the grid to move during the entire exposure. Whenever the grid stops moving during the exposure, an image of the grid appears on the radiograph. Thus, the grid movement should start before the exposure begins, continue during the exposure and end after the exposure is complete.

Making sure that grid motion is out of sequence with the x-ray pulses is also important in preventing grid lines. A grid moving in sequence with the x-ray pulses results in an exposure made of superimposed lead strips. Recall that x-ray production occurs as pulsating photon packets. Thus, if grid movement is in sequence with the photon packets, the later photon packets strike the lead strips in the same place where the adjacent lead strips were exposed by preceding photon packets, superimposing the lead strips.

DISADVANTAGES AND ADVANTAGE OF MOVING GRIDS

There are six disadvantages of using a moving grid.
1. Moving grids increase radiation exposure to compensate for increased absorption of the primary beam.
2. As with all mechanical devices, moving grids are subject to breakdown or failure.
3. Moving grids increase the distance between the patient and the film, which increases the magnification of objects.
4. The motion of the grid can vibrate the table, causing movement of the object.
5. Moving grids are more expensive than stationary grids.
6. The size and weight of moving grids make it impractical to use them for mobile radiography.

The greatest advantage of moving grids is the improved radiographic quality. The improved quality of the radiograph is significant with a moving grid so that it greatly outweighs its disadvantages.

GRID EFFICIENCY

CONTRAST IMPROVEMENT FACTOR

The principal function of a grid is to improve contrast by removing scatter radiation. The amount of improvement is expressed as the contrast improvement factor. A factor of 1 indicates no improvement. Factors greater than 1 reflect an increase in contrast. The usual range is 1.5 to 2.5 (Bushong, 1988, p. 200).

By definition, the contrast improvement factor is the ratio of the contrast of an x-ray film taken with a grid to the contrast of an x-ray film taken without a grid. The mathematical representation of the contrast improvement factor (K) is

$$K = \frac{\text{contrast with grid}}{\text{contrast without grid}}$$

The contrast improvement factor is determined by experimentation with phantoms performed in a laboratory. The human body is different from a phantom, consequently contrast improvement factors should be viewed as a guide to the efficiency of the grid. Other variables affecting the validity of the contrast improvement factor are the many external components, besides grids, that influence contrast. These include, but are not limited to, field size, kilovoltage, patient size and x-ray beam filtration. Because external factors other than grids also influence contrast, to help standardize the contrast improvement factor, the ICRU recommends that tests be performed using 100 kV on a 20 cm phantom.

Tests performed under controlled laboratory conditions by Liebel-Flarsheim yielded the following generalizations relative to contrast improvement with grids (Figure 24–15):
1. Grids improve contrast.
2. There is an increase in improvement with an increase in grid ratio.
3. Increasing kilovoltage decreases contrast.
4. Cross-hatched grids improve contrast more than linear grids of the same ratio.

EXPERIMENTAL CONTRAST VALUES

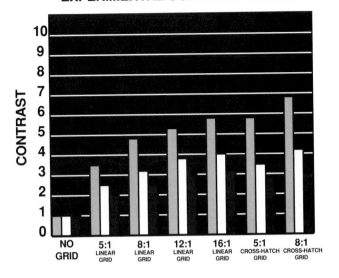

Figure 24–15. Experimental contrast values. (From Liebel-Flarsheim Company.)

SELECTIVITY

Grids absorb both primary and scatter radiation. An ideal grid allows 100% of the primary radiation to be transmitted through the grid while absorbing all the scatter radiation. However, in practice, some of the primary beam is absorbed by the grid and some scatter is transmitted through the grid. The ratio of the amount of primary radiation transmitted through the grid to the amount of scatter radiation transmitted determines the grid selectivity. The mathematical representation of grid selectivity is

$$\Sigma = \frac{T_p}{T_s}$$

where Σ is selectivity, T_p is the amount of primary radiation transmitted and T_s is the amount of scatter radiation transmitted.

Unlike the contrast improvement factor, selectivity is not influenced by external factors. Selectivity is a function of the grid itself.

EXPOSURE FACTOR

The exposure factor (also referred to as the Bucky factor) is an indirect method to measure primary beam absorption. It is used primarily to identify how much of an increase in technical factors is needed to obtain a diagnostically useful radiograph. It is also a measurement of the increase in patient dose. Because the exposure factor measures the grid's absorption rate, it is an indirect method of measuring the efficiency of the grid. The mathematical formula for exposure factor is

$$\text{exposure factor} = \frac{\text{exposure without grid (incident radiation)}}{\text{exposure with grid (transmitted radiation)}}$$

The size of the exposure factor is influenced by the grid ratio and the kilovoltage. Increasing either the grid ratio or the kilovoltage increases the exposure factor.

GRID CUTOFF

Grid cutoff occurs when a grid absorbs a substantial amount of the primary x-ray beam. The increased primary ray absorption occurs because of the misalignment of the x-ray tube and the grid. This misalignment generally occurs in one of five ways, which are
1. Lateral decentering
2. Unlevel grid
3. Tube focus outside the convergence point
4. Inverted focused grid
5. Improper tube angulation.

It is possible to have a combination of different misalignments. For example, grid cutoff may occur because of a lateral decentering of the grid and a tube focus located outside the convergence point.

LATERAL DECENTERING

The central ray should be directed to the middle of the grid. When the central ray is lateral to the center of the grid, there is uniform grid cutoff (Figure 24–16). There are two ways that the central ray becomes directed lateral to the middle of the grid. One method involves a properly directed

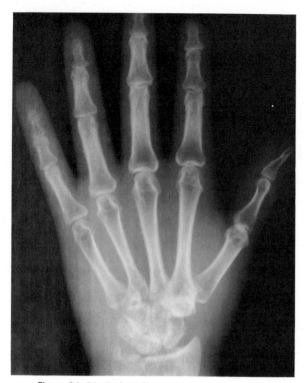

Figure 24–16. Grid cutoff caused by lateral decentering.

central ray relative to the patient but an off-centered grid. The other method of lateral decentering occurs when the anatomical part to be imaged and the grid are centered properly, but the central ray is misaligned (Figure 24–17B).

The amount of loss of the primary beam (in percentage) created by lateral decentering is affected by the grid ratio, the amount of lateral decentering and the convergence point of the grid. The relationship of these factors is mathematically represented (Curry et al., 1984, p. 96) as

$$L = \frac{rb}{f_0} \times 100$$

where L is the percentage of loss of the primary beam, r is the grid ratio, b is the lateral decentering distance and f_0 is the convergence point.
As the numerator (rb) of the formula increases, there is a corresponding increase in the percentage of primary beam absorption. In other words, as the grid ratio or the lateral decentering distance increases, primary beam absorption becomes greater.

UNLEVEL GRID

The grid must be perpendicular to the primary beam. Any angle of the grid to the central ray causes uniform grid cutoff (Figure 24–18). Unlevel grid alignment to the x-ray beam most commonly occurs in mobile radiography. During mobile radiography, it is possible that the patient may exert more pressure on one side of the grid than on the other, tilting the grid. Also, sometimes pillows, traction equipment, etc., hinder the ability to position the grid so that it is perpendicular to the tube. In these instances, the tube should be angled appropriately to redirect the central ray to form a 90 degree angle with the grid.

OUTSIDE CONVERGENCE POINT

The focus of the x-ray tube should be located at the convergence point. Inappropriate tube positioning may locate the tube above or below the convergence point (see Figure 24–8). Positions outside the convergence point increase primary beam absorption.

Radiographs taken outside the convergence point demonstrate grid cutoff on the edges of the film (Figure 24–19). The amount of grid cutoff increases as the grid ratio increases and as the distance from the convergence point becomes greater. However, it should be noted that, below the convergence point, grid cutoff is more significant than above the

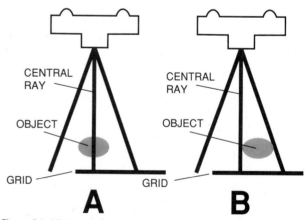

Figure 24–17. Lateral decentering may occur when the grid is off centered relative to the central ray and part (A) or when the x-ray beam is misaligned relative to the part and grid (B).

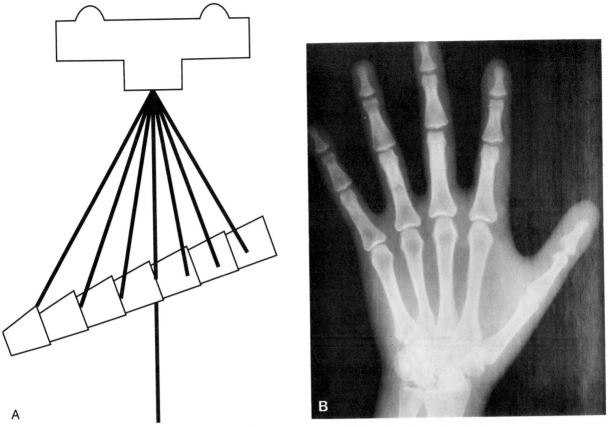

Figure 24–18. Grid cutoff resulting from an unlevel grid *(A)* and resulting radiograph *(B)*.

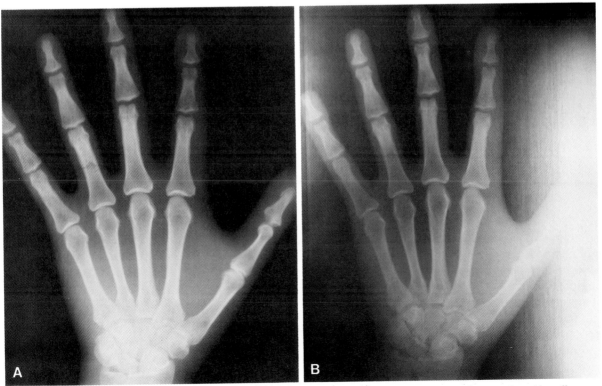

Figure 24–19. Radiographs taken above the convergence point *(A)* and below the convergence point *(B)*, demonstrating grid cutoff.

convergence point, assuming that the distances from the convergence point are equal. For example, if a radiograph is taken 10 inches above the convergence point and another radiograph is taken 10 inches below the convergence point, the film taken above the convergence point has less grid cutoff than the radiograph taken below the convergence point.

It should also be noted that parallel grids have no real convergence point. The effect of having the tube located outside the convergence point occurs on a parallel grid when the tube is centered below the recommended focal distance of the grid.

INVERTED FOCUSED GRID

As stated above (see Focused under Types of Grids), a focused grid has a tube side. Employing the grid upside down causes grid cutoff on the lateral sides (see Figure 24–9).

TUBE ANGULATION

Some x-ray examinations necessitate that the x-ray tube be angled. The direction of tube angulation is determined by the body part being examined and the direction of the length of the lead strips in the grid. Tube angulation is permitted when the beam is angled so that it is parallel to the length of the lead strips. Angling the tube across the lead strips causes uniform grid cutoff (Figure 24–20).

SELECTING A GRID

Selecting a grid involves assessment of many variables. There is no one factor available to determine the best grid needed for an examination. Rather, it is recommended that all factors relating to the examinations be evaluated. The number and type of factors to consider vary with the procedure. For example, the conditions needed to perform an abdominal mobile radiograph are different from those for an abdominal radiograph performed in an imaging department on a three phase x-ray unit. In many cases, the grid selected may necessitate a compromise in another area, e.g., a high absorption grid causes increased radiation exposure to the patient.

To avoid being inundated with numerous variables, the radiographer begins to assess the type of grid specifications needed by considering the amount of scatter radiation produced by the object (the size of the object), the kilovoltage that will be used and the amount of radiation absorbed by the patient.

The nature and thickness of an object determine the amount of radiation needed to penetrate the object. An object that is dense or large usually necessitates high kilovoltages. These objects also tend to produce more scatter radiation than thinner, less dense body parts. Thirteen centimeters (the size of an average adult knee) or greater is a common guideline for the minimum object size for which to use a grid.

Linear grids with low ratios (8:1 or less) are recommended for objects producing moderate amounts of scatter and requiring a kilovoltage no greater than 90 kV. When 100 kV or more is required, high ratio linear grids are in order. Cross-hatched grids are reserved for objects creating a great deal of scatter radiation and for grid-tube alignment that poses no problem. Linear grids with extremely low grid ratios (4:1 and 5:1) are best employed for field sizes no greater than 8 inches, e.g., spot filming devices.

Besides assessing the degree of scatter radiation and kilovoltage range, one should evaluate the amount of radiation absorbed by the patient. It is recommended that a grid that provides an optimum amount of radiographic quality and minimum amount of radiation exposure be employed. Care should be taken to avoid using a highly efficient grid, creating an increase in radiation absorption, if a less efficient grid could have produced similar radiographic results.

QUALITY CONTROL TEST

A common quality control test performed on grids is to determine the alignment of the grid to the central ray, especially whether lateral decentering and an unlevel grid are present.

To perform the test, a thin sheet of lead with several holes is needed (grid alignment tool). This

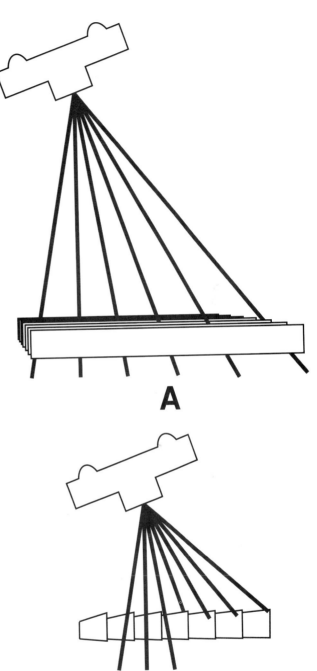

Figure 24–20. No grid cutoff occurs when the x-ray tube is angled parallel to the length of the lead strips (A). However, angling the x-ray tube across the lead strips (B) results in unwanted radiation absorption (grid cutoff).

instrument (Figure 24–21) is available commercially. The tool consists of five large holes 1 inch apart along the longitudinal axis of the lead. A smaller hole is placed above and/or below the large middle hole, and a small hole is located adjacent to one of the large end holes. These small holes are used to demonstrate the position of the grid alignment tool over the film.

The test is performed by placing the tool on the table top so that the long axis is perpendicular to the length of the lead strips of the grid. Five exposures are made, one per large hole. The tube is centered directly over each large hole for the respective exposure. To achieve this, the tube is off-centered.

A properly aligned grid and central ray produce a radiograph in which the center large hole is dark, with the outer holes becoming lighter as one moves to the periphery. Comparison of the holes adjacent to the center hole reveals that they have approximately the same density. The two end holes also have equivalent densities (Figure 24–22). Any variation of this density pattern is indicative of misalignment.

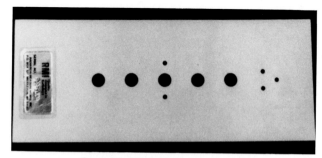

Figure 24–21. Grid alignment test tool.

LABORATORY EXPERIENCE

Two laboratory experiments in *Concepts in Medical Radiographic Imaging: Laboratory Manual* provide an opportunity to apply many of the concepts mentioned in this chapter: Laboratories 39, Grid Lines, and 40, Grid Cutoff.

The Grid Lines laboratory demonstrates the principal causes of grid lines. The experimenter exposes three radiographs. Two radiographs are taken with a motionless grid. One image is produced by employing a stationary grid, while the other radio-

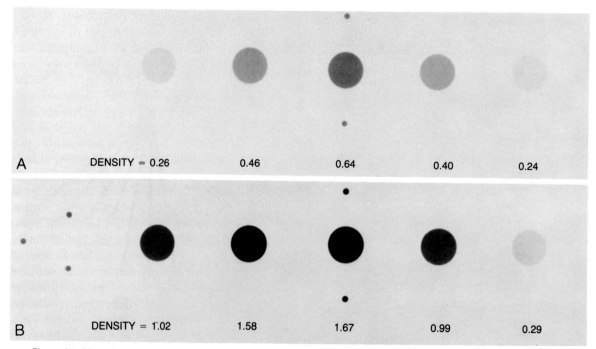

A DENSITY = 0.26   0.46   0.64   0.40   0.24

B DENSITY = 1.02   1.58   1.67   0.99   0.29

Figure 24–22. Radiograph of grid alignment test tool demonstrating properly aligned *(A)* and misaligned *(B)* grid and central ray.

graph is obtained by exposing a film when the knob selecting the Potter-Bucky diaphragm is in the off position (the knob is adjusted so that the grid does not move). The last (third) radiograph is obtained while the grid moves. It is used to compare a radiograph with the lead strips blurred with films having grid lines.

The Grid Cutoff laboratory is designed to demonstrate the various causes of grid cutoff. The effects of the following grid errors are demonstrated: lateral decentering, unlevel grid, outside convergence point, inverted focused grid and improper tube angulation. This laboratory is unusual in that it teaches the experimenter what not to do when using a grid.

Bibliography

Bushong, SC. Radiologic science for technologists (4th edition). St. Louis: Mosby, 1988.

Cullinan, AM. Producing quality radiographs. New York: Lippincott, 1987.

Cullinan, JE and Cullinan, AM. Illustrated guide to x-ray technics (2nd edition). New York: Lippincott, 1980.

Curry, TS, Dowdey, JE and Murry, RC. Christensen's Introduction to the physics of diagnostic radiology (3rd edition). Philadelphia: Lea & Febiger, 1984.

Donohue, DP. An analysis of radiographic quality (2nd printing). Baltimore: University Park Press, 1982.

Gray, JE, et al. Quality control in diagnostic imaging. Baltimore: University Park Press, 1983.

Hendee, WR, Chaney, EL and Rossi, RP. Radiologic physics, equipment and quality control. Chicago: Year Book Medical, 1976.

Kelsey, CA. Essentials of radiology physics. St. Louis: Warren H. Green, 1985.

Liebel-Flarsheim. Characteristics and applications of x-ray grids. Cincinnati: Liebel-Flarsheim, 1983.

Liebel-Flarsheim. Grids and Buckys. Slide/tape. Cincinnati: Liebel-Flarsheim.

Methods of Evaluating Radiological Equipment and Materials. Recommendations of the International Commission on Radiological Units and Measurements (ICRU), Report 10f 1962, National Bureau of Standards Handbook 89, U.S. Dept. of Commerce, issued Aug 23, 1963.

Multi-media. Portable radiography and a study of grids, unit 6-A. Slide/audio tape. Denver: Multi-media, 1977.

McLemore, J. Quality assurance in diagnostic radiology. Chicago: Year Book Medical, 1981.

Selman, J. The fundamentals of x-ray and radium physics (7th edition). Springfield, IL: Thomas, 1985.

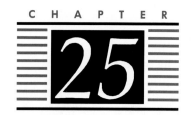

CHAPTER 25

BEAM RESTRICTORS AND QUALITY CONTROL

INTRODUCTION

Imaging departments purchase equipment and develop techniques to obtain an optimum radiographic image with the least amount of radiation exposure to the patient. Several factors affect the amount of radiation exposure to the patient. One important factor is to limit the size of the irradiated field. Limiting the field size is also effective in improving the radiographic image. The image is improved by decreasing radiographic fog. Radiographic fog is unwanted density on the radiograph. There are numerous ways a film becomes fogged, including by scatter radiation.

Scatter radiation is somewhat controllable and may be reduced by using grids (refer to Chapter 24, Grids and Quality Control, for more specific information on grids) and beam restrictors. Grids are positioned between the patient and the film to absorb the scatter radiation produced by the patient. Beam restrictors are located between the tube and the patient, reducing scatter radiation by limiting the size of the irradiated field. Limiting the irradiated field decreases the amount of scatter radiation (Compton effect) and subsequent radiographic fog. Thus, beam restrictors increase radiographic contrast and decrease the radiation exposure to the

patient. This effect is more significant with small field sizes (about 6 inches) than with large exposure fields. Scatter radiation produced from large fields (especially on large patients) is reduced more efficiently with grids. There are three types of beam restrictors. They are aperture diaphragms, cones or cylinders and the variable aperture collimator. This chapter discusses the types, function and quality control tests of beam restrictors.

APERTURE DIAPHRAGMS AND CONES AND CYLINDERS

APERTURE DIAPHRAGMS

The simplest type of beam restrictor is the aperture diaphragm. The aperture diaphragm is a thin sheet of lead or a lead-lined metal diaphragm with a fixed opening in the center (Figure 25–1). The opening determines the size and shape of the x-ray beam field. The size and shape of the opening varies from diaphragm to diaphragm. Because the opening is fixed, field sizes are altered by using different aperture diaphragms (Figure 25–2).

The aperture diaphragm attaches to the x-ray tube. Although the aperture diaphragm restricts the

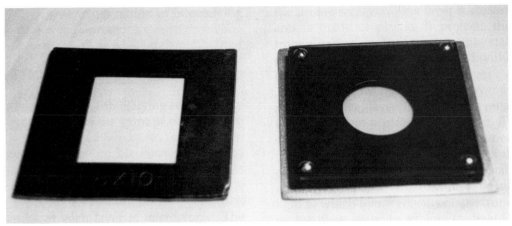

Figure 25–1. Aperture diaphragms with different field sizes.

beam, the edges of the aperture do experience some beam undercutting (Figure 25–3). This undercutting results in penumbra at the edge of the image. Thus, the edges of a coned field have a blurred instead of a sharp border.

In conventional radiography, aperture diaphragms are most commonly employed for specialized units for head radiography. These specialized units have a rod connecting the x-ray tube to the Bucky tray (Figure 25–4). The rod enables the tube to move in an arc while maintaining a fixed source-image distance (SID). Proper adjustment of the Bucky tray to the cassette size centers the x-ray tube to the film regardless of the angle of the central ray (Figure 25–5). Because aperture diaphragms have no method of showing the area to be irradiated

(i.e., light), automatic tube-to-Bucky centering assists in irradiating the correct area. By using the film scale markings located on the plastic head support (Figure 25–6), it is possible to position the patient's head to be centered to the film.

CONES AND CYLINDERS

Cones are metallic tubelike devices (often made of steel or brass) with two fixed circular apertures. One aperture is located at the top or apex of the cone and is closest to the x-ray tube. The other aperture, located at the base of the cone, is larger than the apex aperture.

Cones are usually cylindrical or conical (Figure 25–7). Conical beam restrictors are often referred to as flare cones. Cylindrical beam restrictors are called cylinders. Cylinders often have a telescope-type design. That is, the length of the cylinder may be increased by extending the telescope (Figures 25–7B and C).

The use of two apertures makes cones more efficient than the aperture diaphragm. However, they still permit x-ray beam undercutting (see Figure 25–3). Of the various types of cones, the extended cylinder has the least amount of undercutting.

Like aperture diaphragms, cones have fixed apertures. Thus, to alter the field size, the cone must be changed. Also, cones have no method of demonstrating the field to be irradiated. Consequently, it is difficult to position the patient correctly relative

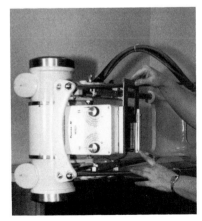

Figure 25–2. Aperture diaphragm being inserted in a Franklin head unit.

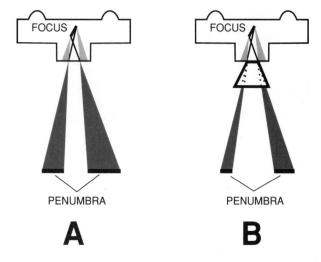

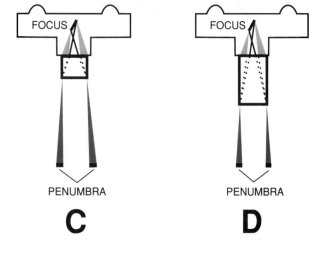

Figure 25–3. Effect of undercutting with aperture diaphragm *(A)*, flare cone *(B)*, unextended cylinder cone *(C)* and extended cylinder cone *(D)*.

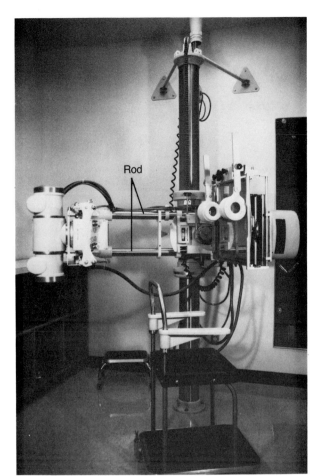

Rod

Figure 25–4. Franklin head unit.

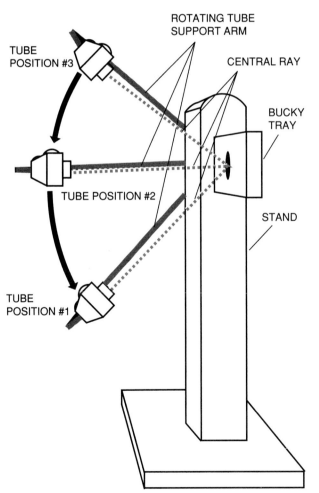

ROTATING TUBE
SUPPORT ARM

CENTRAL RAY

TUBE
POSITION #3

BUCKY
TRAY

TUBE POSITION #2

STAND

TUBE
POSITION #1

Figure 25–5. Proper Bucky tray setting permits the central ray to be directed to the center of the film regardless of the x-ray tube angle.

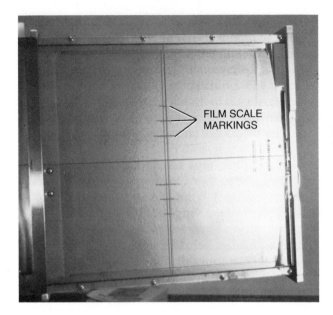

Figure 25–6. Franklin head unit support (located over Bucky tray), demonstrating film scale markings.

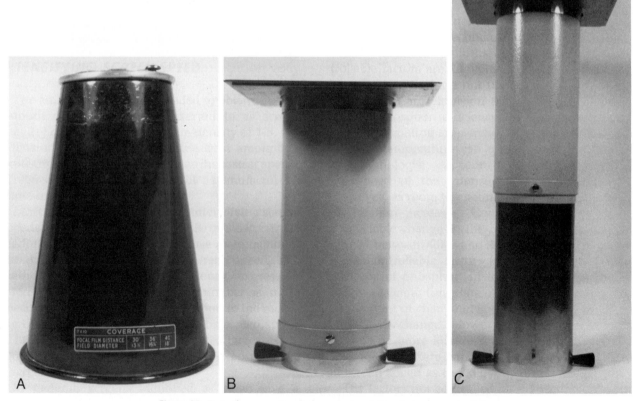

Figure 25–7. *A,* Flare cone; *B,* cylinder cone closed; *C,* cylinder cone extended.

to the field size. Patient positioning is especially critical with small field sizes (10 inches or less).

As mentioned above, cones have circular apertures. Film holders are rectangular. Completely exposing a rectangular film holder with a circular cone results in unnecessary exposure to the patient and increased scatter radiation (Figure 25–8). Thus, to utilize cones correctly, complete irradiation of the film should be avoided.

Cones are rarely used in conventional imaging departments. Cones are most often used in dental radiography. The use of cones in imaging departments is generally limited to examinations of areas entailing small field sizes, e.g., sinuses. This is often achieved by attaching a cylinder cone to a collimator.

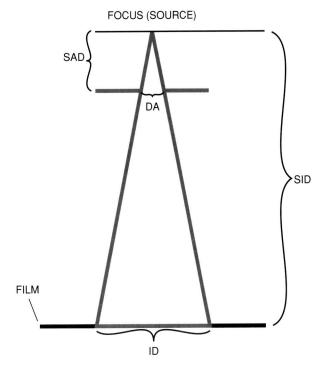

SAD = SOURCE - CONTROLLING APERTURE DISTANCE
DA = DIAMETER OF CONTROLLING APERTURE
SID = SOURCE - IMAGE DISTANCE
ID = IMAGE DIAMETER

Figure 25–9. Similar triangles (from focus to diameter of controlling aperture and from focus to image diameter) are used to determine the size of the irradiated field (image diameter).

CALCULATING IMAGE DIAMETER

Through the use of similar triangles (Figure 25–9), it is possible to determine the diameter of the image (irradiated field). The following information is needed to calculate the diameter of the image:
Source to controlling aperture distance (SAD)
Source-image distance (SID)
Diameter of the controlling aperture (DA).
The controlling aperture is the opening that restricts the beam. In the cylinder cone, this is the lower aperture. The lower aperture of most flare cones tends to taper at a greater angle than the x-ray beam. Consequently, the upper aperture restricts the beam size. The aperture diaphragm has only one opening, which serves as the controlling aperture.

The mathematical expression for determining the image diameter is

$$ID = (SID/SAD)DA$$

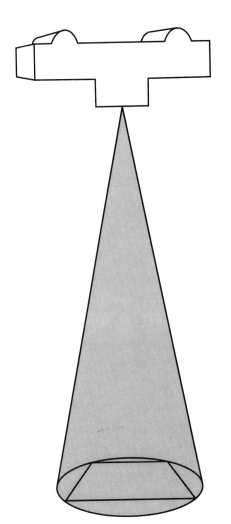

Figure 25–8. Completely exposing a rectangular film holder with a circular cone causes radiation exposure outside the film area.

where ID is the image diameter, SID is the source-image distance, SAD represents the source to controlling aperture distance and DA is the diameter of the controlling aperture. For example, a radiograph is taken at a 40 inch SID using a cylinder cone. The lower aperture of the cylinder is 3 inches and the distance from the target to the lower aperture of the cylinder is 8 inches. The diameter of the image (in inches) is

$$
\begin{aligned}
ID &= (40/8)3 \\
&= (5)3 \\
&= 15
\end{aligned}
$$

By knowing the diameter of the image, it is possible to determine if the irradiated field fits on a specific film size. This is achieved by comparing the shortest distance (width) of the film to the ID (Figure 25–10). For the entire irradiated field to fit on a film, the image diameter must be equal to or less than the width of the film. The image diameter formula is an accurate method for determining the irradiated field. However, in practice, the technologist rarely uses cones, making the application of the formula almost nonexistent.

VARIABLE APERTURE COLLIMATORS

CONSTRUCTION AND FUNCTION

The most common and efficient beam restrictor is the variable aperture collimator, usually referred to as simply a collimator. This type of beam restrictor is a boxlike device that attaches to the x-ray tube (Figure 25–11). Although the specific components may vary, most collimators consist of an entrance shutter, lead leaf shutters, a light source and a mirror (Figure 25–12).

The entrance shutters are located at the top of the collimator. These shutters are useful in decreasing the off-focus radiation (see under Off-focus Radiation). Below the entrance shutters are two sets of paired lead leaf shutters. The sets are located at two different levels (Figure 25–13). Each pair of lead leaf shutters functions as an aperture to restrict the beam. One pair moves in a transverse direction relative to the x-ray table. The other pair moves in a longitudinal direction relative to the x-ray table. The shutter opening (aperture) is adjusted by turning a knob on the front of the collimator. This in turn activates a pulley system that moves the shut-

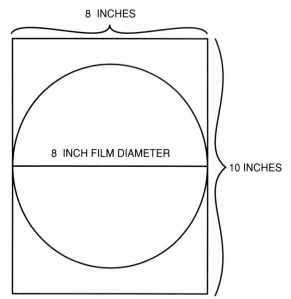

Figure 25–10. To ensure that the irradiated field of the cone is on the film, the shortest part of the film diameter must be compared to the diameter of the irradiated field. In this example, the diameter of the circle cannot exceed 8 inches (film width).

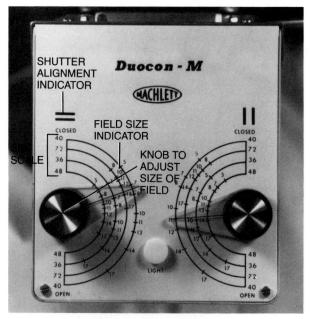

Figure 25–11. Variable aperture collimator.

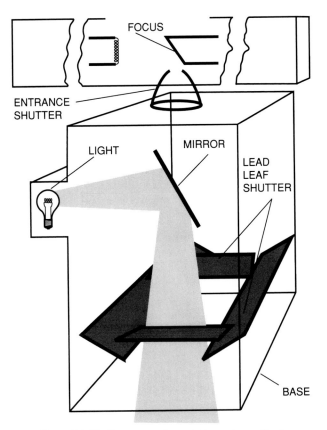

Figure 25–12. Components of a variable aperture collimator.

tor. To project the light toward an object, a mirror (which is radiolucent) is placed below the x-ray tube port at a 45 degree angle to the light source (see Figure 25–12). For proper light projection, the distance from the focus to the mirror must be the same as the distance from the light source to the mirror. The center of the light is usually identified by a plastic sheet with cross lines (Figure 25–14) at the base (port) of the collimator. The lines produce a shadow on the object, identifying the entrance point of the central ray (Figure 25–15).

The mirror and plastic port of the collimator tend to filter some radiation. This does not significantly affect most routine radiographic work. However, it can make a marked difference in radiographic work that uses low kilovoltages, e.g., mammography.

Care must be taken when using a collimator light to properly identify the irradiated field. Recall that a light image is affected by the distance from the light source to the object. The light image provided by the collimator (source) is projected on the top of the patient (object). The closer the patient is to the collimator, the smaller the image of the light field (Figure 25–16). This light image represents the field size of the entrance radiation. The exiting or rem-

ters. Unlike aperture diaphragms and cones, the collimator (via its pulley system) provides an infinite number of field sizes.

The light source and mirror are used to simulate the irradiated field. The light source is a high intensity bulb, which enables the technologist to view its illumination on the object in a well-lit room. To prevent the light bulb from being left on and burning out, it is attached to a timer. The timer allows the light to remain lit for about 30 seconds before it automatically shuts the light off. If the light does burn out, there is a scale on the front of the collimator near the shutter knobs identifying the shutter knob position needed to obtain a specific field size (see Figure 25–11). The scale allows the technologist to set a field size relative to a specific SID.

Because light bulbs are radiopaque, they cannot be placed in the path of the x-ray beam. Rather, they are located on the side or back of the collima-

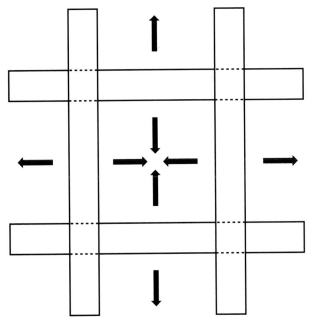

Figure 25–13. Top view of paired lead leaf shutters and the direction of their movement.

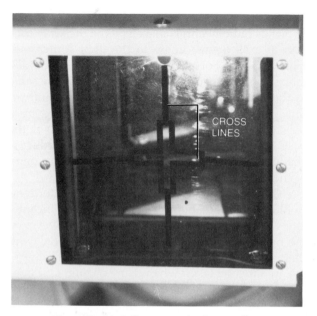

Figure 25–14. Collimator port showing cross lines.

nant radiation field size is larger than the entrance radiation. To avoid unnecessary radiation to the patient, the technologists must never readjust the entrance light image (light seen on the patient) to coincide with the desired remnant radiation field size.

Some collimators have a track at the base to allow the attachment of a cylinder cone. The attachment of a cylinder further improves the efficiency of the collimator. When a cylinder cone is attached to the collimator, it is possible for the collimator shutter to be set larger than the desired field size. This is a result of the opaque metal cylinder attachment's blocking out the collimator light. Consequently, it is recommended that care be taken to ensure that the field size set corresponds to the desired field size. This may be achieved by using the shutter knob scales for field size.

POSITIVE BEAM LIMITING DEVICE

In 1974, U.S. government regulations were implemented requiring x-ray equipment to provide positive beam limiting (PBL) devices. These devices automatically control the beam field size. This is achieved by using sensors in the Bucky tray that detect the size of the film and its orientation (transverse or longitudinal). The sensors are activated when a cassette is locked in the tray. The sensors then send an electronic signal to the collimator. This activates a synchronous motor that adjusts the collimator leaves to correspond to the film size and orientation.

PBL devices have an override switch that allows the technologist to disengage the sensors, enabling the technologist to adjust the field size manually. If the PBL is turned off, the technologist should adjust the field size by decreasing it. Unfortunately, some technologists increase the field size, causing unnecessary radiation exposure to the patient.

OFF-FOCUS RADIATION

Most radiation concepts and theories are explained by identifying the source of radiation as a point on the anode of the x-ray tube called the target or focus. However, in reality, some electrons traveling from the cathode to the anode strike areas outside the target, producing radiation. This type of radiation is called off-focus radiation. Estimates of how much of the primary beam is off-focus radiation range from a low of 8% to a high of 25%. It is estimated that off-focus radiation increases patient exposure by 10–20%. Thus, decreasing off-focus radiation decreases patient exposure. The most efficient method of reducing off-focus radiation is to place a PBL device as close as possible to the target. The collimator achieves this by having the entrance shutters positioned in the tube housing.

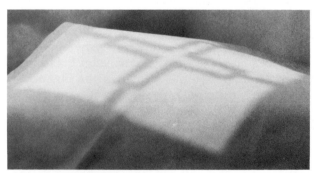

Figure 25–15. Collimator light on object demonstrating how shadows of cross lines identify the central ray.

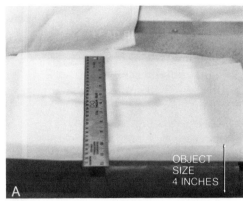

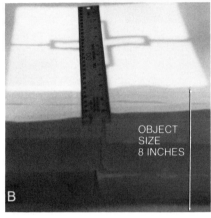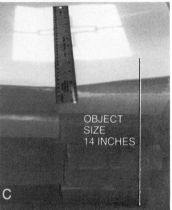

Figure 25–16. For a given source-image distance and field size setting, the larger the object is, the smaller the image of the light projected on the object (assuming the field size setting remains the same).

QUALITY CONTROL TESTS FOR BEAM RESTRICTORS

It is important that the light emitted from the collimator accurately represent the correct irradiated field size and alignment. If the light is larger than the field size, the object of interest may be coned off, requiring a repeated radiograph. Misrepresentation of the irradiated field may be caused by a misaligned mirror, a shift in the light bulb filament or a slippage of the pulley system. These problems can occur if the x-ray tube is hit, e.g., the tube may hit the table during movement, or result from maintenance or repair work on the x-ray tube, tube enclosure or collimator. A template is used to test the accuracy of the light in representing the irradiated field size and alignment.

Besides the accuracy of the light in indicating the irradiated field size and alignment, an important factor is that the angle of the central ray to the image receptor (film) be 90 degrees. Improper align-

ment of the central ray to the film may cause misalignment of the beam to the grid, resulting in unwanted absorption of the primary beam. Thus, to compensate for the primary beam loss, the technical variables are increased, resulting in unnecessary radiation exposure to the patient. Central ray alignment is tested by using a plastic cylinder containing two steel balls.

LIGHT PROJECTION OF IRRADIATED FIELD AND ALIGNMENT

As mentioned above, a template is used to measure the collimator light's ability to represent the irradiated field size and alignment. A template may be homemade or commercially produced. The template is a thin flat plate with two radiopaque rulers (perpendicular to each other) marked in either inches or centimeters (Figure 25–17). The ruler increments begin at zero (usually located in the

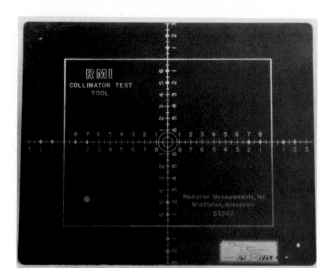

Figure 25–17. Beam template.

center of the template) and increase with the distance from the center of the template. If a template is unavailable, the test may be performed by using any small L-shaped radiopaque objects, e.g., wire or paper clips.

If the test is performed using a template, a cassette is placed on the x-ray table. The table is checked to ensure that it is level. The template is positioned on top of the cassette. A SID commonly employed for examinations, e.g., 40 inches, is set. The light is adjusted so that it coincides with the rectangular outline on the template (this should be smaller than the film size). Lead letters and numbers may be employed on the template to identify the anode side, the date and the room number. If the film is identified with lead, care should be taken to avoid placing the lead too close to the light borders or the center of the light field. After the equipment is properly set up, the cassette is exposed.

The radiographic image of the template demonstrates the location of the irradiated field over the ruler (Figure 25–18). The accuracy of the light is determined by recording where the irradiated field falls on the ruler (penumbra is not included in the measurement). Federal (U.S.) standards require that the light representation be within 2% of the SID employed. For example, for a 40 inch (100 cm) SID, the maximum misalignment of light and irradiated field is 0.8 inch (2 cm).

The procedure to test the relationship of the light

to the field size and alignment using L-shaped radiopaque objects is the same as for the template, with three minor variations. These involve the manner in which the light is set, the placement of the radiopaque object and the number of exposures. The first variation is to adjust the light so that it is about 2 inches smaller than the film. In the absence of a ruler, the second variation requires that an L-shaped object be placed at each corner of the light field. After these alterations are made, the cassette is exposed. After the exposure and without anything being moved, the light is opened to the size of the cassette. A second exposure (double exposure) is made on the cassette. The second exposure is performed to ensure that the radiopaque objects appear on the radiograph. Two exposures are used because a single exposure made of an irradiated field that is smaller than the light projection would result in cone cutting of one or more of the opaque objects (the object would not appear on the radiograph).

The radiographic image demonstrates four L-shaped objects (Figure 25–19). The objects represent the light field. A ruler is used to measure any differences between the light projected and the irradiated field borders.

Regardless of the test instrument used, the radiographic image is also checked for beam alignment. The federal government requires that the central ray be within 2% of the SID of the center of the film. This is determined by drawing diagonal lines from the corner of the film and from the irradiated

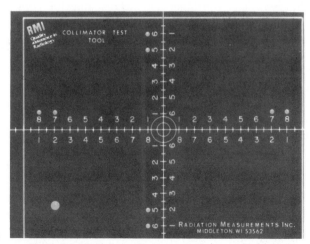

Figure 25–18. Radiographic image of a beam template test.

Figure 25–19. Radiographic image of a beam restrictor test using L-shaped objects.

field (Figure 25–20). The distance between the film lines' intersection and the irradiated field lines' intersection is measured. The measurement should not exceed 2% of the SID.

CENTRAL RAY ANGLE

As stated above, the central ray should make a 90 degree angle with the film. The angle of the central ray is tested by using two radiopaque spheres or balls ($\frac{1}{16}$ inch in diameter) mounted 6 inches apart directly above each other. This type of

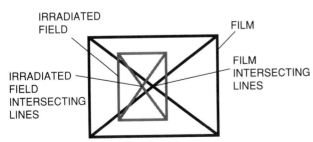

Figure 25–20. To assess the relationship of the center of the irradiated field and the film center, draw diagonal lines from the corners of the film and irradiated field, respectively, and compare the distance between the intersections.

testing tool is available commercially. The instrument has two $\frac{1}{16}$ inch steel balls, one located directly above the other, with both embedded in a 6 inch plastic cylinder (Figure 25–21).

The central ray test may be done separately or in conjunction with the light projection of the irradiated field and alignment tests. If the central ray test is performed with the light test, the cylinder is placed in the center of the template. Otherwise, a cassette is placed on a level x-ray table and the cylinder is positioned on top of the cassette. The center of the projected light is placed over the steel balls. A white piece of paper may be placed under the cylinder to assist in positioning the light so that it is directly over the balls. This is achieved by turning the light on and moving the tube until the shadows from the spheres are superimposed on the paper. After the beam is positioned, an exposure is made.

The radiographic image reveals the steel balls and

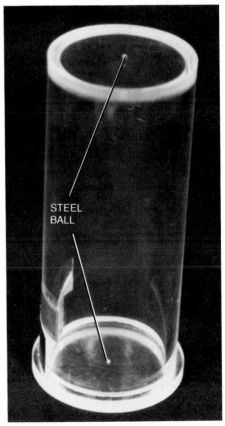

Figure 25–21. Plastic cylinder with steel balls used for testing central beam angle.

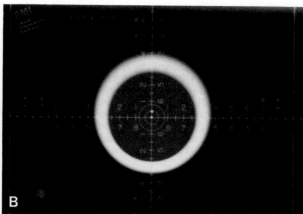

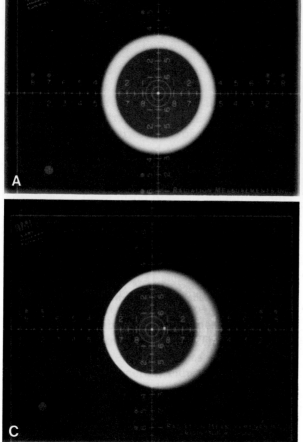

Figure 25–22. Radiograph of central ray angle (alignment) test. *A,* Correct alignment (balls superimposed); *B* 1.5 degree misalignment (ball is on inner circle); *C,* 3 degree misalignment (ball is on outer circle).

two circles (an inner circle and outer circle, if a beam template is also used). A perpendicular beam demonstrates the steel balls superimposed and in the center of the circles (Figure 25–22). If the balls are superimposed, the central ray is perpendicular to within 0.5 degree. If the image of the top ball is located on the line of the inner circle, the central ray is about 1.5 degrees away from the perpendicular. Location of the top ball image on the line of the outer circle indicates that the central ray is misaligned by 3 degrees. Images demonstrating the ball on the second circle or farther away from the center are unacceptable.

LABORATORY EXPERIENCE

Additional laboratory experience relative to beam restrictors may be obtained by performing Laboratory 41, X-ray Beam and Light Projected, in *Concepts in Medical Radiographic Imaging: Laboratory Manual.* This laboratory provides the experimenter with the opportunity to perform three quality control tests. They are the light projection relative to the irradiated field, alignment of the irradiated field and the central ray angle test. These tests are performed in accordance with the procedures described under Quality Control Tests for Beam Restrictors.

Besides obtaining the routine images from the test instruments, after performing the light projection relative to the irradiated field test, the researcher plots the light projected and the irradiated field on graph paper. This provides a visual impression of the relationship of the light to the x-ray beam.

Bibliography

Bushong, SC. Radiologic science for technologists (4th edition). St. Louis: Mosby, 1988.

Carroll, QB. Fuchs's Principles of radiographic exposure, processing and quality control (3rd edition). Springfield, IL: Thomas, 1985.

Chesney, DN and Chesney, MO. X-ray equipment for student radiographers (3rd edition). Boston: Blackwell Scientific Publications, 1984.

Cullinan, AM. Producing quality radiographs. New York: Lippincott, 1987.

Cullinan, JE and Cullinan, AM. Illustrated guide to x-ray technics (2nd edition). New York: Lippincott Co, 1980.

Curry, TS, Dowdey, JE and Murry, RC. Christensen's Introduction to the physics of diagnostic radiology (3rd edition). Philadelphia: Lea & Febiger, 1984.

Donohue, DP. An analysis of radiographic quality (2nd printing). Baltimore: University Park Press, 1982.

Eastman Kodak Company. Fundamentals of radiography (12th ed.) Rochester, NY: Eastman Kodak Company, 1980.

Graham, BJ and Thomas, WN. An introduction to physics for radiologic technologists. Philadelphia: Saunders, 1975.

Gray, JE, et al. Quality control in diagnostic imaging. Baltimore: University Park Press, 1983.

Hendee, WR, Chaney, EL and Rossi, RP. Radiologic physics, equipment and quality control. Chicago: Year Book Medical, 1976.

Hiss, SS. Understanding radiography. Springfield, IL: Thomas, 1980.

McLemore, J. Quality assurance in diagnostic radiology. Chicago: Year Book Medical, 1981.

Selman, J. The fundamentals of x-ray and radium physics (7th edition). Springfield, IL: Thomas, 1985.

Ter-Pogossian, MM. The physical aspects of diagnostic radiology. New York: Harper & Row, 1967.

Thompson, TT. Cahoon's Formulating x-ray techniques (9th edition). Durham, NC: Duke University Press, 1979.

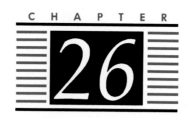

GEOMETRIC IMAGE QUALITY

MICHAEL MIXDORF and MARIANNE TORTORICI

INTRODUCTION

Radiographs contain images of the objects irradiated. In medicine, these objects are the various anatomical parts of the human body. The more accurately the radiographic image reflects the true size and shape of the real object, the better the radiographic quality. Geometric and photographic factors influence radiographic quality. Photographic factors include density and contrast. These are discussed in Chapter 27, Photographic Image Quality. Geometric radiographic quality is affected by magnification, distortion, sharpness and resolution.

Among the geometric factors, magnification (sometimes referred to as size distortion) is the amount of enlargement of an object. Distortion relates to uneven magnification of an object, often observed as a misrepresentation of the object's shape (sometimes called shape distortion). Sharpness is the degree of distinction of the outline (border) of an object. Resolution is the ability of the image to produce clarity (detail) between structures located close to one another (often expressed as the number of line pairs per centimeter seen clearly). Resolution is related to the degree of sharpness and the amount of contrast.

This chapter concentrates on discussions of magnification, distortion, sharpness and resolution. It also considers the technical factors that influence

magnification, distortion, resolution and sharpness (Table 26–1). Each factor is presented separately. However, these topics are related and a change in one factor may alter another or affect photographic image quality. For example, decreasing magnification by the use of a long source-image distance (SID) necessitates an increase in technical variables. This may entail the use of a large focal spot size, causing a decrease in sharpness. As seen by this example, it is not unusual to set a technique that might compromise another factor. Practical experience is the best method of determining how much of a compromise is acceptable.

MAGNIFICATION

DEFINITION

In radiographic magnification, the image recorded on the film maintains the same shape as the object it represents but is larger than the actual object. Sometimes, magnification is preferred (e.g., for cerebral angiography); however, in most clinical radiographic examinations, magnification of an object is undesirable.

The amount of magnification (magnification factor) can be determined by dividing the image size (IS) by the object size (OS), or magnification is equal

Table 26–1. COMMON FACTORS INFLUENCING GEOMETRIC IMAGE QUALITY*

Factor	Original	New	Effect on Geometric Image Quality
Source-image distance	100 cm	180 cm	Increase
Object-film distance	10 cm	20 cm	Decrease
Source-object distance	60 cm	80 cm	Increase
Central ray	90°	45°	Decrease
Focal spot size	1 mm	2 mm	Decrease
Beam restrictor	Diaphragm	Collimator	Increase
Intensifying screen speed	100	200	Decrease
Film crystal size	Large	Small	Increase
Film-screen contact	Good	Poor	Decrease

*All ancillary imaging methods and techniques remain constant from the original factor to the new factor. The only change is represented by the factor listed.

to IS/OS. No magnification exists if the answer is 1. For example, if the image is 15 cm and the object is 15 cm, the magnification is 1, or $^{15}\!/_{15} = 1$. Answers greater than 1 indicate the amount of magnification. For example, if the object is 15 cm and the image is 18 cm, the magnification factor is 1.2, or $^{18}\!/_{15} = 1.2$. Because the number 1 represents the true size of the object, the actual enlargement, relative to the true object, is 0.2. Another method of expressing this concept is as a percentage.

The percentage of magnification is expressed mathematically as

$$\frac{IS - OS}{OS} \times 100$$

For the previous example, the percentage of magnification of the object is 20%, or

$$\frac{18 - 15}{15} \times 100$$

$$^{3}\!/_{15} \times 100$$

$$0.20(100)$$

$$20$$

PRINCIPAL INFLUENCING FACTORS

The principal factors influencing magnification are source-image distance, source-object distance (SOD) and object-film distance (OFD). These are important because they can be used to calculate the amount of magnification. The following is a discussion of the effect of these distances on magnification.

From a clinical standpoint, the object size is usually what is being sought. In the examples above, the object size is unable to be calculated because the formulas would have two unknowns (magnification and object size). However, it is possible to use SID, IS (which can be measured on the film) and SOD (usually able to be estimated with a good deal of accuracy by knowing human anatomy) to determine the object size. The concept of similar triangles provides a means of utilizing this information to calculate the true size of the object (Figure 26–1).

In Figure 26–1, note that from the x-ray tube to the object is one triangle and from the x-ray tube to the film is another triangle. In accordance with the laws of similar triangles, it can be said that the SID divided by the SOD equals the IS divided by the OS, or SID/SOD = IS/OS.

From this formula, it can be seen that, as the ratio of the SID to the SOD increases, the IS increases, assuming a constant OS. To demonstrate this concept, two examples for an object measuring 15 cm follow. In example A, the SID is 100 cm, the SOD is 80 cm for an SID to SOD ratio of 1.25 ($^{100}\!/_{80} = 1.25$). Example B has a SID of 100 cm, an SOD of 50 cm for an SID/SOD ratio of 2 ($^{100}\!/_{50} = 2$). The following mathematical calculations for these examples demonstrate that, as the SID/SOD ratio increases, the IS also increases.

Example A
SID/SOD = IS/OS
$^{100}\!/_{80} = ^{x}\!/_{15}$
$80x = 1500$
$x = 18.75$

Example B
SID/SOD = IS/OS
$^{100}\!/_{50} = ^{x}\!/_{15}$
$50x = 1500$
$x = 30$

Recall that the SID is equal to the sum of the SOD and the OFD (SID = SOD + OFD). In the preceding two examples, the SID was constant (100 cm, or 40 inches), while the SOD changed. This altered the OFD. Thus, in the preceding examples,

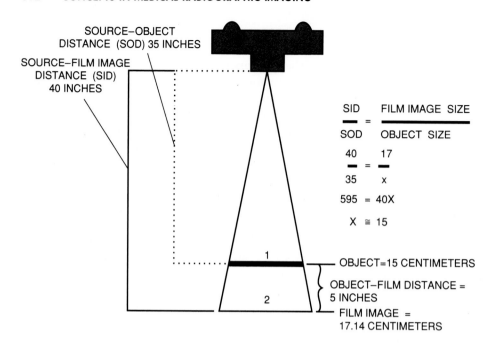

$$\frac{SID}{SOD} = \frac{FILM\ IMAGE\ SIZE}{OBJECT\ SIZE}$$

$$\frac{40}{35} = \frac{17}{x}$$

$$595 = 40X$$

$$X \cong 15$$

Figure 26–1. Similar triangles relationship for determining the magnification of an object. Triangle 1 is formed by tube focus and SOD. Triangle 2 is formed by tube focus and SID.

when the SOD changed from 80 to 50, the OFD changed from 20 cm (or $100 - 80 = 20$) to 50 cm (or $100 - 50 = 50$). Consequently, it can be concluded that, for a constant SID, using a short OFD (in this case 20 cm) decreases the IS or magnification factor. A clinical application is to position the patient so that the object of interest is closest to the film, e.g., to demonstrate the heart, use a posterior-anterior position.

A second method of altering the SID/SOD ratio is to maintain a constant OFD and change the SID. Using the previous examples, to determine the effect of increasing the SID for a 15 cm object at a constant OFD (20 cm), it is necessary to recalculate the IS in example B (example A has a 20 cm OFD and is used as the base). In the new example B, the OFD remains constant (20 cm); if the SID is increased to 180 cm (72 inches) from 100 cm, the new SOD is 160 cm ($180 = SOD + 20$, or $180 - 20 = SOD$, or $SOD = 160$). Thus, the new IS is 16.875, or

New Example B
$$SID/SOD = IS/OS$$
$$180/160 = x/15$$
$$160x = 2700$$
$$X = 16.875$$

The new example demonstrates that increasing the SID while maintaining a constant OFD decreases the IS or magnification factor.

As with IS and OS, it is possible to determine the percentage of magnification by using the SOD and OFD. The formula is OFD/SOD $\times$ 100. For example, if the OFD is 20 cm and the SOD is 80 cm, the percentage of magnification is 25% ($^{20}/_{80} \times 100 = 25$).

In summary, the least amount of magnification occurs when the shortest possible OFD and longest possible SID (which results in a low SID/SOD ratio) is employed. One practical application of this concept is in the case in which a traction setup on a patient creates a large OFD. In this instance, the magnification may be reduced by increasing the SID.

DISTORTION

DEFINITION

Distortion is unequal magnification of different parts of an object or between two objects. Uneven magnification may appear as an enlargement of the object or as a change in the shape of the object.

Distortion is a function of object thickness, the position of the object in the body and the angular relationship among the x-ray beam, the film and the object.

PRINCIPAL INFLUENCING FACTORS

Recall that object thickness influences distortion. Because objects have three dimensions, distortion and magnification occur with all the dimensions within an object. The difference in distortion is minimal for extremely thin objects. However, thick objects have different SID to SOD ratios at the top and base of the object (Figure 26–2). This results in uneven magnification (size distortion) of the object.

Another factor affecting distortion is the position of the object in the body. Any change in the SID/SOD ratio creates uneven magnification. The relationship of two objects to their SID/SOD ratio and position from the central ray affects the amount of

distortion imaged. The distance from the central ray or film of an object relative to that of another object may result in a misrepresentation of the true positions (spatial distortion) of the two objects (Figure 26–3). This false image is a result of the uneven magnification of the objects.

Lastly, the alignment of the object relative to the central ray and the film influences distortion. Objects that are not perpendicular to the central ray or parallel to the film become distorted. This distortion is usually seen as a misrepresentation of the shape of the object. There are several ways that the object may be misaligned relative to the central ray and the film. These include the location of the object relative to the central ray, the angulation of the x-ray tube, the angulation of the object and the angulation of the film.

An object may be located in the body so that it is lateral to (to the side of) the central ray. Figure 26–4 represents the effect of a round object's lateral location relative to the central ray. It can be noted

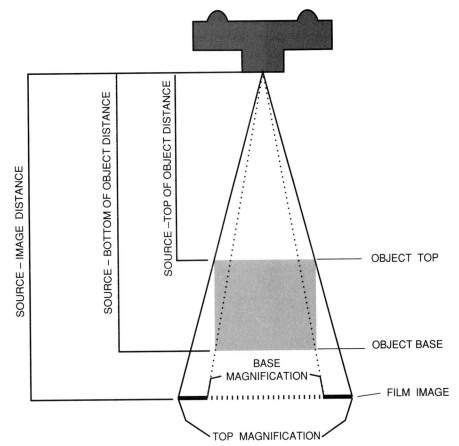

Figure 26–2. Distortion (uneven magnification) of a thick object.

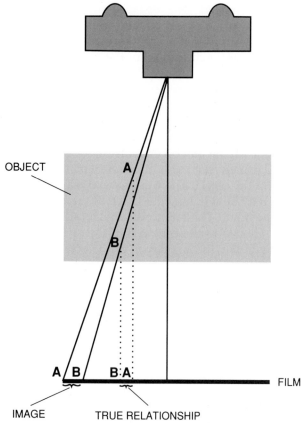

Figure 26–3. Spatial distortion. The true relationship of A to B is that B is more lateral than A. However, the radiographic image of the objects (A, B) demonstrates object A to be more lateral than B.

of an object. The density change may be measured by a microdensitometer (a densitometer designed to measure minor changes in density). It is possible to plot a graph of the measurements obtained from a microdensitometer. The vertical axis of the graph measures density and the horizontal axis records distance in millimeters (measurements taken across the film). For example, an object with perfect sharp-

that, as the object moves lateral to the central ray, the round object is distorted and appears as an ellipse.

When the object is in the path of the central ray, but if the tube, the object or the film is angled (Figure 26–5), there is a misrepresentation of the object's shape.

Although in most radiographic examinations distortion is undesirable, sometimes it is used to visualize objects that may be superimposed. Common methods that use distortion to an advantage are angulation of the object (e.g., an oblique view of the wrist) and tube angulation (e.g., Towne's view of the skull).

SHARPNESS

DEFINITION

The sharpness of an image refers to the variation of density changes visualized on the border (edge)

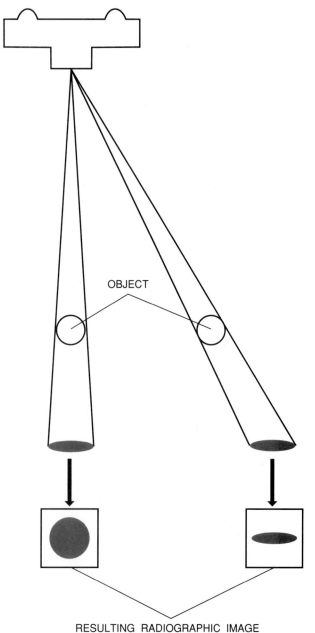

Figure 26–4. The farther an object is from the central ray, the more distorted it becomes.

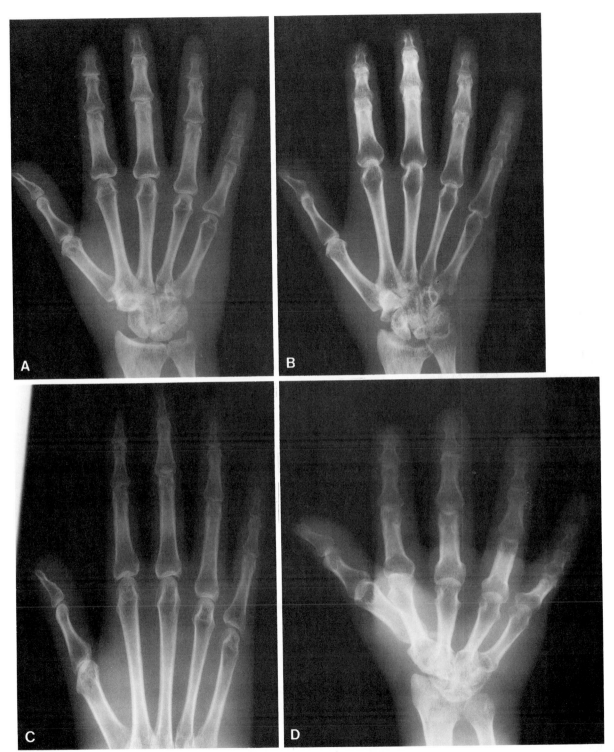

Figure 26–5. The object represented in the normal radiographic image (A) is elongated when the tube is angled (B) or the film is angled (C) and is foreshortened with an angulation of the object (D).

ness has no variation of densities at the edge (Figure 26–6). This results in a perpendicular plot of the edge (Figure 26–7A). As the sharpness decreases (becomes unsharp), the amount of density variations seen at the edge of the object increases, creating a sloped line plot of the edge (Figure 26–7B). The density variation is often referred to as penumbra (edge gradient or unsharpness).

PRINCIPAL INFLUENCING FACTORS

The first item influencing sharpness is focal spot size. The name focal spot is misleading because it leads one to believe that x-rays are emitted from a point (spot). However, the effective focal spot is usually rectangular. Consequently, x-rays are emit-

ted from various points of the focus. Penumbra can be illustrated by extending the ends of the focal spot to produce an image of an object (Figure 26–8). Notice in Figure 26–8 that more penumbra exists toward the cathode end of the x-ray tube (heel effect). Thus, objects that should be imaged with sharpness should be placed toward the anode end of the x-ray tube.

Other factors influencing sharpness are the size of the focal spot, OFD and SOD. Similar triangles can be used to calculate penumbra. This relationship can be expressed mathematically as penumbra (P) divided by the focal spot size (FSS) equals the OFD divided by the SOD, or P/FSS = OFD/SOD. By rearranging the formula algebraically, it is possible to determine the relationship of FSS, OFD and SOD to penumbra. Mathematically, this becomes

$$P/FSS = OFD/SOD$$
$$P(SOD) = FSS(OFD)$$
$$P = \frac{FSS(OFD)}{SOD}$$

The formula reveals that an increase in the numerator (an increase in FSS or OFD) creates an increase in penumbra, assuming that the SOD is constant (Figures 26–9 and 26–10). Also, with a constant numerator (OFD and FSS remain the same), increasing SOD (which results in an increase in SID when OFD is constant) decreases penumbra (Figure 26–11). It can be concluded that, to obtain minimal amount of penumbra, the following should be used:
1. Smallest possible effective FSS
2. Shortest possible OFD
3. Longest possible SID.

Besides FSS, OFD and SOD, beam restrictors also affect penumbra. Beam restrictors limit the area of exposure on the patient. The area of exposure is confined to the anatomical area of interest. Restricting the x-ray beam to the area of interest improves the ability to see the detail of the related anatomical feature.

Currently, there are three types of beam restrictors. From least efficient to most efficient, they are aperture diaphragms, extension cylinder, cones and the most common, the radiographic collimator. All beam restrictors allow some beam undercutting. The less efficient beam restrictors produce more penumbra, decreasing the geometric image quality.

In addition to being caused by technical factors,

Text continued on page 322

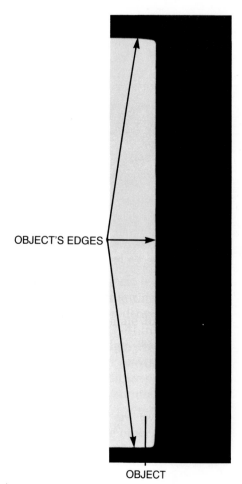

Figure 26–6. A sharp image demonstrating a distinct edge.

OBJECT'S EDGES

OBJECT

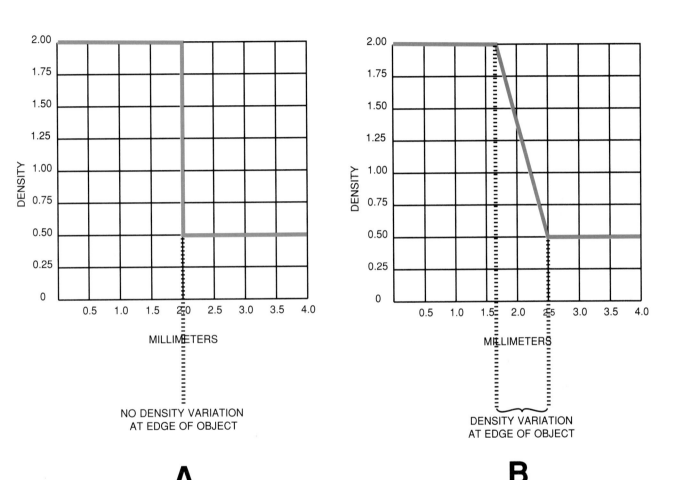

Figure 26–7. Plot of microdensitometer readings for a sharp image (A) and an image with a 1 mm degree of unsharpness (B).

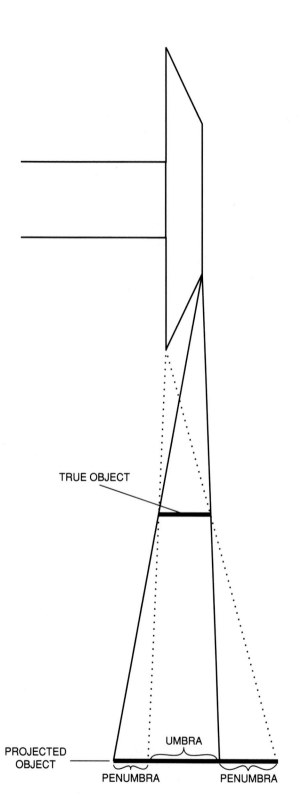

TRUE OBJECT

PROJECTED
OBJECT

UMBRA

PENUMBRA   PENUMBRA

Figure 26–8. Effect of focal spot on penumbra.

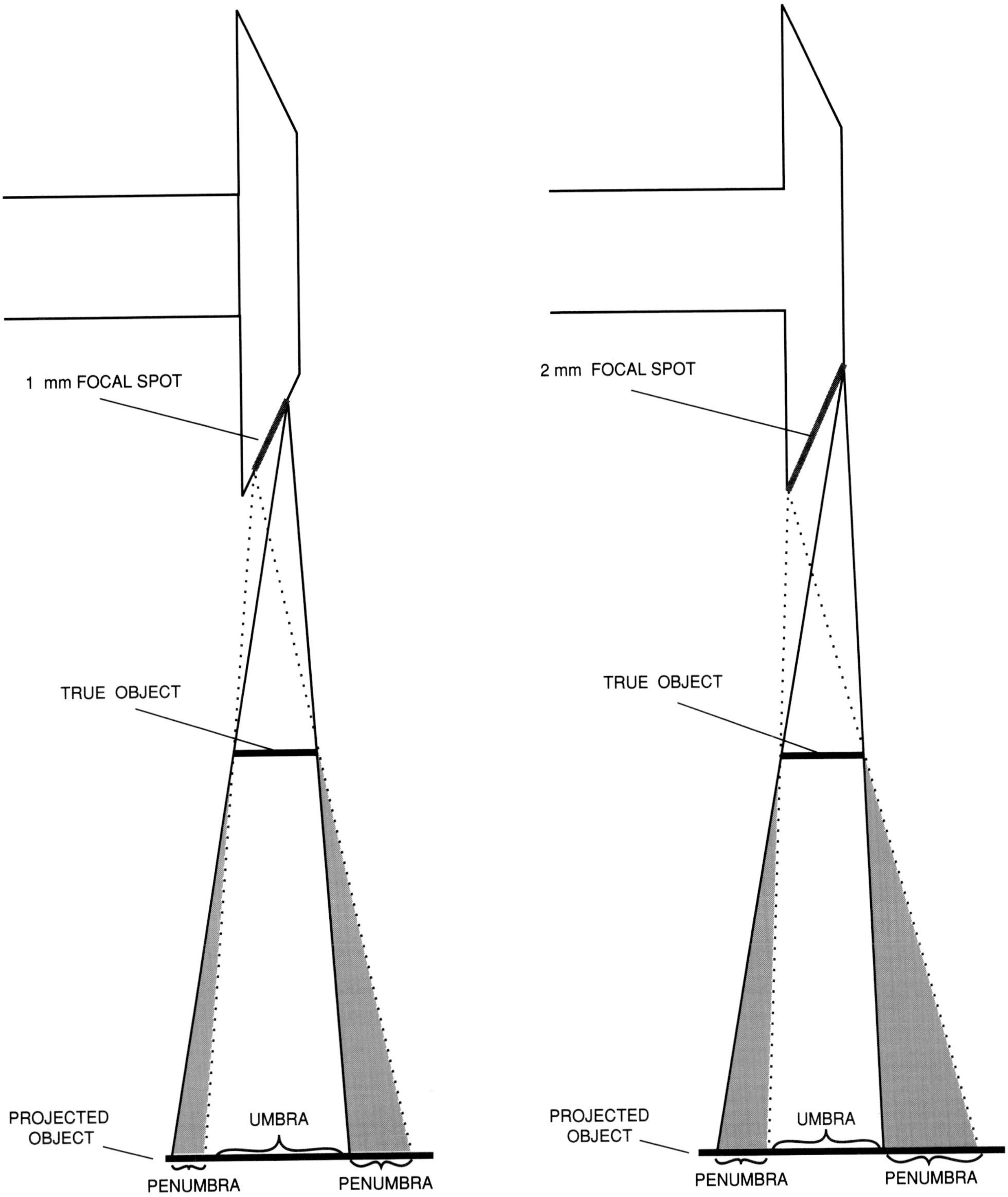

Figure 26–9. Penumbra increases as the effective focal spot size increases.

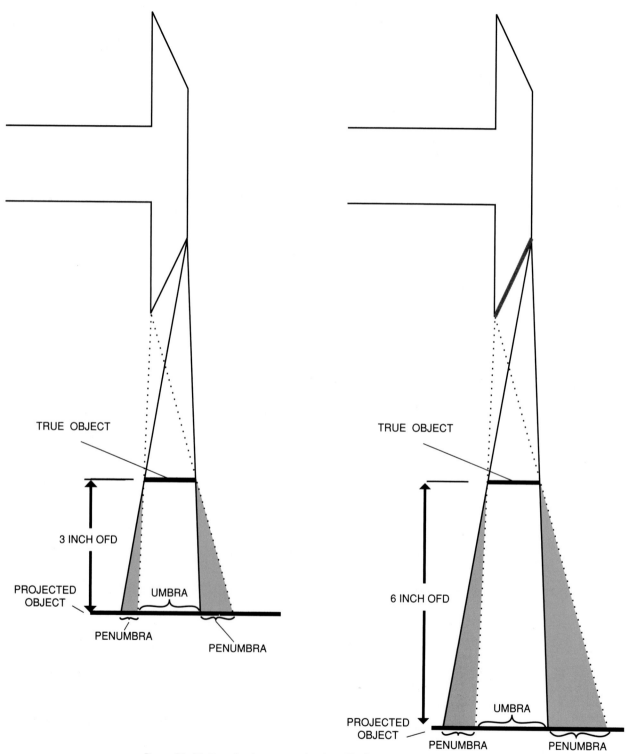

TRUE OBJECT

3 INCH OFD

PROJECTED
OBJECT

UMBRA

PENUMBRA

PENUMBRA

TRUE OBJECT

6 INCH OFD

PROJECTED
OBJECT

UMBRA

PENUMBRA

PENUMBRA

Figure 26–10. Penumbra increases as the object-film distance (OFD) increases.

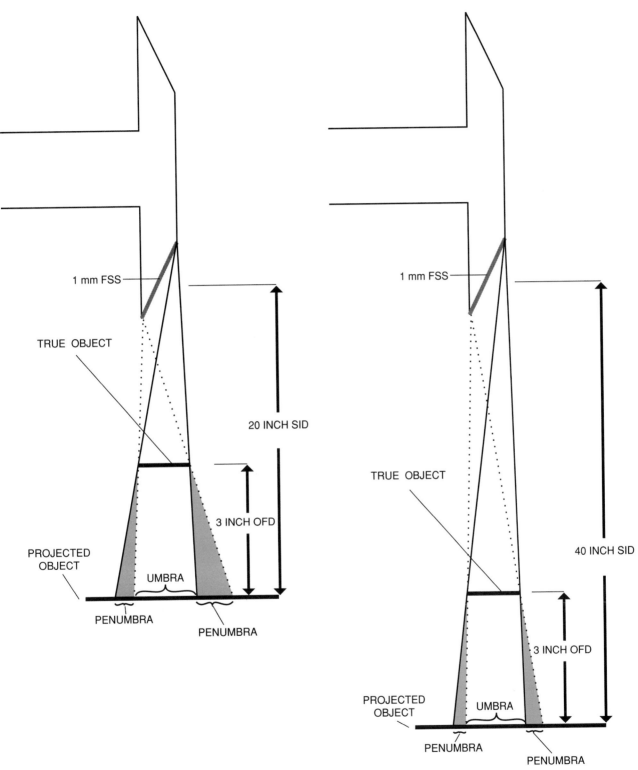

Figure 26–11. Penumbra decreases as the source-image distance (SID) increases.

e.g., FSS, unsharpness may result from the subject itself in the form of motion unsharpness. Motion unsharpness is most often caused by movement of the object. In practical experience, this usually occurs in the form of involuntary organ movement, e.g., heartbeat. As the object moves, the border (edges) of the object becomes blurred (causes penumbra). The amount of penumbra is a function of the amount of movement present, the rate of movement and the length of the exposure. Motion unsharpness may be reduced by immobilizing the anatomical part, providing the patient with proper instructions (e.g., hold breath) and using a short exposure time.

RESOLUTION

DEFINITION

Resolution is the ability to distinguish objects. An image with high resolution enables differentiation of extremely small objects. To do this, the image is sharp and demonstrates a high contrast between the objects. Resolution is often measured or described in line pairs per centimeter (or millimeter). One line pair per centimeter represents one radiopaque line (usually lead) and an adjacent radiolucent line (an air space).

Resolution is measured using a resolution grid. The grid contains several different line pairs per centimeter (see Figure 23–8). The more line pairs per centimeter visualized, the higher the resolution of the image is.

PRINCIPAL INFLUENCING FACTORS

Intensifying screens play an important role in resolution. Four primary factors influence the image sharpness resulting from intensifying screens: screen speed, crossover, screen contact and quantum mottle. Image sharpness decreases as the speed of the screen increases. This is due to an increase in diverging light rays that strike the film, creating more penumbra and decreasing the sharpness of the image. Conversely, decreasing screen speed by adding a yellow dye decreases the angle of the diverging light rays striking the film and increases image sharpness.

Divergent rays also play a role in decreasing image sharpness in crossover. Crossover is a term used when light emitted from one intensifying screen passes through the film, strikes the other intensifying screen and is reflected back to the film (see Figure 23–10). Crossover occurs when double emulsion film and two intensifying screens are used. Some detail cassettes employ one intensifying screen and single emulsion film to eliminate crossover.

To have good image sharpness, there must be a good film-screen contact. When there is a space (no matter how small) between the film and the screen, the light emitted from the screen diverges, creating a blurring effect on the film. This decreases image sharpness.

Image sharpness is also affected by quantum mottle or noise. Quantum mottle appears on a radiograph as irregular film densities, or blotches. Quantum mottle results because the random distribution of x-ray quanta to produce the image is too small. In general, quantum mottle increases as screen speed or kilovoltage increases. In practical experience, quantum mottle is most apt to be a problem with extremely fast (1200 speed) intensifying screens.

Closely associated with intensifying screens and image blur is the type of film selected for a particular screen speed. Insofar as film-screen combination is concerned, better recorded detail results from a fast film and medium screen speed combination than from the reverse (Selman, 1985, p. 348). Also, film with small crystals tends to provide a high resolution. This occurs because less divergence of light results in a decrease in penumbra.

LABORATORY EXPERIENCE

Magnification and distortion are demonstrated by experimentation in *Concepts in Medical Radiographic Imaging: Laboratory Manual* in Laboratories 43, Effect of Magnification on Radiographic Quality, and 42, Effect of Distortion on Radiographic Quality, respectively.

The Effect of Magnification on Radiographic Quality laboratory contains two experiments. One experiment alters the SOD by varying the SID (maintaining a constant OFD). The other experiment changes the SOD by varying the OFD (SID remains the same). In both procedures, the experimenter calculates the magnification factor. There is a section in each experiment for the researcher to record his/her visual observations of the radiographs.

In the Effect of Distortion on Radiographic Quality laboratory, the experimenter takes four radiographs. One radiograph is exposed with the tube angled, another radiograph is taken with the anatomical part angled and a third radiograph is irradiated while the film is angled. The last radiograph is exposed with the anatomical part perpendicular to the tube and parallel to the film. The experimenter reviews all radiographs and summarizes the effect of distortion on radiographic quality.

Sharpness and resolution are demonstrated in Laboratories 37, Intensifying Screen Resolution, and 44, Effect of Motion on Radiographic Quality. The Intensifying Screen Resolution laboratory employs a resolution grid to demonstrate the line pairs per centimeter for intensifying screens of various speeds. Also, a resolution test is performed on a direct film holder. The results obtained with all film holders are compared for resolution.

The Effect of Motion on Radiographic Quality laboratory involves two exposures. One exposure is taken of a stationary guitar string, the other of a guitar string in motion. The string images are compared for sharpness.

Bibliography

Bushong, SC. Radiologic science for technologists (4th edition). St. Louis: Mosby, 1988.

Chesney, DN and Chesney, MO. Radiographic imaging (4th edition). Boston: Blackwell Scientific Publications, 1981.

Curry, TS, Dowdey, JE and Murry, RC. Christensen's Introduction to the physics of diagnostic radiology (3rd edition). Philadelphia: Lea & Febiger, 1984.

Donohue, DP. An analysis of radiographic quality (2nd printing). Baltimore: University Park Press, 1982.

Eastman Kodak Company. Fundamentals of radiography (12th edition). Rochester, NY: Eastman Kodak Company, 1980.

Lauer, OG, Mayes, JB and Thurston, RP. Evaluating radiographic quality. Mankato, MN: Burnell Company, 1990.

Selman, J. The fundamentals of x-ray and radium physics (7th edition). Springfield, IL: Thomas, 1985.

Sprawls, P. Physical principles of medical imaging. Rockville, MD: Aspen, 1987.

Sprawls, P. Principles of radiography for technologists. Rockville, MD: Aspen, 1990.

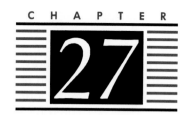

CHAPTER 27

PHOTOGRAPHIC IMAGE QUALITY

MICHAEL MIXDORF and MARIANNE TORTORICI

INTRODUCTION

The photographic quality of a radiographic image refers to the visibility of the image. One of the goals of a serious and competent radiographer is to produce the proper photographic quality for a particular examination. This is desirable because the correct photographic quality in a radiograph heightens detail in the recorded image. The two primary elements of photographic image quality are density and contrast. Images that are too light or too dark (reduced or increased density, respectively) hinder radiographic interpretation. It is also important to be able to distinguish one object from another (contrast). In general, the optimum radiograph has a density range between 0.25 and 2 and has a fairly high contrast. This chapter defines density and contrast. It also identifies the factors that influence density and contrast.

DENSITY

A simplified definition of density is the amount of blackness on the radiograph. There are degrees, or shades, of blackness. The amount of blackness is directly related to the amount of metallic silver on the radiograph (the more metallic silver, the darker the radiograph). A more formal definition of density is the logarithm of opacity.

By definition, opacity (O) is incident light (I_o) divided by transmitted light (I_t), or $O = I_o/I_t$. The incident light is the light beam entering the radiograph (light source of a densitometer). The various tones (degrees of blackness) of the radiograph absorb some of the incident light and allow some of the incident light to pass through the radiograph. The amount of incident light passing through the radiograph is called the transmitted light. Recall that the formal definition of density is the logarithm of opacity. Thus, the mathematical expression for density (D) is

$$D = \log O$$

If $O = I_o/I_t$, then by substitution, the mathematical representation of density becomes the logarithm of the incident light divided by the transmitted light, or

$$D = \log I_o/I_t$$

Many factors affect the density, including

Milliamperage
Exposure time
Source-image distance

Kilovoltage
Intensifying screens
Grids
Processing
Scatter radiation
Field size (beam restrictors)
Atomic number of object
Thickness of object
Density of object
Type of film
Filtration
Heel effect
The relationship of these factors to density is discussed under Factors Affecting Photographic Quality.

CONTRAST

Radiographic contrast is the difference between two densities (it should be noted that a film that is completely black or clear has no contrast because there is only one density imaged). In Chapter 11, Kilovoltage and Quality Control, it was mentioned that contrast may be expressed in terms of short or long scale. A short scale is referred to as high contrast. Long scale contrast is said to be low contrast. Decreasing contrast (going from a short scale of contrast to a long scale) results in an image with fewer density differences between penetrometer steps (more shades of gray). Conversely, increasing contrast (going from a long scale of contrast to a short scale) produces an image with a greater difference between densities (fewer shades of gray).

There are at least three kinds of contrast in radiology. They are subject, film and radiographic (or image). Subject contrast refers to the ability of an object to absorb radiation. Film contrast is inherent in the film and is expressed by the sensitometric curve (refer to Chapter 21, Sensitometry and Processor Quality Control). Radiographic contrast refers to the variety of densities found on the radiographic image and is influenced by both subject and film contrast.

Generally speaking, the same factors that influence density also influence contrast, the exceptions being milliamperage and source-image distance, which have essentially no effect on contrast.

Before a discussion of the effect of these factors, it is important to understand the differences between subject, film and radiographic contrast (see below).

SUBJECT CONTRAST

Subject contrast is determined by the geometry and the resultant x-ray attenuation properties of the subject being radiographed. The amount of radiation absorbed by an object depends on the object's thickness, density and atomic number (composition). The human body contains many different objects (e.g., organs) with different thicknesses, densities and atomic numbers. For example, the femur bone is thicker than the ulna bone, yet it has the same atomic number, and they have comparable densities. Examples of organs with different densities but with the same thickness and atomic number are a normal lung and a lung containing a pathologic change, e.g., fluid. Examples of organs with different atomic numbers are the kidney and lung. These organs also tend to have different densities and thicknesses.

As mentioned above, thickness, density and atomic number influence the amount of radiation absorbed. When objects have the same density and composition, the thicker objects absorb more radiation. The higher the atomic number, the more radiation is absorbed by objects with equal thicknesses and densities. Denser objects absorb more radiation, assuming that the thickness and atomic numbers are the same.

The more radiation absorbed by an object, the less remnant radiation exits the object for film exposure. Consequently, objects absorbing a greater amount of radiation (e.g., bone) have a lighter density on the radiograph than objects absorbing a lesser amount, e.g., lungs.

FILM CONTRAST

Film contrast is the amount of sensitivity of the film to radiant energy intensity. The amount of film contrast is determined by the film's manufacturer. Some films provide higher contrast than other films. The relationship of contrast and film is expressed by the sensitometric curve (see Chapter 21).

RADIOGRAPHIC CONTRAST

Radiographic contrast describes the amount of density range observed on the film. This may be expressed as a ratio of the lightest area (maximum amount of light transmitted) to the darkest area (minimum amount of light transmitted). This is expressed mathematically as

$$K = I_{min}/I_{max}$$

where K equals the contrast, I_{min} is the lightest density and I_{max} represents the darkest portion of the film.

Both subject contrast and film contrast influence radiographic contrast. The technologist cannot directly alter the subject or film contrast. However, there are indirect methods of influencing subject and film contrast. Subject contrast is influenced by the technical factors selected by the technologist. Selecting an appropriate film type helps to regulate the effect of film contrast on the radiographic image.

FACTORS AFFECTING PHOTOGRAPHIC QUALITY

Numerous factors affect photographic quality. The following presents a description of the individual factors. The description includes the effect of the factor on density and contrast. However, it

should be noted that these factors are related and a change in one may compromise another. Table 27–1 provides some examples of the effect of these factors on photographic quality.

OBJECTS BEING IMAGED

Three elements of an object being radiographed influence the photographic quality of the image. They are the thickness, the density and the atomic number of the object. These elements are inherent in the patient and their effect on photographic quality cannot be controlled by the technologist. However, knowledge of the anatomy of the human body and the effect of thickness, density and atomic number are useful in allowing the technologist to control the photographic quality indirectly by adjusting technical factors. The following describes the effect of object thickness, density and atomic number on density and contrast.

In objects with similar densities and atomic numbers, but varying tissue thicknesses, the thicker areas absorb more of the x-rays than the thinner sections. Thus, more remnant radiation occurs with thinner sections. Consequently, the thinner sections produce more density on the radiograph than the thick sections. Also, contrast is highest where the thickness difference of two adjacent objects is the greatest.

Along with tissue thickness is the contribution of tissue density to the photographic image quality.

Table 27–1. COMMON FACTORS INFLUENCING THE PHOTOGRAPHIC IMAGE*

Factor	Original	New	Effect On Density	Effect On Contrast
Object thickness	10 cm	20 cm	Decrease	Increase
Object density	3	5	Decrease	Increase
Atomic number	10	20	Decrease	Increase
Kilovoltage	60 kV	85 kV	Increase	Decrease
Field size	5 inches	12 inches	Increase	Decrease
Grid ratio	5:1	16:1	Decrease	Increase
Grid frequency	60 lines/cm	80 lines/cm	Decrease	Increase
Filtration	1 mm	2 mm	Decrease	Decrease
Milliampere-seconds	20 mAs	40 mAs	Increase	No effect
Source-image distance	40 inches	72 inches	Decrease	No effect
Intensifying screen speed	100	200	Increase	Decrease

*All ancillary imaging methods and techniques remain constant from the original factor to the new factor. The only change is represented by the factor listed.

Consider a radiologic examination of a normal tibia and that of a tibia with osteoporosis. The normal tibia has the same thickness and atomic number as the diseased tibia but differs in density. The diseased tibia is less dense than the normal tibia. Thus, more remnant radiation exits the diseased tibia and strikes the film. Consequently, the radiograph of the diseased tibia has more density and a lower contrast than that of the normal tibia.

The effective atomic number of the tissue under examination also influences the photographic image. The higher the atomic number of an object, the greater the radiation absorption. Radiographic density is directly related to atomic number. The lower the atomic number, the greater the radiographic density. If the difference in atomic number of two adjacent objects is high, e.g., bone and tissue, the contrast is also high.

Sometimes the density, the thickness or the atomic number of adjacent objects is similar, e.g., soft tissue in the abdomen. In these instances, it is possible to increase the contrast by introducing some type of medium (iodinated agents, barium sulfate) in the body.

FILM TYPE AND PROCESSING CONDITIONS

The manufacturer determines the amount of contrast that a film produces. Although the technologist cannot control the film's sensitivity, it is possible to examine a particular film's response to certain exposure conditions by analyzing its characteristic curve (see Chapter 21). The technologist's job is to produce an exposure between 0.25 and 2 on the density scale of the characteristic curve. A film produced in this range is considered diagnostically acceptable in terms of density and contrast. Films produced with less than 0.25 optical density (toe portion) or greater than 2 optical density (shoulder portion) are unacceptable because, in those areas, film contrast is not apparent. Curves demonstrating a steep slope reflect film with a high contrast.

A staff radiographer, while probably not exercising direct control over the type of film employed in an imaging department, should at least be familiar with the sensitivity of the film used as expressed by the manufacturer's characteristic curve.

One item that is under the control of the technologist is regulating the processing conditions. Most imaging departments use automatic processors. This has standardized the manner in which films are developed. However, the automatic processor should be monitored daily to ensure proper operation. Two important items to monitor are the developer temperature and the length of time that the film is in the developer. If the developer temperature becomes too high, it increases the density and decreases the contrast on the film by developing unexposed crystals. Also, increasing the developing time increases the density and decreases the contrast on the film. A variety of things can go wrong with the processor and adversely affect the photographic image. To discuss them all is beyond the scope of this text.

KILOVOLTAGE

Kilovoltage regulates the amount of penetration of the object. The higher the kilovoltage, the greater the x-ray penetration of the object. The kilovoltage selected is often a function of patient exposure factors and x-ray tube limitations. As kilovoltage increases, the density increases and contrast decreases. Probably the greatest influence on contrast is kilovoltage selection.

Utilizing low kilovoltage for a particular milliampere-seconds setting produces a film of an anatomical structure that has short scale contrast (a high degree of contrast). This could be particularly useful in radiography of an extremity, such as a hand (when seeking a subtle fracture line). Although low kilovoltage is desirable, there are times when it may be inappropriate. For instance, chest radiography is done at extremely high kilovoltage settings (115–120 kV and sometimes 150 kV). In chest radiographs, a long scale of contrast, which incorporates more shades of gray in revealing pathologic features, is more efficacious for proper diagnosis. Low kilovoltage often necessitates a high milliampere-seconds setting to obtain a diagnostic radiograph. The combination of low kilovoltage and high milliampere-seconds increases the radiation absorption by the patient. Thus, low kilovoltage radiography should be performed in conjunction with appropriate film and intensifying screen combinations to reduce, as much as possible, the higher dose that is administered with this type of technique.

SCATTER AND FOG

Scatter and fog serve no useful purpose. They degrade the radiographic image. Both result in an increase in density and a decrease in contrast. Scatter radiation and fogging may be considered a noise factor that contributes to the dullness of the image.

Scatter radiation is weak radiation that either reaches the film from interaction with the patient or is generated from the source (x-ray tube) directly. It increases the patient exposure and the magnification of the radiograph. The amount of scatter is a function of patient size, field size and kilovoltage. Increasing any of these items increases the interaction of the x-ray and the patient and increases the amount of scatter radiation. Several methods are used to decrease scatter. These include limiting the field size, employing a kilovoltage range between 70 and 90 kV and using grids.

Fogging can occur a variety of ways. Some common examples are improper methods of handling film, storage of film at too high a temperature or in an area with too much humidity, chemical contamination, radiation and improper development. Most fog can be eliminated by implementing proper imaging practices.

BEAM RESTRICTORS

Beam restrictors regulate the size of the field irradiated. Beam restrictors affect the photographic image quality by controlling the amount of scatter radiation. The greater the field size, the more scatter radiation occurs. This increases density and decreases contrast. The methods of beam restriction employed in radiography today consist of the collimator, cones, extension cylinder and aperture diaphragms. Of these, collimators are the most common and efficient.

Collimators restrict the x-ray beam's total area of exposure while reducing the penumbra, or the area of unsharpness. Because they are constructed of lead, they are able to absorb some of the weaker x-rays generated and emitted at the source. These weaker x-rays, if they are allowed to interact with the patient and the film, degrade the image by contributing to a loss of contrast. In equipment purchased after 1976, a sensing device is connected

from the collimator to the Bucky tray. This device senses the size of film placed in the Bucky tray, and the collimation or exposure field size is automatically adjusted to the size of the film used.

An extension cylinder is sometimes attached to a collimator. Employing such a device, in addition to the collimator, further filters the x-rays to remove the weaker rays. The extension cylinder is most commonly used in radiography of small structures that are surrounded by dense areas of tissue. For example, the skull is an excellent area in which to employ an extension cylinder.

Aperture diaphragms are a much simpler version of a collimator. They are attached, manually, just below the port or sometimes to the bottom of the collimator. Aperture diaphragms are most commonly employed with polytomographic and skull radiographic units.

GRIDS

A grid is a device used to filter out unwanted scatter and secondary radiation *after* the x-ray beam has interacted with the patient but before the beam reaches the intensifying screen and film. Modern x-ray tables are built with grids; therefore, the technologist does not need to add a grid to the cassette being inserted in the Bucky tray. However, performing mobile examinations or examinations on patients who cannot move onto the x-ray table (e.g., patients in a gurney) necessitates that a stationary grid be attached to the front of the cassette for imaging of anatomical parts measuring 13 cm or more.

Grids work by absorbing *scatter* or *primary* rays that *intersect* with a portion of the lead strips. Ideally, all scatter should be absorbed while allowing only the primary beam to reach the image receptor. In reality, *most* of the scatter is cleaned up, while *some* of the primary beam is lost.

The efficiency of a grid is measured by grid frequency and grid ratio. The number of strips per centimeter is called the grid frequency. Grids are manufactured with a frequency from as low as 20 lines per centimeter (50 lines/inch) to as high as 43 lines per centimeter (110 lines/inch). The higher the grid frequency, the more scatter radiation is absorbed. Consequently, there is a decrease in density and an increase in contrast. In general, as the grid frequency increases, the radiographic technique (milliampere-seconds, kilovoltage) must be increased to obtain a radiograph of proper density and contrast.

Grid ratio is the ratio of the height of the individual strips to the distance between the strips. Grid ratios range from a low of 5:1 to a high of 16:1. When the grid ratio is high (16:1), more scatter radiation is absorbed. Thus, increasing the grid ratio decreases density and increases contrast. However, with high grid ratios, e.g., 16:1, care must be taken to be as precise as possible in aligning the tube with the grid. The primary x-rays must enter the grid almost parallel to the lead strips. When the grid ratio is high, the entrance angle of the primary ray is small (5 degrees or less). If the tube is angled even slightly, in relationship to the grid, the examination might be compromised by the grid's absorbing too much of the primary ray, producing grid cutoff. Also, the higher the grid ratio, the higher are the radiographic technical factors needed to obtain diagnostic density and contrast.

FILTERS

Filters are designed to harden the x-ray beam (make the x-ray beam more homogeneous). They perform their function by absorbing weak x-rays. The more homogeneous the beam, the more even the penetration of the object. Thus, increasing the amount of filtration decreases density and contrast.

There are several types of filters. One type, the flat thin filter, can be added to the collimator housing, just below the port. This is the most common type of filter and is employed for the majority of imaging procedures. This type of filter is used for body parts with similar thicknesses.

A second type of filter is attached to the collimator head. This device is thin in the middle and thick at the sides. This type of filter is commonly referred to as a trough. It is employed for an area in which the thickness of an object is greatest in the center, e.g., the chest. Recall that thin areas permit more remnant radiation than thick parts. Thus, the radiograph is darker over the thin areas and lighter under the thick parts. Proper use of the filter necessitates that the technologist align the thin anatomical section under the thick portion of the filter. For example, for a chest examination, the lungs are aligned under the portion of the collimator with the greatest filter thickness. In this example, the radiographic contrast is improved because the filter evens out the densities in the thin and thick areas of the chest.

A third type of filter is the wedge filter. This filter is designed so that it increases in thickness from one end to the other end. A common use of the wedge filter is for the foot. Proper use of the wedge filter necessitates that the thickest part of the aluminum filter be placed over the thinnest part of the object. For example, in the foot the thick end of the filter is placed over the toe area.

HEEL EFFECT

The anode heel effect produces more radiation toward the cathode end of the x-ray tube. Thus, when an object of uniform thickness is imaged, there is more radiographic density under the anatomical part that was located closest to the cathode. This increase in density results in a decrease in contrast. The anode heel effect can be used to advantage. For example, when performing a thoracic spine examination, place the patient so that the head is toward the anode end and the feet are near the cathode. This results in a more uniform photographic image.

MILLIAMPERE-SECONDS

Milliampere-seconds represents the quantity of x-rays. As the milliampere-seconds value doubles, the quantity of radiation also doubles. The quantity of radiation is directly proportional to the density on a film. Thus, the milliampere-seconds value has a linear, or direct, relationship to density; increasing the milliampere-seconds increases density. Because the milliampere-seconds amount has a direct relationship to density, doubling the milliampere-seconds value doubles the density. Recall that radiographic contrast is a ratio of the minimum density to the maximum density. For example, if object A has a density of 1 and an adjacent object, B, has a density of 5, or a contrast of 1:5, doubling the milliampere-seconds value results in a density of 2 for object A and a density of 10 for object B. The contrast would be 2:10, which is the same as 1:5. Consequently, the effect of the normal ranges of milliampere-seconds on contrast is negligible.

SOURCE-IMAGE DISTANCE

Recall that x-rays originate from a point and emerge in a fanlike configuration from the x-ray tube. Thus, as the distance from the source of the x-rays (tube) increases, the irradiated area becomes larger. Consequently, the same amount of radiation must spread over a larger area, or is thinner. Assuming that the technical factors remain the same, increasing the source-image distance decreases the density. As in the case of milliampere-seconds, the rate of attenuation for SID is proportional; therefore the effect on contrast is minimal.

INTENSIFYING SCREENS

Intensifying screens convert x-ray energy to light. They are used to increase the rate of exposure on the film. Increasing the exposure rate enables the technologists to employ lower technical factors and to image thick anatomical parts. The rate of increasing the exposure is a function of the intensifying screen speed. There are several speeds available. The faster the intensifying screen speed, the larger the exposure to the film. Thus, the faster the intensifying screen speed, the darker (increase in density) the radiograph. The increased density will decrease contrast.

LABORATORY EXPERIENCE

Five laboratory experiments in *Concepts in Medical Radiographic Imaging: Laboratory Manual* are related to this chapter: Laboratories 17, Heel Effect; 46, Added Filtration; 24, Effect of Milliampere-seconds on Density; 21, Effect of Kilovoltage on Contrast; and 45, Inverse Square Law.

The first four laboratories listed are cited in earlier chapters. Thus, it is possible that the investigator has already completed these experiments. The following is a brief description of all five experiments.

The Heel Effect laboratory is designed to demonstrate the intensity difference of the x-ray beam. This laboratory is performed at two different source-image distances and field sizes to illustrate the decreasing influence of the heel effect at longer source-image distances and small field sizes.

The Added Filtration laboratory portrays the effect of increasing filtration on density and exposure rate. Five exposures are made of a penetrometer and over a dosimeter pencil. The filtration is increased for each exposure. Density differences are measured on the radiograph. The effect of filtration on the exposure rate is determined by reading the dosimeter pencil.

The Effect of Milliampere-seconds on Density laboratory provides the investigator with the laboratory experience to demonstrate the relationship between milliampere-seconds and density. In this laboratory, six exposures are made of a penetrometer at increasing milliampere-seconds values. The six penetrometer images are compared for density changes.

A penetrometer is used in the Effect of Kilovoltage on Contrast experiment. In this procedure, several radiographs are taken at different kilovoltage values (all other factors remain the same). The radiographs are compared for differences in the number of steps visualized on the penetrometer (contrast).

Assessment of the effect of source-image distance on x-ray intensity is performed in the Inverse Square Law laboratory. This experiment employs a dosimeter pencil or other radiation monitoring device to measure the x-ray intensity emitted at varying source-image distances.

Bibliography

Bushong, SC. Radiologic science for technologists (4th edition). St. Louis: Mosby, 1988.

Cahoon, JB. Formulating x-ray techniques (8th edition). Durham, NC: Duke University Press, 1974.

Carroll, QB. Fuchs's Principles of radiographic exposure, processing and quality control (3rd edition). Springfield, IL: Thomas, 1985.

Chesney, DN and Chesney, MO. Radiographic imaging (4th edition). Boston: Blackwell Scientific Publications, 1981.

Curry, TS, Dowdey, JE and Murry, RC. Christensen's Introduction to the physics of diagnostic radiology (3rd edition). Philadelphia: Lea & Febiger, 1984.

Donohue, DP. An analysis of radiographic quality (2nd printing). Baltimore: University Park Press, 1982.

Hiss, SS. Understanding radiography. Springfield, IL: Thomas, 1980.

Kelsey, CA. Essentials of radiology physics. St. Louis: Warren H. Green, 1985.

Lauer, OG, Mayes, JB and Thurston, RP. Evaluating radiographic quality. Mankato, MN: Burnell Company, 1990.

Selman, J. The fundamentals of x-ray and radium physics (7th edition). Springfield, IL: Thomas, 1985.

Sprawls, P. Physical principles of medical imaging. Rockville, MD: Aspen, 1987.

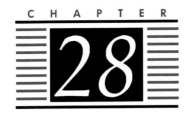

REJECT FILM

ANALYSIS

MICHAEL MIXDORF

INTRODUCTION

Reject film analysis is a systematic procedure designed to catalog and determine the causes of repeat films (radiographs not of diagnostic quality requiring another exposure to the patient) and reject films (repeat radiographs plus any scrap film, e.g., black, green or clear films). The advantage of knowing the reason for film rejection is to implement solutions. The information gained and the solutions derived from a reject film analysis provide the following:

1. The reduction of unnecessary x-ray exposure to the patient by decreasing the number of repeats
2. The savings of a considerable amount of money in film and processing chemistry by using and processing less film
3. The improvement in the efficiency of the department because less time is spent on repeat radiographs and processing problems.

Several methods are used to conduct a reject film analysis. The methods and standards may vary significantly from institution to institution. Consequently, it is extremely difficult and inadvisable to compare the results of reject film analysis among institutions. Rather, a reject film analysis is best used as a tool for assessing and improving the effectiveness within an imaging department.

A common application of a reject film analysis is as an index for departmental quality control effectiveness. When performed before the implementation of a quality control program, reject film analysis provides baseline information to compare with a second analysis conducted after the program's inception. The first analysis reveals problem areas in need of solutions; the second analysis demonstrates the effectiveness of the solutions.

This chapter presents common methods for reject film analysis. After completing the chapter, the reader will be able to determine the method most relevant for his/her institution or to modify a method to accommodate specific needs.

PRECAUTIONS

To accomplish an accurate reject film analysis, the cooperation of radiologists and technologists is essential. Radiologists accepting less than diagnostic films are discouraged from continuing the practice. It is important that radiologists be consistent in the quality of radiographs that they accept. This consistency helps maintain the established standards of the quality control program. Besides the radiologists, technologists must be active participants in the reject film analysis program. This is especially important because some repeat radiographs are a result of human error and technologists may perceive a reject film analysis as intimidating. Consequently, it is vital that the results of a reject film analysis never be used as the basis for a punitive action against anyone or to compare the work of one technologist with that of another technologist. If technologists perceive a reject film analysis as a means of discipline or comparison, they tend to inhibit the collection of poor quality radiographs (e.g., smuggling their nondiagnostic radiographs out of the department). Such practices invalidate the results of a reject film analysis.

Before the implementation of an analysis program, to alleviate technologists' fears and elicit cooperation, managers/supervisors should explain the goals and benefits of an analysis to the technologists. There is some controversy whether to inform the technologists of the date a reject film analysis will be implemented. Advocates of advising the technologists believe that the technologist will cooperate with the process, facilitating the analysis. Those opposed to informing the technologist believe that the technologists will unconsciously sabotage film collection, invalidating the results. If the department managers/supervisors elect not to tell their staff the exact time periods when a reject film analysis will be conducted, they should at least advise the technologists that an analysis will take place sometime in the future.

INITIATING A REJECT FILM ANALYSIS PROGRAM

ESTABLISHING GUIDELINES AND STANDARDS

To provide consistency, standards and guidelines for collecting and assessing radiographs are established. The guidelines and standards should be easy to implement and should describe the methods needed to perform a successful analysis. Some of the more important areas needing written guidelines or standardization include

1. Definition of terms
2. Identification of individuals responsible for the program
3. The method of film collection
4. Types of films to be included or excluded in the analysis
5. The process for categorizing the films
6. The acceptable rejection rate.

In radiography, some terms have a variety of meanings. Thus, to avoid misunderstanding created by semantics, the first reject film analysis guideline is to identify terms that need to be defined. The number of terms defined is determined by the institution writing the guidelines. It is recommended that terms that are used often, have multiple meanings or are key terms be defined. Some examples are the terms reject film, repeat film and positioning error.

Another reject film analysis guideline is to identify the individuals responsible for the program. It is best to identify the individual by job title instead of by personal name. This is helpful because jobs tend to be consistent, whereas individuals filling the positions are apt to change. It is common practice to have the quality control person be responsible for the reject film analysis. An ideal situation is to have the quality control technologist and a radiologist be mutually responsible for the reject film analysis. However, in many institutions, it is impractical for a radiologist to help in film analysis. Whoever is responsible for the analysis must be objective and accurate in the analysis.

The individual performing the analysis may use a variety of methods to collect the reject films. Consequently, included among the guidelines is a description of the film collection method. Common methods used are collection of film by room, department specialty or technologist (see under Film Collection for more detailed information regarding these methods).

Because an imaging department produces a variety of films, the types of films included for a reject film analysis are identified and listed in the guidelines. Some examples of the type of films produced in an imaging department include, but are not limited to, sensitometry films, scout radiographs, black films and green films.

After collection, each film is identified and categorized as to the cause for rejection. The guidelines should identify the categories to be used for classifying reject films. Most lists are unable to include all the reasons for rejecting films. Consequently, the most reliable method of classifying reject films is to develop a list of categories that is capable of classifying a minimum of 95% of the reject films. It is appropriate to have a catchall category (e.g., miscellaneous) to include films with no specific listing of their reason for rejection. The following is an example of a list of reasons for rejecting films:

Too dark
Too light
Motion
Wrong position
Static
Fog
Clear film
Green film
Black film
"Goofs" (examples include failure to have the patient remove radiopaque items such as jewelry and the double-exposed radiograph).
Miscellaneous
Acceptable

When developing a list of reasons for rejecting films, it is also appropriate to have a category for acceptable films. The intent of having a classification for acceptable films is to determine the number of diagnostic radiographs that should not have been repeated. Some institutions place acceptable films under the category of miscellaneous.

After all films have been categorized, the number in each category is recorded on a reject film analysis form for assessment. Several types of forms may be used for analysis (see Figures 28–1 to 28–4 for example forms). To determine the amount of reject films, a percentage of the reject rate is calculated. Interpretation of the meaning of the percentage depends on the standards established by the quality control team. There is no universal standard for an acceptable or unacceptable rate. The diversity among imaging departments does not lend itself to a universal standard. Thus, departments should establish a realistic standard rate (usually in the form of a percentage) of reject films relative to their respective work environment. For example, imaging departments with a large number of trauma cases or student radiographers can expect a higher rate of reject film than do institutions dealing with ambulatory patients and experienced radiogra-

phers. In general, the range of acceptable reject rates tends to be from 5 to 10%.

START-UP EFFECT

The people who should be actively involved in a reject film analysis include the designated reject film analysis technologist and preferably a radiologist. It is appropriate at the start-up of a reject analysis to have the radiologist meet with supervisors and staff to identify the standards for diagnostic radiographs. This helps to minimize what has been termed the start-up effect. This effect is simply a higher or lower rate of rejection often seen during the initial implementation of the standards for acceptable radiographs. Historically, this has been caused by a strengthening of standards relative to the initiation of the program as well as the technologists' anxiety regarding the use of analysis findings. Because of this effect, the data gathered during the first month tend to be erratic, resulting in erroneous conclusions. To reduce errors, it is recommended that data are not used during the first 2 months of analysis. This allows time for the start-up effect to dissipate, being replaced by more reliable results.

REJECT FILM ANALYSIS PROCESS

FILM COLLECTION

The reject film analysis process involves counting reject films, categorizing the reject films and performing calculations. When an analysis program is first implemented, all waste films within the department are removed. After all waste film is removed, a process of collecting reject films is implemented. There are several methods to collect film. All methods involve having the technologists place the reject films in a container.

Common methods of collecting reject films include gathering waste film from each room, specialty area (e.g., ultrasound and radiography) or technologist. In each of these methods, films may be collected as a unit or according to the cause of rejection. In the former collection method, technol-

REJECT FILM ANALYSIS BY SPECIALTY AREA

Facility _____

From _____ to _____
                    date   date

Cause	Number of Films	Percent (see H)
1. Sensitometry films	_____	_____
2. Green films	_____	_____
3. Clear films	_____	_____
4. Positioning	_____	_____
5. Patient motion	_____	_____
6. Too light	_____	_____
7. Too dark	_____	_____
8. Black films	_____	_____
9. Static	_____	_____
10. Fog	_____	_____
11. Miscellaneous	_____	_____
12. Acceptable films	_____	_____
13. Films passed (not rejected)	_____	

A. Total repeats (sum of columns 4–12) _____

B. Total rejects (sum of columns 2–12) _____

C. Total waste (sum of columns 1–12) _____

D. Total films used (C + films passed) _____

E. Percent repeats $= \dfrac{\text{total repeats (A)}}{\text{total films used (D)}} \times 100$ _____

F. Percent rejects $= \dfrac{\text{total rejects (B)}}{\text{total films used (D)}} \times 100$ _____

G. Percent total waste $= \dfrac{\text{total waste (C)}}{\text{total films used (D)}} \times 100$ _____

H. Percent for specific cause $= \dfrac{\text{number of films/cause}}{\text{total films used (D)}} \times 100$ _____

STANDARDS

Percent repeats (E) = 6% or less

Percent rejects (F) = 8% or less

Percent total waste (G) = 10% or less

Percent for a specific cause (H) = 5% or less

Prepared by _____

Date _____

Figure 28–1. Reject film analysis by specialty area.

ogists put all rejected films in one container. In the latter method, technologists place the reject film in a container according to the reason for rejection, e.g., too dark and too light. The specific procedure used to gather reject films is decided by the individual department. It is possible that a department may utilize a method other than the ones mentioned here. The type of method is not as important as having the method designed to support the objectives and goals of the analysis.

FILM CATEGORIZING

After the reject films are collected, they are categorized. Films collected by having the technologists discard the radiographs according to the reason for rejection are already presorted and need only be counted by the reject film analysis individual. However, if films are collected as a unit, the individual responsible for the reject film analysis must review each radiograph to determine the reason for its being discarded.

Most reasons for film rejection are readily apparent, e.g., motion. Yet, some reasons for film rejection are difficult to determine. For example, a radiograph demonstrating an off-centered part could be categorized as poor positioning. However, it is also possible that the Bucky tray was not properly positioned, resulting in the radiograph's belonging in the goofs category. Consequently, it is possible that the person categorizing the films may need to consult the technologist for more information. The process of third party categorizing of radiographs has the disadvantage of being more time consuming than collection of films by reason for rejection.

After all radiographs are sorted, the number of films per category is tallied and recorded on a reject film analysis form. (Figures 28–1 to 28–4 represent examples of forms.) These forms are used to calculate the reject rate.

REJECT FILM RATE CALCULATIONS

To determine percentages of rejections, the individual conducting the assessment needs the following information:

1. The number of reject films for each category
2. The total amount of film used
3. The formulas needed to obtain the required percentages.

After the reject films are categorized, a count is taken of the number of radiographs in each category. This figure is recorded in the appropriate place on the reject film analysis form. It is important to review each category to ensure that the number of reject films has been recorded (the number zero is recorded in categories without any reject films).

Another figure necessary for calculating percentages is the total number of films used during the film collection period. The total of films used includes the sum of the reject films and the radiographs passed, or good films. Three methods are commonly used to determine the total number of films. All the methods provide a close estimate of the total number of films used. The simplest method is to install a film counter on the processor. In this method, the films are counted as they enter the processor. The disadvantage of using a processor film counter is that, when two films enter the processor simultaneously (e.g., by placing two 8 × 10 inch films side by side), they are recorded as one film. To determine the total number of films used with this system, the film counter number is added to the number of films rejected. For example, with a film counter reading of 12,874 and a reject film count of 677, the total number of films used is 13,551 (12,874 + 677 = 13,551). The second method of tabulating the total number of films involves counting the number of film boxes used. In this technique, the total number of films is determined by multiplying the number of film boxes used during the reject film collection period by the number of films in each box. For example, if 140 boxes of film are used and each box contains 100 films, the total number of films used is 14,000 (140 × 100 = 14,000). The last method for finding the total number of films used employs the number of examinations performed. This method entails three steps. The first step is to obtain the number of procedures performed during the reject film collection period. The next step is to multiply the average number of films per examination by the number of procedures performed, e.g., two films per chest x-ray procedure × 2000 chest examinations = 4000 films. The final step is to add the sum of the films used for all examinations to the total number of

Text continued on page 342

REJECT FILM ANALYSIS BY EXAMINATION

Facility _____

From _____ to _____

                 date   date

REJECTS (REPEATS)

| | Column Number | | | | | | |
Examination	1 Dark	2 Light	3 Motion	4 Wrong Position	5 Goofs*	6 Examina- tion Total	7 Percent (H)
Abdomen							
Extremity							
Upper							
Lower							
Barium enema							
Upper gastrointestinal tract							
Chest							
Hip							
IVP							
Mandible							
Nasal bones							
Pelvis							
Rib							
Shoulder							
Sinuses							
Skull							
Spine							
Cervical							
Dorsal							
Lumbar							
Sacral							
$\% = \dfrac{\text{column sum}}{\text{total (D)}}$							

Films passed (not rejected) _____

*Errors such as failure to remove necklace and double exposures.

A. Total repeats (column total for column 6) _____

Figure 28–2. Reject film analysis by examination.

REJECTS (SCRAP)

Type of Film   Number

Green _____

Clear _____

Black _____

B. Total rejects (sum of green, clear and black films) _____

OTHER

Number of sensitometry films _____

C. Total waste (sum of A, B and sensitometry film) _____

D. Total films used (C + films passed) _____

E. Percent repeats $= \dfrac{\text{total repeats (A)}}{\text{total films used (D)}} \times 100$ _____

F. Percent rejects $= \dfrac{\text{total rejects (B)}}{\text{total films used (D)}} \times 100$ _____

G. Percent total waste $= \dfrac{\text{total waste (C)}}{\text{total films used (D)}} \times 100$ _____

H. Percent per examination $= \dfrac{\text{examination total (column 6)}}{\text{total films used (D)}} \times 100$ _____

STANDARDS

Percent repeats (E) = 6% or less

Percent rejects (F) = 8% or less

Percent total waste (G) = 10% or less

Percent for specific examination (H) = 5% or less

Prepared by _____

Date _____

Figure 28–2 *Continued* Reject film analysis by examination.

REJECT FILM ANALYSIS BY ROOM

Facility _____

From _____ to _____
        date   date

REJECTS (REPEATS)

Column Number

Room	1 Dark	2 Light	3 Motion	4 Wrong Position	5 Goofs*	6 Examination Total	7 Percent (H)
1	_____	_____	_____	_____	_____	_____	_____
2	_____	_____	_____	_____	_____	_____	_____
3	_____	_____	_____	_____	_____	_____	_____
4	_____	_____	_____	_____	_____	_____	_____
5	_____	_____	_____	_____	_____	_____	_____
6	_____	_____	_____	_____	_____	_____	_____
7	_____	_____	_____	_____	_____	_____	_____
$\% = \dfrac{\text{column sum}}{\text{total (D)}}$	_____	_____	_____	_____	_____	_____	_____
Films passed	_____						

*Errors such as failure to remove necklace and double exposures.

A. Total repeats (column total for column 6) _____

Figure 28–3. Reject film analysis by room.

REJECTS (SCRAP)

Type of Film — Number

Green _____

Clear _____

Black _____

B. Total rejects (sum of green, clear and black films) _____

OTHER

Number of sensitometry films _____

C. Total waste (sum of A, B and sensitometry film) _____

D. Total films used (C + films passed) _____

E. Percent repeats $= \dfrac{\text{total repeats (A)}}{\text{total films used (D)}} \times 100$ _____

F. Percent rejects $= \dfrac{\text{total rejects (B)}}{\text{total films used (D)}} \times 100$ _____

G. Percent total waste $= \dfrac{\text{total waste (C)}}{\text{total films used (D)}} \times 100$ _____

H. Percent per examination $= \dfrac{\text{examination total (column 6)}}{\text{total films used (D)}} \times 100$ _____

STANDARDS

Percent repeats (E) = 6% or less

Percent rejects (F) = 8% or less

Percent total waste (G) = 10% or less

Percent for specific examination (H) = 5% or less

Prepared by _____

Date _____

Figure 28–3 *Continued* Reject film analysis by room.

REJECT FILM ANALYSIS BY TECHNOLOGIST

Facility _____

From _____ to _____
        date   date

REJECTS (REPEATS)

Column Number

Technologist	1 Dark	2 Light	3 Motion	4 Wrong Position	5 Goofs*	6 Examination Total	7 Percent (H)
1	_____	_____	_____	_____	_____	_____	_____
2	_____	_____	_____	_____	_____	_____	_____
3	_____	_____	_____	_____	_____	_____	_____
4	_____	_____	_____	_____	_____	_____	_____
5	_____	_____	_____	_____	_____	_____	_____
6	_____	_____	_____	_____	_____	_____	_____
7	_____	_____	_____	_____	_____	_____	_____
$\% = \dfrac{\text{column sum}}{\text{total (D)}}$	_____	_____	_____	_____	_____	_____	_____
Films passed	_____						

*Errors such as failure to remove necklace and double exposures.

A. Total repeats (column total for column 6) _____

Figure 28–4. Reject film analysis by technologist.

REJECTS (SCRAP)

Type of Film   Number

Green _____

Clear _____

Black _____

B. Total rejects (sum of green, clear and black films) _____

OTHER

Number of sensitometry films _____

C. Total waste (sum of A, B and sensitometry film) _____

D. Total films used (C + films passed) _____

E. Percent repeats $= \dfrac{\text{total repeats (A)}}{\text{total films used (D)}} \times 100$ _____

F. Percent rejects $= \dfrac{\text{total rejects (B)}}{\text{total films used (D)}} \times 100$ _____

G. Percent total waste $= \dfrac{\text{total waste (C)}}{\text{total films used (D)}} \times 100$ _____

H. Percent per examination $= \dfrac{\text{examination total (column 6)}}{\text{total films used (D)}} \times 100$ _____

STANDARDS

Percent repeats (E) = 6% or less

Percent rejects (F) = 8% or less

Percent total waste (G) = 10% or less

Percent for specific examination (H) = 5% or less

Prepared by _____

Date _____

Figure 28–4 *Continued* Reject film analysis by technologist.

reject films. Figure 28–5 demonstrates the process of calculating the total number of films by examination.

The total number of films used and the amount of films rejected for each category are used to determine the reject films rates (usually in percentage form). The department's guidelines and standards identify the specific rates to be calculated. In general, most reject analysis programs include the following:

1. The percentage of repeat films relative to the total films used
2. The percentage of reject films relative to the total films used
3. The percentage of reject films per category.

Figure 28–6 is an example of a completed reject film analysis form and illustrates the process of calculating the percentage for repeat films, for reject films and by categories. In Figure 28–6, the percentage of repeat films is calculated by dividing the number of repeat films (767) by the total films used (12,012) and multiplying by 100, or 767/12,012 × 100 = 6.38. The percentage of reject films is determined by dividing the total reject films (926) by the total films used (12,012) and multiplying by 100, or 926/12,012 × 100 = 7.7. The category percentage is calculated by dividing the number of films per category (cause) by the total number of films used and multiplying by 100. For example, the percentage for the category too light is 124/12,012 × 100 = 1.03. It should be noted that the percentage figures used here are rounded off.

INTERPRETING THE RESULTS

The interpretation of the results from a reject film analysis is useful in identifying problems and determining the costs of reject films. The identification of problems enables solutions to be implemented,

CALCULATION PROCESS OF TOTAL FILMS BY EXAMINATION

Procedure	Number Performed	Average Number of Films	Total
Abdomen	318	1	318
Extremity			
Upper	40	2	80
Lower	70	2	140
Barium enema	1026	5	5130
Upper gastrointestinal tract	1248	6	7488
Chest	2329	2	4658
Hip	65	2	130
IVP	510	8	4080
Mandible	50	3	150
Nasal bones	63	2	126
Pelvis	791	1	791
Rib	67	4	268
Shoulder	44	2	88
Sinuses	70	4	280
Skull	137	4	548
Spine			
Cervical	121	5	605
Dorsal	40	2	80
Lumbar	189	4	756
Sacral	33	2	66
TOTAL			25,782

Total rejects   =   1,034
"Good" films (films passed) = 25,782
Total films   = 26,816

Figure 28–5. Calculation process of total films by examination.

REJECT FILM ANALYSIS BY SPECIALTY AREA

Facility _____ Example Hospital _____

From _____ Sept. 1, 1991 _____   to   _____ Sept. 30, 1991 _____
　　　　　　　　　　date　　　　　　　　　　　　　　　　　　　　　　　　date

Cause	Number of Films	Percent (see H)
1. Sensitometry films	35	0.29
2. Green films	126	1.05
3. Clear films	33	0.27
4. Positioning	78	0.65
5. Patient motion	9	0.07
6. Too light	124	1.03
7. Too dark	249	2.07
8. Black films	19	0.16
9. Static	85	0.71
10. Fog	68	0.57
11. Miscellaneous	46	0.38
12. Acceptable films	89	0.74
13. Films passed (not rejected)	11,051	

A. Total repeats (sum of columns 4–12) _____ 767 _____

B. Total rejects (sum of columns 2–12) _____ 926 _____

C. Total waste (sum of columns 1–12) _____ 961 _____

D. Total films used (C + films passed) _____ 961 + 11,051 = 12,012 _____

E. Percent repeats $= \dfrac{\text{total repeats (A)}}{\text{total films used (D)}} \times 100 = \dfrac{767\,(100)}{12,012} = 6.38\%$

F. Percent rejects $= \dfrac{\text{total rejects (B)}}{\text{total films used (D)}} \times 100 = \dfrac{926\,(100)}{12,012} = 7.70\%$

G. Percent total waste $= \dfrac{\text{total waste (C)}}{\text{total films used (D)}} \times 100 = \dfrac{961\,(100)}{12,012} = 8\%$

H. Percent for specific cause $= \dfrac{\text{number of films/cause}}{\text{total films used (D)}}$ as $\times\ 100$ _____

STANDARDS

Percent repeats (E) = 6% or less

Percent rejects (F) = 8% or less

Percent total waste (G) = 10% or less

Percent for a specific cause (H) = 5% or less

Prepared by _____ Jane Smith, R.T. _____

Date _____ October 5, 1991 _____

Figure 28–6. Example of completed analysis by specialty area.

which resolves the problem. The cost data are useful in assessing the effectiveness of the department.

IDENTIFYING PROBLEMS

Interpretation of the results is performed by comparing the findings with the established departmental standards. For example, in Figure 28–6, the department established the following standards:
Repeats—6%
Rejects—8%
Total waste—10%
Specific cause—5%

Comparing the findings in Figure 28–6 with the standards, it is noted that
1. The repeat rate is slightly higher than the standard
2. The reject rate is approaching the standard
3. The total film waste and category percentages (specific cause) are within acceptable limits.

Because the repeat rate exceeds the standard, it becomes necessary to interpret the meaning of the percentage. It is not unusual for there to be several reasons for a percentage increase. Consequently, as in this example, when interpreting the excess repeat rate, the more information available to the individual assessing the results (investigator), the more the accuracy of the conclusion/solution increases. Thus, the investigator may have to look in other areas to obtain added information. In this example, it would be wise for the investigator to review past reject analysis results (assuming that the program has been in operation for a while and that previous reports are available) to see if the current rate differs significantly from previous figures. The information obtained by comparing current and previous reports helps to determine the specific approach of the investigator. If the results for the previous 6 months demonstrate similar findings, it is possible that the standard is set too low and needs to be readjusted. If the previous reports differ significantly from the current report, the investigator may wish to research further. One area that might be researched is what, if any, changes might have occurred in the department (e.g., the hiring of new technologists and an increase in the number of students).

The process described above represents an abridged summary of one possible approach to analyzing data from a reject film program. It can readily be seen that film assessment is a complex issue with no one answer. It should also be noted that the interpretation of the results is directly related to the work environment. Thus, it is impractical and inadvisable to attempt to compare the results of one facility with those of another facility. It is important to avoid using the results of a reject film analysis to punish the technologist or compare one worker with another worker.

COSTS

The data obtained from a reject film analysis are used to calculate the costs of the rejected films. Cost assessment may be in the form of a close estimate or exact costs. The most common method used to estimate costs is to multiply the average cost of one film by the number of films rejected. The average cost of one film is obtained by finding the sum of the cost per film of all sizes of films and dividing by the number of films. For example,

Cost of 8×10 inch film = $1.60
Cost of 10×12 inch film = $1.70
Cost of 11×12 inch film = $1.80
Cost of 14×17 inch film = $\underline{\$2.00}$
$$\$7.10$$

$7.10/4 = $1.775, or $1.78

Employing the data from Figure 28–6 and using the example average film cost of $1.78, the estimated cost of rejected films (926) is $1648.28, or $1.78 \times 926 = 1648.28$

If the department is interested in obtaining an exact dollar figure for reject films, the cost of each size of film is multiplied by the number of films discarded per size. The total cost is calculated by adding the dollar figure for all film sizes. For example, assume that the number of reject films for Figure 28–6 is

Number of 8×10 inch films = 224
Number of 10×12 inch films = 270
Number of 11×12 inch films = 189
Number of 14×17 inch films = 243

Using the cost per film size above, the total reject film cost becomes
   8×10 inch film: $224 \times \$1.60$ = $ 358.40
10×12 inch film: $270 \times \$1.70$ = $ 459.00
11×12 inch film: $189 \times \$1.80$ = $ 340.20
14×17 inch film: $243 \times \$2.00$ = $\underline{\$ 486.00}$
$$\$1643.60$$

These techniques are also used to determine the cost per cause of rejection (for each category). Film counts are determined for the specific category instead of for the total number of reject films. Also, when using the estimated cost method, the number of reject films for the category is substituted for the total number of reject films. For example, in Figure 28–6, assume that the following film sizes constitute the category static:

Number of 8 × 10 inch films = 22
Number of 10 × 12 inch films = 27
Number of 11 × 12 inch films = 18
Number of 14 × 17 inch films = 18
                               ——
                               85

Using the estimated cost method, the cost of film rejection for the static category is $151.30 (1.78 × 85 = 151.30). The specific cost for the static category is $149.50 (see the following calculations):

 8 × 10 inch film: 22 × $1.60 = $ 35.20
10 × 12 inch film: 27 × $1.70 = $ 45.90
11 × 12 inch film: 18 × $1.80 = $ 32.40
14 × 17 inch film: 18 × $2.00 = $ 36.00
                                 ———————
                                 $149.50

LABORATORY EXPERIENCE

Laboratory 47, Reject Film Analysis, in *Concepts in Medical Radiographic Imaging: Laboratory Manual* provides the learner with experience in reject film analysis. This experiment enables the investigator to perform a reject film analysis to determine if there are areas of an imaging department needing improvement. The laboratory allows the learner to select one of four different charts for tabulating and categorizing reject films. Also, the laboratory allows the instructor the option of having students collect their own reject films or providing students with a stack of reject films.

Bibliography

Gray, JE, et al. Quality control in diagnostic imaging. Baltimore: University Park Press, 1983.
Jenkins, D. Radiographic photography and imaging processes. Baltimore: University Park Press, 1980.
McLemore, JM, Quality assurance in diagnostic radiology. Chicago: Year Book Medical, 1981.

RESISTOR COLOR CODE

The majority of resistors used in electronics are cylindrical, with a wire lead projecting from each end. The outer case of the cylinder is made of nonconductive plastic or ceramic material. The material providing the electrical resistance is contained inside the outer case and is connected at each end to a lead wire.

The resistance (ohms) and tolerance (accuracy in terms of percentage) of a cylindrical resistor are indicated by the color coded bands on the outer case. There are either three or four bands around the resistor. The band location is important when determining the ohms range. The band closest to an end of a resistor indicates the first significant figure of the resistor's ohms. The second band represents the second significant figure. The third band indicates the number of zeros to be added to the first two figures. The number of zeros is determined by either multiplying or dividing the first two figures by a specific power of 10. The last band, the fourth, identifies the tolerance. This band may or may not be present. If it is present, the color code indicates the percentage of tolerance. In the absence of a band, the tolerance is plus or minus 20%. Table A–1 presents the color coded numerical

values of resistors. Figure A–1 contains two examples of how to calculate the range of a resistor.

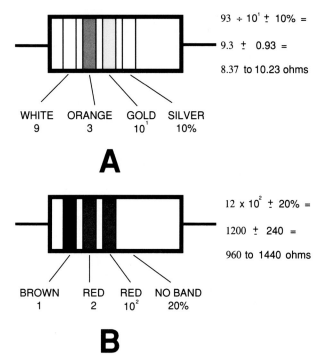

$93 \div 10^1 \pm 10\% =$

$9.3 \pm 0.93 =$

8.37 to 10.23 ohms

WHITE   ORANGE   GOLD   SILVER
9   3 10^1 10%

A

$12 \times 10^2 \pm 20\% =$

$1200 \pm 240 =$

960 to 1440 ohms

BROWN   RED   RED   NO BAND
1   2 10^2 20%

B

Figure A–1. Examples of how to calculate the ohms range of a resistor with tolerance band *(A)* and without tolerance band *(B)*.

Table A–1. RESISTOR COLOR CODED NUMERICAL VALUE

1st and 2nd Band	Significant Figure of Resistance	3rd Band	Power of 10	4th Band	Tolerance of Resistor
Black	0	Black	$\times 10^0$	Gold	± 5%
Brown	1	Brown	$\times 10^1$	Silver	±10%
Red	2	Red	$\times 10^2$	None	±20%
Orange	3	Orange	$\times 10^3$		
Yellow	4	Yellow	$\times 10^4$		
Green	5	Green	$\times 10^5$		
Blue	6	Blue	$\times 10^6$		
Violet	7	Silver	$\div 10^2$		
Gray	8	Gold	$\div 10^1$		
White	9				

SUMMARY OF FORMULAS

BEAM RESTRICTOR IMAGE DIAMETER

Beam Restrictor Image Diameter—the diameter of an image for a specific cone or aperture.

$$ID = (SID/SAD)DA$$

where ID is image diameter, SID represents source-image distance, SAD is source to controlling aperture distance and DA is the diameter of the controlling aperture.

COULOMB'S LAW

Coulomb's Law—the formula used to determine the force of electrical charges.

$$F = \frac{kq_1q_2}{d^2}$$

where F is force, k is the type of medium, q stands for charge and d represents distance.

DENSITY

Density—the amount of blackness on the film.

$$Density = \log O$$
$$or$$
$$Density = I_o/I_t$$

where O is opacity, I_o is incident light and I_t is transmitted light.

FILTRATION

Filtration—the total amount of x-ray tube filtration.

$$F_t = F_i + F_a$$

where F_t is the total filtration, F_i represents inherent filtration and F_a is the added filtration.

GEOMETRIC IMAGE QUALITY

Percentage of Magnification—the amount of magnification of an object.

Using distance to determine magnification,

$$Percentage\ of\ magnification = OFD/SOD \times 100$$

where OFD is object-film distance and SOD is source-object distance.

Using the object and image to determine magnification,

$$Percentage\ of\ magnification = \frac{IS - OS}{OS} \times 100$$

where IS is image size and OS is object size.

The effect of the ratio of source-image distance to source-object distance on magnification is determined by

$$SID/SOD = IS/OS$$

where IS is image size, OS is object size, SOD is source-object distance and SID is source-image distance.

Sharpness—the amount of penumbra of an image.

$$P = \frac{FSS\ (OFD)}{SOD}$$

where P is penumbra, FSS is focal spot size, OFD is object-film distance and SOD is source-object distance.

GRIDS

Grid Ratio—the relationship of the height of the lead strips to the distance between the lead strips.

Grid ratio = height of lead strips/interspace width

Contrast Improvement Factor—how much improvement is obtained by using a grid.

$$K = \frac{contrast\ with\ grid}{contrast\ without\ grid}$$

where K is the contrast improvement factor.

Selectivity—the amount of primary beam absorption compared with the secondary absorption of the grid.

$$\Sigma = \frac{T_p}{T_s}$$

where Σ is selectivity, T_p is the amount of primary radiation transmitted and T_s is the amount of scatter radiation transmitted.

Exposure Factor—an indirect method of determining the amount of primary beam absorbed by grid.

Exposure factor =
$$\frac{exposure\ without\ grid\ (incident\ radiation)}{exposure\ with\ grid\ (transmitted\ radiation)}$$

Loss of Primary Beam—the amount of loss of primary beam created by lateral decentering of grid.

$$L = \frac{rb}{f_o} \times 100$$

where L is the percentage loss of the primary beam,

r is the grid ratio, b is the lateral decentering distance and f_o is the convergence point.

HEAT UNITS

Heat Units—the measurement of the amount of heat at the anode.

Single phase:

$$HU = kVp \times mA \times s$$

Six pulse, three phase:

$$HU = kVp \times mA \times s \times 1.35$$

Twelve pulse, three phase:

$$HU = kVp \times mA \times s \times 1.41$$

where HU is heat units, kVp is kilovoltage, mA is milliamperes and s is seconds.

IMAGE INTENSIFICATION

Conversion Factor—a variable used to determine the brightness output of the image intensifier.

$$Conversion\ factor = \frac{candela/m^2}{mR/s}$$

where m is meters, mR indicates milliroentgens and s is seconds.

Minification Gain—the brightness gain due to minification.

$$Minification\ gain = \frac{(D_i)^2}{(D_o)^2}$$

where D_i is the input screen diameter and D_o is the output diameter.

Brightness Gain—the brightness gained by using an image intensifier.
Brightness gain = minification gain × flux gain

INTENSIFICATION FACTOR

Intensification Factor—a factor used to estimate screen speed.

$$IF = \frac{\text{exposure without screens}}{\text{exposure with screens}}$$

where IF is the intensification factor.

INVERSE SQUARE LAW

Inverse Square Law—the formula that determines x-ray intensity at a given distance.

$$I = 1/d^2$$

where I is intensity and d represents distance.

KILOVOLTAGE

Kilovoltage—determines the kilovoltage for variable kilovoltage chart.
Single phase:

$$\text{Size of object} \times 2 + 30 \text{ kVp}$$

Three phase:

$$\text{Size of object} \times 2 + 20 \text{ kVp}$$

Kilovoltage Compensation—a method of calculating new kilovoltage with a change in the milliampere-seconds value.
The 13% rule is used when doubling the milliampere-seconds value.

$$kVp_1 \times 0.13 = \text{amount of kVp to subtract}$$

$$kVp_2 = kVp_1 - \text{amount of kVp to subtract}$$

The 15% rule is used when decreasing the milliampere-seconds value by half.

$$kVp_1 \times 0.15 = \text{amount of kVp to add}$$
$$kVp_2 = kVp_1 + \text{amount of kVp to add}$$

where kVp_1 is the original kilovoltage and kVp_2 is the new kilovoltage.

MILLIAMPERE-SECONDS

Milliampere-seconds—a value used to calculate the quantity of x-rays.

$$mAs = mA \times s$$

where mAs indicates milliampere-seconds, mA is milliamperes and s is the exposure time in seconds.

Milliampere-seconds Compensation—the determination of a new milliampere-seconds value when the source-image distance is changed.

$$mAs_2/mAs_1 = (SID_2)^2/(SID_1)^2$$

where mAs_2 is the milliampere-seconds value, mAs_1 is the old milliampere-seconds value, SID_2 is the new source-image distance and SID_1 is the original source-image distance.

OHM'S LAW

Ohm's Law—the formula used to calculate current, voltage or resistance of an electrical circuit.

$$I = E/R$$

where I is the current in amperes, E represents electromotive force in volts and R is the resistance in ohms.

PARALLEL CIRCUIT

Resistance—calculates the ohms of a parallel circuit.

$$1/R_t = 1/r_1 + 1/r_2 + \ldots 1/r_n$$

where R_t is total resistance in ohms and r represents resistance over an individual component.

Current—determines the amperes in a parallel circuit.

$$I_t = i_1 + i_2 + \ldots i_n$$

where I_t is the total current in amperes and i represents current over an individual component.

PHOTON ENERGY

Photon Energy—calculates the quality of a photon.

$$E = h\upsilon$$

where E is the photon energy, h is Planck's constant and υ is the frequency of x-rays measured in hertz.

REJECT FILM ANALYSIS

Percentage of Repeats—the percentage of repeats.

$$\text{Percent repeats} = \frac{\text{total repeats}}{\text{total films used}} \times 100$$

Percentage of Rejects—the percentage of reject films.

$$\text{Percent rejects} = \frac{\text{total rejects}}{\text{total films used}} \times 100$$

Percentage of Total Waste—the percentage of waste of all film.

$$\text{Percent total waste} = \frac{\text{total waste}}{\text{total films used}} \times 100$$

Percent for Specific Cause—the amount of loss in percentage owing to a specific cause.

$$\text{Percent for specific cause} = \frac{\text{number of films/cause}}{\text{total films used}} \times 100$$

RELATIONSHIP OF FREQUENCY AND X-RAY WAVELENGTH

Frequency and X-ray Wavelength—demonstrates the mathematical relationship of the size of the wavelength to the number of cycles per second.

$$c = \lambda \upsilon$$

where c represents the speed of x-rays, λ is wavelength and υ is frequency.

RESISTANCE OF CONDUCTOR

Resistance—relationship of factors affecting electrical resistance.

$$R = \rho \frac{L(T)}{A}$$

where ρ is the medium, L is length, T represents temperature and A is the cross section.

SERIES CIRCUIT

Resistance—determines the ohms of a series circuit.

$$R_t = r_1 + r_2 + \ldots r_n$$

where R_t is the total resistance in ohms and r is the resistance over an individual component.

Voltage—determines the voltage in a series circuit.

$$E_t = e_1 + e_2 + \ldots e_n$$

where E_t is the total electromotive force in volts and e is the electromotive force over an individual component.

SPINNING TOP TEST

Spinning Top Test—calculates the quantity of dots that should appear on a radiograph for a specific time setting on a single-phase x-ray unit.

$$\text{Number of dots on radiograph} = \text{time} \times \text{useful impulses}$$

TOMOGRAPHY

Object Movement—the distance an object moved on film.

$$\text{Movement} = 2d \tan \theta/2$$

where d is the distance of an object from a fulcrum and θ represents the exposure angle.

Section Thickness—image thickness.

$$h = B/(\tan \theta/2)$$

where h is the section thickness, B is the maximum permissible blur and θ represents the exposure angle.

TRANSFORMERS

Turns Ratio—a ratio that determines if the transformer is step-up or step-down.

$$N_s/N_p$$

where N_s is the number of turns on the secondary side and N_p is the number of turns on the primary side.

Transformer Ratio—a ratio that determines voltage in transformer.

$$E_s/E_p = N_s/N_p$$

where E_s is the voltage in the secondary side, E_p is the primary side voltage, N_s is the number of turns on the secondary side and N_p is the number of turns on the primary side.

Transformer Efficiency—the degree of efficiency for separate primary and secondary sides

$$E_pI_p = E_sI_s$$

where I_p is the current on the primary side, I_s is the current on the secondary side, E_s is the voltage in the secondary side and E_p is the primary side voltage.

Autotransformer—a ratio that determines voltage in an autotransformer

$$E_s/E_p = N_t/N_p$$

where E_s is the voltage in the secondary side, E_p is the primary side voltage, N_t is the number of turns tapped on the secondary side and N_p is the number of turns in the primary side.

WATTS

Watts—the power of an electrical circuit.

$$W = EI$$
or
$$W = (IR)I$$
or
$$W = I^2R$$

where W is watts, E is electromotive force in volts, I is the current in amperes and R is the resistance in ohms.

PROCESSOR

TROUBLESHOOTING

CHECKLIST

Table C–1. TRANSPORT SYSTEM

Section A: Components

Roller subsystem (film handling problems)	Motor subsystem (speed, drive problems)
Roller size, hardness driven, nondriven squeegee; roller pins, studs, shafts, bearings; guide shoes—adjustable, nonadjustable; deflector plates, wires, bars; face plates; tie bars, support bars; feed tray	Electrical power supply; switch, fuses, relays; motor brushes, controller gears; gears, sprockets, pulleys; chains, belts; bearings; shafts

Section B: Location of Causes of Transport Problems

1. Misaligned gears, sprockets
2. Misaligned chains, belts
3. Misaligned turnarounds, crossovers
4. Misaligned racks
5. Misaligned guide shoes, deflector plates
6. Misaligned drive shafts
7. Misaligned support bars
8. Misaligned feed tray
9. Worn, broken gears, sprockets
10. Worn, broken chains, belts
11. Worn, broken bearings, shafts
12. Tension springs too tight, too loose
13. Roller gear ends loose
14. Dryer drive alignment
15. Roller studs binding
16. Time delay on feed too short
17. Dirty rollers
18. Fuses, breaker, protectors
19. Slipping gears, sprockets
20. Slipping chains, belts
21. Broken electrical conductor, terminal, connector
22. Damaged switch
23. Electrical power source
24. Drive motor gears damaged
25. Drive motor starter circuit damaged
26. Drive motor run circuit damaged
27. Damaged rollers
28. Damaged drive shafts
29. Chemical failure—developer, fixer, hardeners
30. Film characteristics—size, type, sides
31. Lubrication
32. Wrong parts used
33. Cleanliness
34. Film feeding procedure

From E. I. DuPont de Nemours & Co. (Inc.), Wilmington, DE.

Table C–1. TRANSPORT SYSTEM

Section C: Transport Problems	Section D: Common Causes	Section E: Less Common Problems
Film jams	1–8	9–17, 19, 20, 24, 27–34
Abrasions	1–4	5, 7–15, 17, 19, 20, 27–33
Overlapped films	16, 34	3–5, 7–15, 19, 20, 27, 28, 30, 32
Cocked films	8, 34	3–5, 11–15, 17, 27–28, 31
Detector switch activation	8, 22	1, 2, 5–7, 9–13, 15, 17, 19, 20, 27–28
Unusual noise	1, 2	4, 6, 7, 9–15, 19–20, 24, 27, 28, 31–34
Film dropping in dryer	14, 32	1, 2, 4, 6, 9–13, 15, 19–20, 27, 28, 30
Film retained in dryer	29	1, 2, 4, 7, 9–12, 14–17, 19, 20, 27, 28, 30–33
Increased density	27, 31	1, 3–5, 9–15, 19, 20, 29, 33
Decreased density	29	4, 14, 23, 30–32
Rapid gear, sprocket wear	31, 33	1–7, 14, 15, 17, 19, 20, 27–29
Component not turning	1, 9	2–7, 10–15, 18–28, 31–33
Scratches	5, 29	1–4, 6–15, 19, 20, 27–34
Gelatin pick-off deposits	17, 29	3–7, 9–15, 19, 20, 27, 28, 30, 32, 33
Pressure marks	4	3, 5–7, 9–13, 15, 17, 19, 20 27, 29, 33, 34

From E. I. DuPont de Nemours & Co. (Inc.), Wilmington, DE.

Table C–2. REPLENISHMENT SYSTEM

Section A: Components

Detector switch (microswitch); detector assembly—airflow, rollers; main switch, fuses relays; pump head, motor, gearbox; lines—tubing, fittings; gauges—flow indicators, meters; tanks—outside processor; check valves; needle valves; filters

Section B: Location of Causes of Replenishment Problems

1. Detector switch malfunction
2. Detector switch adjustment
3. Detector assembly malfunction
4. Cleanliness of detector assembly, switch
5. Electrical supply
6. Pump setting
7. Pump accuracy
8. Pump reproducibility
9. Pump leak
10. Pump malfunction
11. Lines kinked, blocked
12. Lines—air leak, air block
13. Lines—solution leak
14. Lines—fittings damaged
15. Gauges not calibrated
16. Filters or strainers clogged
17. Tanks not calibrated
18. Check valves stuck
19. Check valves deteriorated
20. Check valves installed incorrectly
21. Adjustment valve failure
22. Replenishment tanks empty
23. Frequency of mix
24. Absence of floating lid
25. Water supply problems

Section C: Replenishment Problems	Section D: Common Causes	Section E: Less Common Problems
Chemical volume low	6–8	1–5, 9–24
Chemical volume high	6–8, 18	1, 2, 4, 15, 17, 19–20, 23
Chemical activity low	6–8	1–5, 9–24
Chemical activity high	6–8, 18	1, 2, 15, 17, 19, 20, 23
Increased density	6–8	1–4, 15, 17–21, 23
Unclear films	6–8	1–5, 9–24
Unwashed film (mixing valve)	6–8	1–5, 9–24
Undry films	25	1–24
Scratches, abrasions	6–8	1–5, 9–24
Film jams	6–8	1–5, 9–24
Decreased density	6–8	1–5, 9–24
Chemical breakdown	6–8	1–5, 9–24
High consumption	6, 24	1–5, 9–24
Leaks	13, 14	9, 11, 12, 16, 17–21
Variable sensitometry	7, 8	1, 4, 17

From E. I. DuPont de Nemours & Co. (Inc.), Wilmington, DE.

Table C–3. ELECTRICAL SYSTEM

Section A: Components

Power supply; lockout box, fuses, terminals; processor switches; processor relays; processor terminals; processor fuses, circuit breakers; motor protectors; motors—pump, drive; heaters—developer, dryer; indicator lights; conductors

Section B: Location of Causes of Electrical Problems

1. No supply at source
2. Half normal supply (one line)
3. Wrong phase
4. Variable supply
5. Line voltage fluctuation
6. Loaded line (e.g., elevator on same line)
7. Fuses burned
8. Fuses corroded
9. Fuses broken
10. Wrong size fuse
11. Circuit breaker blown (open)
12. Circuit breaker broken
13. Relay stuck closed
14. Relay stuck open
15. Burned contacts
16. Welded contacts
17. Bent contacts, rocker plates
18. Broken switch open
19. Broken switch closed
20. Jammed switch open
21. Jammed switch closed
22. Motor started switch defective
23. Motor starter windings burned, shorted
24. Motor running windings burned, shorted
25. Heater element burned, shorted
26. Thermostat switch malfunction
27. Indicator light burned out
28. Loose connections
29. Short circuit in conductors
30. Corroded connectors
31. Heat
32. Lack of lubrication

Section C: Electrical Problems	Section D: Common Causes	Section E: Less Common Problems
Nothing runs	1–3	6, 11, 12, 14, 15, 17, 18, 20, 29, 30
Drive motor will not start	22, 23	1–9, 11, 12, 14, 15, 17, 18, 20, 28–32
Drive motor will not run	24	
Drive motor will manual start, will run	22, 23	1–9, 11, 12, 15, 17, 18, 20, 28, 30, 32
Pump motor will not start	22, 23	1–9, 11, 12, 14, 17, 20, 28–31, 33
Pump motor will not run	24	
Motor speed changes	4, 32	3, 5, 6, 24, 28
Motor fails annually	2–6	10, 30–32
No circulation	22, 26, 32	1–9, 11, 12, 14, 15, 17, 18, 20, 23, 24, 28–31
No heat	7, 25, 26	1–6, 8, 9, 11, 12, 14, 15, 17, 18, 20, 27–30
Too much heat	10, 13, 26	3–5, 16, 17, 19, 21, 27
Too little heat	26	2–9, 11, 12, 14, 27–31
Insufficient replenishment	14	2–9, 17, 24, 28–32
Heater will not turn off	13	10–12, 16, 17, 19, 21, 26, 29
Motor will not turn off	13, 16, 21	3–5, 17, 19, 29
Insulation burned	6, 13	3–5, 10, 29–31
Insulation crumbling	6, 13	3–5, 10, 29–31

From E. I. DuPont de Nemours & Co. (Inc.), Wilmington, DE.

Table C–4. CIRCULATION/FILTRATION SYSTEM

Section A: Components

Circulation	Filtration
Electrical power supply; switch, fuses, relays; pump motor starter; pump motor; heat exchanger; tubing, fittings	Filter type; filter size

Section B: Location of Causes of Circulation and Filtration Problems

1. Line voltage fluctuations	14. Air blockage of filters
2. Pumps not lubricated	15. Blocked tubing
3. Failure of pump motor thermostat	16. Improper flow, e.g., backward
4. Burned motor starter	17. Filter clogged
5. Burned motor starter windings	18. Filter caked
6. Dirty magnets and shafts	19. Filter channels
7. Worn bearings	20. Filter micron size too small
8. Loose pump-motor linkage	21. Filter micron size too large
9. Warped pump head	22. Filter missing
10. Leaking pump head	23. Heat exchanger leaking
11. Leaking tubing	24. Heat exchanger clogged
12. Leaking fittings	25. Dirty pump
13. Air blockage of pumps	26. Defective switch

Section C: Circulation and Filtration Problems	Section D: Common Causes	Section E: Less Common Problems
No circulation	4, 17	2, 3, 5–16, 18, 20, 25–26
Reduced flow	26	1–18, 20, 24, 25, 26
Variable flow	1–3	6–9, 26
Pump not running	2, 3	1, 4, 7, 9, 13–18, 20, 25–26
Pump running, no flow	13, 14	10–12, 15–18, 20, 25
Pump motor will not start	3, 4	1, 2, 5, 26
Pump runs after manual start	4, 5	
Loud, noisy pump	6, 26	7–9, 13
Leaks at pump	9	10–12, 16
General leaks	10	11–18, 20
Foam	13, 14	9–12, 19, 21, 23
Increased temperature of chemicals	17, 25	9–16, 17, 20
Frequent filter changes, e.g., weekly	20	17, 18, 24–26
Lower density	2, 3	1, 4–18, 20, 24–26
Unclear films	2, 3	1, 4–18, 20, 24–26
Reduced or no replenishment	17	11, 12, 14, 18
Dirt on films	21	17, 19, 26

From E. I. DuPont de Nemours & Co. (Inc.), Wilmington, DE.

Table C–5. TEMPERATURE CONTROL SYSTEM

Section A: Components

Thermostat; thermometers; switch, fuses, relays; water supply; electrical power supply; heaters; indicator lights; circulation pump; mixing valve (if used); heat exchanger

Section B: Location of Causes of Temperature Problems

1. Electrical power fluctuations
2. Water supply fluctuations
3. Loss of cold water
4. Loss of hot water
5. Loss of volume
6. Loss of pressure
7. Mixing valve malfunction
8. Clogged filters and strainers
9. Clogged heat exchanger
10. Clogged tubing
11. Thermostat stuck open
12. Thermostat stuck closed
13. Thermostat uncalibrated
14. Thermometer uncalibrated
15. Thermometer broken
16. Heater broken
17. Heater relay stuck open
18. Heater relay stuck closed
19. Indicator light burned out
20. No circulation
21. Switch or fuse failure

Section C: Temperature Problems	Section D: Common Causes	Section E: Less Common Problems
Decreased temperature and density	11	1, 2, 4–7, 13–17, 19–21
Increased temperature and density	3, 18	1, 2, 5–10, 12–15, 19–21
Unclear films	3 or 4	5–7
Unwashed films	3 or 4	1, 2, 5–15
Undried films	17	11, 13–16, 19–21
Streaks on films	20	8–10
Unequal development	8, 9, 20	1–7, 10, 20
Unequal clearing	10, 20	1–9
Unequal washing	7, 9, 20	1–6, 8, 10, 20
Unequal drying	16, 20	1–10
Temperature fluctuations	1, 2	7–10, 13, 14, 20
Developer gets hotter, heater off	2	3, 5–7, 19
Developer does not heat	2, 21	1, 4–11, 13–17, 19–20
Indicator light cycles on/off slowly	20	8–10, 13
Hot water heats developer	7	2, 3, 5, 6, 8–10

From E. I. DuPont de Nemours & Co. (Inc.), Wilmington, DE.

Table C–6. DRYER SYSTEM

Section A: Components

Electrical supply; blower/motor; thermostat; safety thermostat; air tubes; sheaves (pulleys and belts); main switch, fuses, relays; heater(s); thermometer; indicator light; exhaust; receiver bin

Section B: Location of Causes of Dryer Problems

1. Electrical supply fluctuations
2. Insufficient electricity
3. Broken (open) switch, relay, or fuse
4. Broken (closed) switch, relay, or fuse
5. Stuck switch or relay
6. Blower fins clogged with dirt
7. Blower bearings worn or broken
8. Blower drive belt misaligned
9. Blower drive belt broken
10. Motor starter windings burned
11. Motor starter relay broken
12. Motor running windings burned
13. Motor circuit breaker open
14. Heater burned open
15. One of heaters burned open
16. Thermostat stuck closed
17. Thermostat stuck open
18. Safety thermostat open
19. Too high setting for safety thermostat
20. Thermostat not calibrated
21. Thermometer not functioning
22. Indicator light broken
23. Air tubes dirty
24. Air tubes installed wrong
25. Exhaust tube too small
26. Exhaust tube blocked
27. Exhaust too small
28. Exhaust too great
29. Room intake air too cool
30. Rollers dirty
31. Rollers allow film slippage
32. Squeegee roller function
33. Developer depleted
34. Fixer depleted
35. No wash water
36. Transport speed too fast
37. Ambient conditions

Section C: Drying Problems	Section D: Common Causes	Section E: Less Common Problems
Overall wet, cool, soft films	3, 17, 19, 33, 34	1, 2, 5–15, 18, 20, 21, 23–27
Above trailing edge	15, 33, 34	1, 2, 6–8, 19–21, 23–27, 29–32, 36
Film cool, barely dry	15, 19, 20, 33	1, 2, 6–8, 21, 23, 24
Film hot, damp	19, 20, 37	6–10, 15, 21–34, 36
Overall moist, warm, hard films	27	6, 25, 28, 37
Above trailing edge	27	6, 25, 26, 28, 37
6th–10th film becomes damp	27, 33	34, 37
14 × 17 inch film dry, 8 × 10 inch film damp	31	
8 × 10 inch film dry, 14 × 17 inch film damp	3, 17, 19, 33, 34	1, 2, 5–15, 18, 20, 21, 23–27
Serial films become damper	27, 33	19–22, 25, 26, 28–30, 34, 37
Marginal drying, high heat	19, 20, 25, 28	15, 18, 21–24, 26, 27, 30–37
Water spots	32, 33	6, 10, 14, 15, 17–21, 30, 31
Cross-hatched pattern	6, 30, 33	10, 15, 17–21, 23, 24, 31, 32, 34
Waveform pattern	19, 20	4–6, 10, 15, 16, 21–27
Baked, glossy surface	19, 20	4, 16, 21, 22
"Light" area streaks	23, 24	
Jams	31, 33	3, 6–14, 17–30, 32, 34–37
Film cocking	31, 33	
Dirt on films	30	23, 24, 33, 34
No heat	3, 14	1, 2, 5, 9–12, 17–22, 28, 29, 37
No air	9–11	1–3, 5–8, 12, 13, 23, 24

From E. I. DuPont de Nemours & Co. (Inc.), Wilmington, DE.

INDEX

Note: Numbers followed by an i indicate illustrations;
those followed by a t indicate tables.